# RESPIRATORY PATIENT CARE

# Respiratory

# Patient

# Care

**KANUTE P. RAREY, B.S., R.R.T.**
*Education Consultant*
*International Health Educators, Inc.*

**JOHN W. YOUTSEY, Ed. S., R.R.T.**
*Associate Professor and Chairman*
*Department of Respiratory Therapy*
*College of Allied Health Sciences*
*Georgia State University*
*Atlanta, Georgia*

PRENTICE-HALL, Inc., *Englewood Cliffs, New Jersey 07632*

*Library of Congress Cataloging in Publication Data*

Rarey, Kanute P
   Respiratory patient care.

   Includes bibliographies and index.
   1. Inhalation therapy.  I. Youtsey, John W.,
joint author.  II. Title.  [DNLM: 1. Respiratory
tract diseases—Therapy. WF 145 R221r]
RC735.I5R37    615.8′36    80-39946
ISBN  0-13-774604-0

Editorial/production supervision
  and interior design by *Virginia Huebner*
Cover design by *Frederick Charles, Ltd.*
Manufacturing buyer: *Anthony Caruso*

Printed in the United States of America

10  9  8  7  6  5  4  3  2

Prentice-Hall International, Inc., *London*
Prentice-Hall of Australia Pty. Limited, *Sydney*
Prentice-Hall of Canada, Ltd., *Toronto*
Prentice-Hall of India Private Limited, *New Delhi*
Prentice-Hall of Japan, Inc., *Tokyo*
Prentice-Hall of Southeast Asia Pte. Ltd., *Singapore*
Whitehall Books Limited, *Wellington, New Zealand*

To our families. . . .

*Gaila, Heather, and Amanda Youtsey*

*Anita and Allen Rarey*

To *Andrew M. Switzer* (my grandfather). . . .

for that part of his life that he shared with me,
*K. Rarey*, and for his influence upon my life.

"Imagine a single breath having started."

*Gustav Eckstein*

# CONTENTS

# 7 AIRWAY MANAGEMENT 160

# 10  PULMONARY FUNCTION TESTING

# Preface

*Respiratory Patient Care* is the end-product of study, clinical experience, education, and management in respiratory care. Respiratory care information is organized here in a concise, comprehensive presentation of information necessary for safe, effective respiratory patient therapy. The objective of the book is to present practical clinical material that aids in the day-to-day provision of respiratory care.

This book is written for all health care professionals: therapists, technicians, nurses, emergency medical technicans, and physicians. It is a reference, a resource, and a guide that can be useful in reviewing specific techniques, in developing new procedures and procedure manuals, in preparing in-service programs and, in guiding patient care. Its comprehensive design provides a useful tool for students and graduates in preparing for the certification and registry examinations.

The material is not presented as a final study of respiratory therapy, nor an all-encompassing manual never to be supplemented; the book is designed to act as a base upon which the reader can organize the clinical and technical concepts of cardiopulmonary care and to aid in the daily patient care in which each individual is involved.

## ACKNOWLEDGEMENTS

Any project that requires time and energy also requires the tolerance and support of those around. This book was one of those projects and we would like to acknowledge those individuals who supported our efforts. We are grateful for the support of the faculty of the Department of Respiratory Therapy in the College of Allied Health Sciences and the Educational Media Department at Georgia State University, Atlanta, Georgia; the Respiratory Therapy Department and Allied Health Education Department at Memorial Medical Center, Savannah, Georgia; and the Respiratory Therapy Department at Georgia Baptist Medical Center, Atlanta, Georgia.

The following friends and associates have also influenced and supported the writing of the book: Linda Kirkland, R.N., Charles Tuggle, M.A., Herb Douce, M.Ed., R.R.T., Craig Barfield, C.R.T.T., Robert Churchill, R.R.T., for many of the photographs in the text, and Joseph Rau, R.R.T., for his technical support during the manuscript preparation. Sincere appreciation is given to them for their kind and steadfast support. Special thanks is also given to Ms. Faye Waldhour and Ms. Sharon Johnson who patiently and expertly completed numerous typings of the manuscript and corrected the many spelling errors that we overlooked.

KANUTE P. RAREY, B.S., R.R.T.

*Atlanta, Georgia*

JOHN W. YOUTSEY, Ed.S., R.R.T

# CHAPTER 1

# Medical Gas Administration

Medical gas administration is a fundamental part of respiratory patient care and is used to treat cardiopulmonary disease. Table 1-1 lists common medical gases administered in respiratory therapy and anesthesia. Medical gases are prescribed by a physician, and they should be evaluated periodically for effectiveness and the need to continue therapy. The physician's order for gas therapy should include the following:

Date and time therapy is to start
Percent concentration of gas to be delivered (i.e., 21–100 percent $O_2$)
Type of humidity or aerosol
Type of administration equipment to be used (i.e., cannula, nonrebreathing mask)
Liter flowrate
Duration of therapy (i.e., continuous, p.r.n., h.s., q4h)
Signature of prescribing physician

In the following section we will discuss the administration of oxygen, oxygen-carbon dioxide, and helium-oxygen. These gases and gas mixtures are used in respiratory therapy to relieve certain specific pulmonary and systemic complications of disease. Their safe, effective use requires an understanding of the therapeutic considerations and possible hazards of each gas or gas mixture.

## OXYGEN THERAPY

Oxygen is administered to treat and prevent the symptoms of hypoxia. An increase above 20.95 percent oxygen in the inspired gas concentration provides an increase of molecular oxygen for diffusion from ventilated, perfused alveoli into the pulmonary arterial blood. The goal is to provide an adequate oxygen content in the arterial blood to meet the metabolic needs of all body tissues. The treatment of hypoxia with supplemental oxygen will decrease the work of the cardiopulmonary system that normally compensates for hypoxia. The body initially compensates with an increased cardiac output (both volume and rate), followed by increased ventilation and peripheral vasoconstriction leading to an elevated blood pressure.

### ARTERIAL OXYGEN SATURATION

Hypoxemia and hypoxia are two distinct physiological phenomena. Hypoxemia refers to a decreased oxygen content in the arterial blood, whereas hypoxia refers to the lack of oxygen in body tissue. Oxygen entering the arterial blood is primarily transported to the cell in a loose chemical bond with hemoglobin. If the hemoglobin does not combine with oxygen in the pulmonary circulation, it is described as reduced hemoglobin. Each gram (g) of hemoglobin can combine with 1.34 ml (milliliter) of oxygen. The normal amount of hemoglobin is 12–16 g/100 ml of blood. Hypoxemia will occur with a decrease in the oxygen carrying capacity of arterial blood and/or a decrease in the partial pressure of oxygen in the arterial blood (normal range is 80–100 torr in patients under 60 years old with no chronic respiratory disease). The relationship between the arterial oxygen saturation and the partial pressure of oxygen in arterial blood is graphically described on a sigmoid shaped curve, called the oxygen-hemoglobin dissociation curve (see Fig. 1-1).

The chemical attraction of hemoglobin for oxygen is altered by clinical changes in the patient that may occur with the process and treatment of disease. These changes are illustrated in Figure 1-1.

## TABLE 1-1
### Common Medical Gases

| | Oxygen | Carbon Dioxide | Helium | Cyclopropane | Air | Nitrous Oxide |
|---|---|---|---|---|---|---|
| Physical state in cylinder at 70° F. | Gas | Liquid and Gas Gas* | Gas | Liquid and Gas | Gas | Liquid and Gas |
| Molecular Weight | 16 | 44 | 4 | 42 | 29 | 44 |
| Chemical Formula | $O_2$ | $CO_2$ | He | $C_3H_6$ | Air | $NO_2$ |
| Color, Odor, Taste | Colorless Odorless Tasteless | Colorless Odorless Slightly acid taste | Colorless Odorless Tasteless | Colorless Odor resembling petroleum benzine Pungent Taste | Colorless Odorless Tasteless | Colorless Odorless Tasteless |
| Cylinder Color Code (E and Smaller) | Green | Gray Gray and Green | Brown Brown and Green | Orange | Yellow | Light Blue |
| Density (lb/ft³) | 0.083 | 0.115 | 0.013 | 0.109 | 0.079 | 0.115 |
| Combustion Characteristics | Nonflammable Support combustion | Nonflammable** —does not support combustion | Nonflammable** —does not support combustion | Flammable | Nonflammable Supports combustion | Nonflammable Supports combustion |
| Approximate Full Cylinder Pressure at 70° F. | 1900–2200 psig | 835 psig +68% of weight of water cylinder can hold 1800–2200 psig* | 1600 psig | 75 psig +55% | 1950 psig | 750 psig +68% |
| Critical Temperature (° F.) | -181.9 | 88 | -450 | 256 | -220 | 98 |
| Critical Pressure (psia) | 737 | 1072 | 33 | 797 | 547 | 1054 |
| Boiling Point (° F. 760 torr) | -297 | -109.3 | -452 | -27 | -317 | -127 |

*Oxygen and carbon dioxide therapeutic mixtures
**Support combustion when mixed with oxygen
+Filling density of gas that exists as liquids in a cylinder

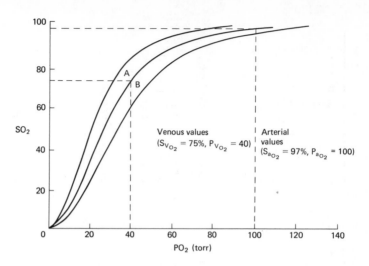

FIG. 1-1. Oxygen-hemoglobin dissociation curve. Area A represents an increase in arterial saturation due to increased pH, decreased $pCO_2$, decreased temperature, and/or decreased 2,3 DPG. Area B represents a decreased arterial oxygen saturation caused by a decreased pH, increased $pCO_2$, increased temperature, or increased 2,3 DPG.

## A Decrease in Arterial Oxygen Saturation

Changes that cause a decrease in the chemical attraction of hemoglobin for oxygen result in a decreased arterial oxygen saturation. This, in turn, results in an overall decrease in the amount of oxygen available to the tissues, since less oxygen is combined with hemoglobin as it moves through the pulmonary circulation. The following factors cause a decrease in the attraction of hemoglobin for oxygen:

1. Increased temperature (above $37°C$), such as with increased body metabolism in infection, tissue trauma, or organ damage.
2. Acidemia (decreased pH below 7.35), caused by an increase in the hydrogen-ion concentration in the blood, such as increased carbonic acid production with carbon dioxide retention, lactic acid produced with tissue hypoxia, and/or keto acid produced with diabetes.
3. Hypercapnia (increased $PaCo_2$ above 45 torr), caused by ineffective ventilation of the lung producing hypoventilation, such as with acute or chronic ventilatory failure.
4. Increased 2,3 DPG (2,3-diphosphoglycerate). This does not naturally occur, since 2,3 DPG is an intracellular enzyme within the red blood cell that speeds the chemical release of oxygen from hemoglobin.

4

An Increase in Arterial Oxygen Saturation

Clinical changes that increase the chemical attraction of hemoglobin for oxygen will also increase the saturation of arterial blood with oxygen. This increased attraction will allow more oxygen to combine with hemoglobin as it passes through the pulmonary circulation. However, due to this stronger chemical bond, less oxygen than normal will be released to the cells. Factors that increase the strength of the bond between hemoglobin and oxygen include the following:

1. Decreased temperature (below 37°C), such as with a decrease in body-cell metabolism with hypothermic therapy or exposure to a cold gas atmosphere or environment.
2. Alkalemia (increased pH above 7.45) caused by a decrease in the hydrogen-ion concentration in the blood, such as with the loss of body acid through severe vomiting and diarrhea, decreased carbon dioxide levels, or an abnormal increase in body bicarbonate in the blood caused by drug therapy or kidney failure.
3. Hypocapnia (decreased $PaCO_2$ less than 35 torr) caused by hyperventilation of the lungs such as with anxiety, hypoxemia, or improper adjustment of continuous mechanical-ventilation rate or tidal volume.
4. Decreased 2,3 DPG (2,3-diphosphoglycerate). This decrease in the intracellular enzyme may appear in transfused blood stored for a prolonged period of time in the clinical laboratory prior to use. This will inhibit the release of oxygen from hemoglobin within the red blood cell, preventing its delivery to the tissue.

TABLE 1-2

**Normal Arterial and Venous Values**

|  | *Arterial* | *Venous* |
|---|---|---|
| pH | 7.35–7.45 | 7.35–7.45 |
| $PCO_2$ (torr) | 35–45 (40) | 46 |
| $HCO_3^-$ (meq/L) | 21–25 | 21–25 |
| B.E. | +2 to –2 | +2 to –2 |
| $PO_2$ (torr) | 80–100* | 40 |
| $SaO_2$ (percent) | 97% | 75% |
| Oxygen content (ml/100 ml) 15g Hb | 19.8 ml | 15.4 ml |

*Arterial oxygen tension decreases in patients over 65 years old and with chronic cardiopulmonary disease.

The pick up and release of oxygen by hemoglobin in the blood and the amount available to the tissue will be altered with any changes in these factors. (See Table 1-2 for normal values.)

## HYPOXIA

Hypoxia means a reduced amount of oxygen available at the tissue level regardless of cause or location. Hypoxia may alter normal arterial oxygen saturation and tension as listed in Table 1-3. Hypoxia can be divided into four categories:

1. *Hypoxic hypoxia.* The blood supply to the tissue has a decreased oxygen tension ($PaO_2$ below 80 torr) and, therefore, a decreased saturation ($SaO_2$ below 97 percent). This condition occurs with acute and chronic cardiopulmonary disease. It may be due to a mismatching of effective alveolar ventilation and pulmonary perfusion, a decrease in the inspired oxygen concentration such as with suffocation or high altitude (ambient hypoxia), or thickening of the alveolar-capillary membrane caused by interstitial fluid or fibrosis inhibiting diffusion.

2. *Anemic hypoxia.* The arterial oxygen tension will be normal and the saturation of hemoglobin may be normal, but the carrying capacity of oxygen in the blood will be decreased because of a decrease in the amount of hemoglobin available to transport oxygen. A decrease in available hemoglobin will lower the arterial oxygen content. The amount of hemoglobin transporting oxygen will be reduced by the loss of red blood cells caused by hemorrhagic disease of the red bone marrow which limits red blood-cell production, or carbon monoxide or methemoglobinemia poisoning. Carbon monoxide has an affinity for hemoglobin that is 210 times greater than that of oxygen.

3. *Circulatory hypoxia.* The amount of oxygen available to the tissues is lowered by a decrease in the blood supply to the tissues or inadequate amounts of blood to supply oxygen to meet increased metabolic demands.

### TABLE 1-3

#### Changes in $PaO_2$ and $SaO_2$ With Hypoxia

| Types of Hypoxia | $PaO_2$ | $SaO_2$ |
| --- | --- | --- |
| Hypoxic hypoxia | Decreased | Decreased |
| Anemic hypoxia | Normal | Normal or higher than normal |
| Circulatory hypoxia | Decreased | Decreased |
| Histotoxic hypoxia | Normal | Normal |

This is also called stagnant hypoxia. It is caused by a decrease in cardiac output as seen with congestive heart failure or cardiac arrest, or with decreased arterial vascular tone leading to arterial hypotension such as with shock.

4. *Histotoxic hypoxia.* Arterial oxygen saturation and oxygen tension levels would be normal. This form of hypoxia is caused by toxic substances inhibiting oxygen use by the tissues and blocking normal cell metabolism, such as with cyanide poisoning.

Oxygen therapy is prescribed to provide the patient with an adequate amount of oxygen for normal tissue metabolism and thus prevent tissue hypoxia. Changes in partial pressure and arterial oxygen saturation are indications of hypoxia. A decrease in normal values represents a decrease in arterial oxygen content (see Table 1-2 for normal values).

## PHYSIOLOGICAL HAZARDS OF OXYGEN THERAPY

The following are physiological hazards of oxygen therapy:

1. *Absorption atelectasis.* The major gas concentrations of room air are 20.95 percent oxygen and 78.08 percent nitrogen. When breathing high oxygen concentrations, the level of nitrogen in the lungs decreases. Unlike inert nitrogen, oxygen is continually being consumed in body metabolism and also has a faster diffusion rate than nitrogen. If an alveolus becomes occluded, such as with secretions or aspiration, the oxygen will diffuse more rapidly than the inert nitrogen it replaced, thus allowing the collapse of the alveoli leading to atelectasis.

2. *Retrolental fibroplasia.* If the $PaO_2$ is allowed to remain at abnormally high levels (greater than 150 torr) for a prolonged period of time, retinal damage may occur causing permanent vision loss. The high $PaO_2$ causes retinal arterial vasoconstriction and tissue scarring. This occurs more frequently in newborns and infants when retinal growth is most rapid and sensitive to arterial oxygen changes. The severity and rate of occurrence is dependent on individual tolerance, length of exposure, and level of oxygen concentration. The hazard is reduced by monitoring the arterial oxygen tension to maintain it within a normal physiological range (40–60 torr) for newborns.

3. *Oxygen toxicity.* Long-term exposure to high inspired oxygen concentrations also can cause topical damage to alveolar tissue. The destruction and scarring of this tissue may lead to the development of a thickened alveolar-capillary membrane, previously described in infant respiratory distress syndrome as hyaline membrane. This also has been observed in

adult lungs. Such changes cause the reduction of gas diffusion from the alveoli and result in an inflammatory response of the lung and central nervous system to the high oxygen concentration. Again, arterial oxygen tension should be monitored and inspired oxygen concentration limited to maintain the arterial oxygen tension within the patient's normal range. Symptoms of headaches, chest pain, and shortness of breath may be observed. Their occurrence is based on patient tolerance, exposure time, and gas concentration.

4. *Oxygen induced hypoventilation.* This is a complication observed in patients with chronic lung disease. Because of increased carbon dioxide tensions with chronic hypoventilation, these patients' respiratory centers become insensitive to normal fluctuations in carbon dioxide tension. Their respiratory stimulus is low oxygen tension, described as hypoxic drive. The delivery of elevated oxygen concentrations which increases the $PaO_2$ beyond the normally low arterial tension of these patients may cause apnea. This hazard must always be considered with patients who are known or suspected to have a chronic lung disease and a compensated respiratory acidosis.

5. *Psychological dependence.* Patients requiring oxygen therapy for a long period of time may come to associate oxygen gas flow with the relief of their "shortness of breath." Some have been observed to develop a psychological, rather than a physiological, need for oxygen. This may occur in the treatment of chronic lung diseases during the terminal stages. Such a patient may require weaning from gas therapy with a gradual reduction of oxygen to room air.

6. *Drying of the respiratory mucosa.* All medical oxygen in bulk or cylinder systems is dry (less than 6ppm) when released from the system. Humidity must be added to the gas before it is delivered to the patient, otherwise it will place an increased physiological demand on the patient's respiratory system. Mucosal drying is even more of a potential problem if the normal humidification by the nasal cavity has been bypassed by an endotracheal or tracheostomy tube. This results in the thickening of respiratory secretions and possible mucosal bleeding. The humidity deficit between the required 100 percent relative humidity at body temperature in the lungs and the dry oxygen should be relieved by the addition of humidity to the therapeutic oxygen delivered to the patient. Humidity should always be added to dry medical gases. (See Chapter 2.)

## PHYSICAL HAZARDS OF OXYGEN THERAPY

Physical hazards of oxygen therapy include:

1. *Fire.* Oxygen supports combustion. At 20.95 percent in the atmosphere, oxygen provides a chemical base for fire described as rapid oxidation. The higher the concentration of oxygen in an atmosphere, the lower

**TABLE 1-4**

**Safety Systems for Medical Gases**

| | $O_2$ | $O_2/CO_2$ | $He/O_2$ | $C_3H_6$ | $C_2H_4$ | $He$ | $CO_2$ | $NO_2$ | $Air$ |
|---|---|---|---|---|---|---|---|---|---|
| Color Code (E cylinders) | green | green with gray shoulder | green with brown shoulder | orange | red | brown | gray | blue | yellow |
| Pin index Safety System (200 psig or greater) | 2-5 | 2-6 (<7% $CO_2$) 1-6 (>7% $CO_2$) | 2-4 (<80% He) 4-6 (>80% He) | 3-6 | 1-3 | — | — | 3-5 | 1-5 |
| Diameter Index Safety Systems Connection Number (200 psig or less) | 1240 | 1200 (<7% $CO_2$) 1080 (>7% $CO_2$) | 1180 (<80% He) 1060 (>20% He) | 1100 | 1140 | 1060 | 1080 | 1040 | 1160 |
| American Standard Safety Connections (threaded outlet no., diameter and no. per inch, thread turn) | CGA-541 0.903-14 NGO RH-Ext. | CGA-541 0.903-14 NGO RH-Ext. | CGA-541 0.903-14 NGO RH-Ext. | CGA 921 | CGA-351 0.825-14 NGO LH-Ext. | CGA-351 0.825-14 NGO LH-Ext. | CGA-321 0.825-14 NGO RH-Ext. | CGA-321 0.825-14 NGO RH-Ext. | — |

the ignition point of substances within that atmosphere. For this reason, when increased oxygen concentrations are in use, great care must be taken to prevent fires. What is a small match flame at normal oxygen concentration may act as a torch in a high oxygen concentration.

Warning signs must be posted on the patient's door to warn of the fire hazard and smoking should not be permitted in the room. Also, all spark producing appliances or highly combustible materials, such as electric razors, rubbing alcohol, static producing toys, transistor radios, and the nurse call bells should be removed from the immediate vicinity of the patient receiving oxygen therapy. Such items should never be permitted inside oxygen tents or oxygen-enriched infant isolettes.

2. *Explosion.* The use of compressed gas cylinders creates a potential hazard of explosion. The pressures in many compressed gas cylinders exceed 2200 psig. Heating of cylinders or rupture of cylinder valves or casings can create a powerful explosion. These high-pressure gas cylinders should never be exposed to temperatures greater than 125°F. Cylinder transport and handling require care to prevent dropping and damaging the cylinders and valves. Cylinder stands or wall chains should be used to support the gas cylinders. Attachments should be used that match the type of valve on the cylinder (see Table 1-4) and valve caps should be used during transport to prevent damage to the valve.

3. *Malfunction of equipment.* Oxygen-administration and humidification equipment should be checked at least every four hours for proper placement on the patient and proper functioning of the equipment. All patient-care personnel should be aware of proper equipment placement and function when in the patient's room. The oxygen concentration should be monitored with a gas analyzer at least once every eight hours to check the delivery of the prescribed oxygen concentration.

## EVALUATION OF OXYGEN THERAPY

Physiological considerations when administering oxygen should be continually evaluated.

1. Arterial blood gas analysis will indicate the partial pressure of oxygen and the arterial oxygen saturation. The relationship between $PaO_2$ and arterial saturation is illustrated in Fig. 1-1. With these values and the patient's hemoglobin, the actual arterial oxygen content and capacity can be calculated by using the following formula:

Arterial oxygen capacity = amount of hemoglobin (grams) $\times$ 1.34
ml $\times$ 100% arterial saturation

+ 0.003 ml $\times$ measured partial pressure
of arterial oxygen.

Arterial oxygen content = amount of hemoglobin (grams) × 1.34 ml × measured saturation

+ 0.003 × measured arterial partial pressure of oxygen.

1.34 is the amount of oxygen that can combine chemically with 1 g of hemoglobin under normal physiological conditions. 0.003 ml is the amount of oxygen dissolved in 100 ml of arterial blood for each torr $PaO_2$.

> EXAMPLE: 11 g of hemoglobin, 85% saturated with oxygen at a $PaO_2$ of 50 torr:
>
> 11 g × 1.34 ml × 100% + 0.003 ml × 50 torr
> (11 × 1.34 × 1.0) + (0.003 × 50)
> 14.74 + 0.15
> = 14.89 vol% arterial oxygen capacity
>
> 11 g × 1.34 ml × 85% + 0.003 ml × 50 torr
> (11 × 1.34 × .85) + (0.003 × 50)
> 12.53 + 0.15
> = 12.68 vol % arterial oxygen content

2. Tachypnea, tachycardia, shortness of breath, and dyspnea and cyanosis are clinical symptoms and signs associated with hypoxemia, but analysis of arterial blood is necessary to measure actual presence and degree of hypoxemia. Other clinical signs include a reduction of peripheral vision, dizziness, mental clouding, and personality and behavior changes. Cyanosis, a blue skin color in areas where blood capillaries lie near the surface, such as the lips, nailbeds, tear ducts, and tongue, may be a false or late indication of hypoxemia. It occurs late in the patient with anemia and early in the patient with polycythemia. Cyanosis occurs when there are more than 5 g of reduced (unsaturated) hemoglobin in the arterial blood; therefore, this sign alone is a poor estimate of hypoxemia and should be considered only with other information when evaluating patient oxygenation.

Analysis of arterial blood oxygen content is the most effective evaluation of adequate oxygen administration. This is combined with monitoring of pulse and blood pressure. A decrease in cardiac output estimated by a decrease in the cardiac rate indicates that the increased work of the cardiopulmonary system has been relieved by the prescribed oxygen therapy.

3. Patients with chronic respiratory disease have a resting $PaO_2$ which is below the range of 80-100 torr of a healthy individual. Their $PaO_2$ may range from 40-80 torr depending on the length and severity of their chronic respiratory problem. This low range $PaO_2$ will be associated with a compensating respiratory acidosis. When treating those patients with oxygen, care must be taken to return their $PaO_2$ to their own "normal"

resting level. This prevents the elimination of their potential hypoxic drive. (See oxygen induced hypoventilation in this chapter.)

## CARBON DIOXIDE-OXYGEN THERAPY

Carbon dioxide is the physiological chemical that stimulates the central nervous system to regulate the ventilation of the lung. An increased carbon dioxide level in the blood has multiple effects on the body. It causes an increased rate and depth of ventilation, increased heart rate and blood pressure, and cerebral vasodilation. Common therapeutic mixtures of carbon dioxide and oxygen include 5% $CO_2$/95% $O_2$ and 10% $CO_2$/90% $O_2$ (see Table 1-1). Carbon dioxide should always be delivered in combination with oxygen.

### PHYSIOLOGICAL EFFECT OF $CO_2$-$O_2$ THERAPY

**Physiological Effects of Carbon Dioxide-Oxygen Therapy:**   The patient must have a responsive respiratory center for therapy to be effective. Without this, therapy will be very dangerous and of no real therapeutic value. The physiological effects of carbon dioxide-oxygen therapy are:

1. *Improvement of cerebral blood flow.*  Increased levels of carbon dioxide in the blood plasma cause dilation of cerebral blood vessels, leading to an increase in blood flow to the brain. It can be used to improve cerebral circulation of stroke patients.

2. *Stimulation of deep breathing.*  Increased carbon dioxide levels stimulate the medullary respiratory center, increasing the rate and depth of ventilation. An increased depth of ventilation will improve inflation of alveoli and may prevent post-operative atelectasis resulting from shallow breathing.

3. *Treatment of singulation (hiccups).*  Hiccups are the result of spasms occurring in the diaphragmatic muscles. Increased carbon dioxide can be used to stimulate the medullary respiratory center to override the uncontrolled spasms of the diaphragm.

### THERAPEUTIC CONSIDERATIONS OF $CO_2$-$O_2$ THERAPY

**Therapeutic Considerations and Possible Hazards of Carbon Dioxide-Oxygen Therapy:**

1. Prolonged use of carbon dioxide-oxygen therapy can cause central nervous-system depression. Carbon dioxide mixtures also stimulate the cardiovascular centers in the brain, leading to an increase in heart rate

and blood pressure. With changes of greater than 20 beats per minute in heart rate or greater than 40 torr increase in blood pressure, therapy should be discontinued.

2. Therapy should not be given for more than 4–6 minutes with a 5 percent mixture and no more than 1–2 minutes with a 10 percent mixture. The heart rate, ventilatory pattern, and blood pressure should be monitored continuously throughout the treatment. Therapy should be given with a tight, closed system such as nonrebreathing mask, but it should be handheld to facilitate rapid removal from the patient, as necessary.

3. Carbon dioxide-oxygen therapy should not be administered to chronic lung disease patients with a compensating respiratory acidosis. For these patients the carbon dioxide stimulation of the brain to ventilate the lungs is no longer the strongest respiratory stimulant in their system. Therefore, the patient's respiratory centers do not respond to the increased carbon-dioxide levels.

4. Potential side effects of carbon dioxide-oxygen mixtures include headache, nausea, dyspnea, tachycardia, blurred vision, high blood pressure, mental clouding, unconsciousness, and convulsions.

## HELIUM-OXYGEN THERAPY

Physiologically, helium is an inert gas. It is not used in body metabolism and normally exists only as a trace element in the atmosphere. Next to hydrogen, it is the lightest known gas (see Table 1-1). Because of helium's low density it is used in the management of airway obstruction. It is inhaled in a mixture with oxygen to replace nitrogen and decrease the density of the total mixture. Common mixtures of helium and oxygen gases are 80 percent He and 20 percent $O_2$; and 70 percent He and 30 percent $O_2$.

### PHYSIOLOGICAL EFFECTS OF He-$O_2$ THERAPY

With the low density of their gas mixture, He-$O_2$ therapy may decrease the amount of turbulent gas flow around airway obstructions associated with bronchospasms and with asthma. The density of an 80 percent He and 20 percent $O_2$ mixture is 0.429 g/l. The separate densities of oxygen and helium are 1.43 g/l and 0.1785 g/l respectively. Their combined density as an 80 percent–20 percent mixture is approximately one-third of the density of air.

The effect on the patient is a decrease in the effort required to ventilate his lungs. Comparing the density of helium mixtures and air, the same work of breathing would move three times as much helium-oxygen mixture as air. This causes more effective ventilation in the presence of large airway obstruction. This mixture effectively reduces turbulent gas but is no more effective than air if turbulence does not exist.

## THERAPEUTIC CONSIDERATIONS OF He-O₂ THERAPY

1. Helium-oxygen therapy must be delivered by a tight-fitting closed system because the smallest leak will allow the helium to diffuse to the atmosphere. A nonrebreathing mask is recommended.
2. A compensated Thorpe tube flowmeter calibrated to the helium-oxygen should be used because a compensated oxygen flowmeter will register a lower than actual flowrate. If a helium-oxygen flowmeter is not available, a conversion factor can be used. For each 1 l/min flow reading on an oxygen flowmeter, 1.8 l/min will actually be delivered. The helium-oxygen mixture is also a poor gas vehicle for aerosols. A benign side effect of helium is its temporary distortion of a patient's voice. This side effect should be explained to the patient prior to therapy. It will only last a few minutes following the therapy.

# GAS DELIVERY EQUIPMENT

## PRINCIPLES OF OPERATION

Gas-delivery equipment is classified as low-flow gas systems and high-flow gas systems. The accuracy of the delivered oxygen concentration depends on the type of gas-flow system used.

A.  Low-Flow Gas System

This system delivers less than the minimum peak inspiratory flowrate required by the patient. The system does not provide all the gas that the patient needs each breath. Therefore, the gas that is not delivered by the system, but required by the patient on inspiration, is entrained from the surrounding room air. This dilutes the gas concentration delivered to the patient and can cause the available oxygen concentration to vary. The gas concentration delivered with a low-gas flow system depends on these factors:

1. *Size of reservoir in the system.* The size of the gas reservoir may range from the 50–70 ml in the patient's nasal cavity to a 1–2 liter anesthesia bag attached to a mask. The greater the size of the area that can be filled with reserve oxygen for the patient to inhale, the lesser the amount of gas that

will be drawn from room air. Examples are the nasal cannula that uses the nasal cavity and the standard partial rebreathing mask with a 500–1000 ml reservoir bag. The greater the size of the reservoir, the higher the gas concentration that can be delivered. A limitation of the low-flow system is that it depends on increasing the size of the gas reservoir to increase the amount of gas available (see Fig. 1-2).

2. *Flowrate of gas into the system.* The gas flowrate in the low-flow system is not adequate to meet the inspiratory demands of the patient. To increase the oxygen concentration, the flowrate of the source gas must be increased. The gas flowrate during inhalation goes to the patient and during exhalation it will fill the gas reservoir in the system. The filling of the mask reservoir or the nasal cavity is limited to the last 25 percent of the expiratory phase when most expiratory flow has stopped. The greater

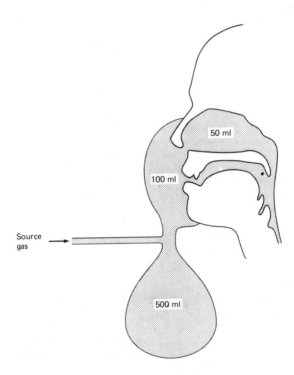

**FIG. 1-2.** Reservoirs in low flow gas systems. Low flow gas systems are dependent on a reservoir to increase the range of gas concentrations that can be delivered. The gas reserve is necessary because the gas flowrate in these systems is less than the minimum peak inspiratory flowrate of the patient.

the gas flowrate into the system, the larger the reservoir that the gas could fill while the patient exhales and the more gas that could be available to the patient during the next inhalation.

3. *Ventilatory pattern.* If the patient's tidal volume or respiratory rate decreases, the inspired gas concentration of a low flow system increases. There is an increase in the patient's inspiratory time that allows more source gas to be delivered to the patient, thus increasing the total gas concentration because less room air will be entrained. An increase in tidal volume or respiratory rate decreases the total gas concentration. In this case inspiratory time is decreased.

Low-flow gas systems deliver an estimated range of gas concentrations at specific gas flowrates (see Table 1-5). The percentage of gas delivered can be increased depending on the size of the reservoir in the system and whether or not the source-gas flowrate can fill that reservoir during the patient exhalation phase. Examples of the low-flow gas system include the nasal cannula, aerosol mask, and partial rebreathing mask. Low-flow gas system equipment is used in respiratory care because it is familiar, easy to assemble and use, and economical to use.

TABLE 1-5

**Approximate Gas Concentrations Delivered by Low Flow Gas Delivery Equipment***

| *Delivery Equipment* | *Range of Gas Concentration Delivered Patient* | *Range of Flowrate (liters per minute)* |
|---|---|---|
| Nasal catheter | 24–44% | 1–6 |
| Nasal cannula | 24–44% | 1–6 |
| Simple mask | 44–68% | 6–10 |
| Partial rebreathing mask | 52–80% | 8–15 |
| Nonrebreathing mask | 100% | 12–15** |
| Tent croupette | 30–50% | 10–15 |
| Aerosol mask | 30–100% | 10–15 |
| Briggs adaptor (T tube) face tent | depending on the source gas concentration and the amount of air being entrained into the nebulizer system that is used with this equipment | |

*Gas concentration delivered by these apparatus will depend on the size of the reservoir, the gas flowrate, and the ventilatory pattern of the patient. The above gas concentration ranges were calculated with the following values: TV 500 ml, respiratory rate 20, I:E ratio 1:2, atmospheric $F_IO_2$ .2

**Calculated on the following values: TV 500 ml, respiratory rate 15, I:E ratio 1:2, atmospheric $F_IO_2$ .2

## B. High-Flow Gas System

This system delivers a total gas flowrate that will supply the patient's required peak inspiratory flowrate. The patient receives all the gas from the system; therefore, the concentration of the gas delivered to the patient is exact and does not vary. The variables that affect the low-flow gas system do not affect the gas concentration of the high-flow system.

1. *Gas reservoir size.* The high-flow gas system does not depend on a gas reservoir to increase the desired gas concentration. A reservoir may be placed in the system as a gas reserve, but it is not necessary to increase the oxygen concentration.

2. *System gas flowrate.* In a high-flow gas system the flowrate is adequate to provide the peak inspiratory demand of the patient at any time he inhales. For example, if the patient's peak inspiratory flowrate is 800 ml/sec, then minimum flowrate through the system would have to be 48,000 ml/min or 48 l/min. The actual flowrate through a high-flow system should be higher than the patient's peak inspiratory flowrate to meet any excessive inspiratory demands. Three to four times the patient's minute ventilation can be used as a guide.

CALCULATION OF THE MINIMUM GAS FLOWRATE REQUIRED
IN A HIGH-FLOW GAS SYSTEM

The minimum flowrate is calculated from the estimated peak inspiratory flowrate of the patient. For example:

A patient with the following clinical measurements:

| | |
|---|---|
| Respiratory rate | 15 |
| Tidal volume | 600 ml |
| I:E (normal adult) | 1:2 |

Length of respiratory cycle = 60 sec/min ÷ 15 breaths/min = 4 sec

Inspiratory time = 4 sec ÷ 3 (based on the I:E ratio of 1:2) = 1.33 sec

Inspiratory flowrate = 600 ml/1.33 sec (amount of tidal inhaled during the inspiratory time)

Patient's peak inspiratory flowrate = 450 ml/sec

450 ml/sec × 60 sec. = 27300 ml/min = 27.3 l/min

Minimum flowrate into a high flow system to meet the above patient's inspiratory demands = 27.3 l/min

3. *Ventilatory pattern.* Since the total gas requirements of the patient are provided by the system, there will be no variation in the gas concentra-

TABLE 1-6

**Specific Gas Concentrations Delivered by High-Flow
Gas Delivery Equipment**

| Delivery Equipment | Gas Concentration Delivered | Oxygen/Air Ratio | Total Gas Flowrate Delivered |
|---|---|---|---|
| Masks or equipment with a venturi | 24% | 1:20 | @ 4 L/min. 84 l/min |
| | 28% | 1:10 | 44 l/min |
| | 35% | 1:5 | @ 8 L/min. 48 l/min |
| | 40% | 1:3 | 32 l/min |
| | 70% | 1:.6 | @ 15 L/min. 24 l/min |
| Mechanical ventilator-patient circuit | 21–100% | — | Patient's peak inspiratory flowrate |
| Intermittent Mandatory Ventilation Circuits | 21–100% | — | Patient's peak inspiratory flowrate |
| Continuous Positive Airway Pressure Circuit | 21–100% | — | Patient's peak inspiratory flowrate |

tion received by the patient with changes in respiratory rate or the tidal volume inhaled. High-flow gas systems deliver constant, specific gas concentrations to the patient (see Table 1-6). This delivery equipment must attach to the patient so that the patient cannot entrain room air during inhalation and so that he or she receives only the gas from within the system. Such equipment is sometimes expensive and complex to assemble and to adjust on the patient, but it does provide an exact gas concentration to the patient, making it the safer and more efficient delivery equipment. Examples of high-flow gas systems include masks using the venturi principle, mechanical ventilator circuits, and CPAP patient circuits.

## LOW-FLOW GAS EQUIPMENT

This equipment delivers less than the minimum peak inspiratory flowrate required by the patient and therefore delivers a varying range of gas concentrations. The equipment is economical, familiar, and commonly used in respiratory care medical gas administration (see Table 1-5).

### Nasal Cannula (see Fig. 1-3)

A nasal cannula is a small bore, green plastic tube with two one-half-inch tips that are shaped to fit into the nares of the patient. It wraps

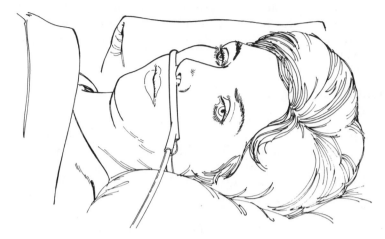

**FIG.** 1-3. Nasal cannula.

around the patient's face and is secured by an elastic band that fits around the back of the patient's head. Because of the limited area of the nasal cavity to act as a reservoir (50-70 ml) this equipment delivers a low range of gas concentration (24-44 percent $O_2$ at 1-6 l/min). It provides minimal discomfort to the patient and does not inhibit access to the mouth and face.

The following are therapeutic considerations for use of the nasal cannula:

1. Gas flowrates greater than 6 l/min will not increase the delivered gas concentration because the nasal cavity is the only reservoir for oxygen with the cannula and will generally be filled by 6 l/min flowrate.
2. The nasal cannula may deliver less oxygen to the patient when the nasal cavity is obstructed, such as with a severe deviated nasal septum, nasal mucosa edema, nasal polyps and excessive nasal secretion drainage.
3. The cannula can be easily dislodged and may become plugged with nasal secretions. It should be checked periodically for placement and patency of the prongs (tips) entering the nares. A check at least every four hours is recommended.
4. If needed, the tips of the nasal prongs may be trimmed with scissors to fit more comfortably into an individual patient's nares.
5. The cannula may be irritating and cause bleeding from the nasal

mucosa. It can also cause irritation and ulceration on the top of the ear lobes due to the elastic band. The cannula delivers only a limited amount of humidity to the patient using standard humidification equipment. (See Chap. 3.)

## Nasal Catheter (see Fig. 1-4)

This is a single small bore, green plastic tube with perforations at the distal end. It is inserted through a nare and the nasal cavity into the oropharynx until it lies behind the uvula (the membranous extension of the soft palate). Since the nasal cavity is also the only reservoir for oxygen with this equipment, it delivers a low range of gas concentrations (24-44 percent $O_2$ at 1-6 l/min). After insertion, the catheter is secured to the patient's nose and/or forehead with nonabrasive tape.

The following are therapeutic considerations for use of the nasal catheter:

1. The catheter may be used with patients that cannot keep a cannula properly in place and with patients having facial trauma or facial burns. It is not the best choice in any case where a mask or cannula can be used.
2. It is contraindicated with nasal obstruction or nasal bleeding. If resistance is met on insertion of the catheter, it should never be forced.
3. Proper position of the catheter is important. Over insertion into the esophagus can lead to gastric insufflation. Its presence in the nasal cavity may also be uncomfortable and cause nasal mucosal drying and hemor-

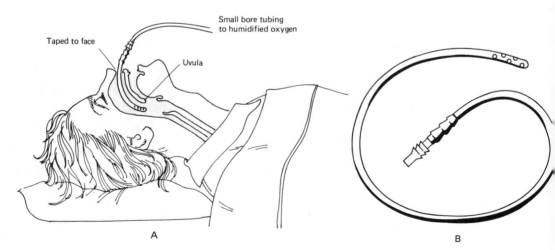

Taped to face

Small bore tubing to humidified oxygen

Uvula

A

B

FIG. 1-4. A. Nasal catheter inserted through the nasal cavity. B. Nasal catheter.

rhaging. Placement should be checked periodically and the catheter should be changed to the opposite nare every eight hours to prevent tissue necrosis.

4. To approximate the length of the catheter to be inserted into the nasal cavity for proper placement, measure the distance of the tube from the tip of the patient's nose to the top of the earlobe. Mark the length from the distal end with a piece of tape.

5. To keep the perforations on the catheter patent during insertion, attach the catheter to connecting tubing and run a low-oxygen flowrate through it.

6. Method of placement.

a) Lubricate the tip of the catheter with a water soluble lubricating jelly (i.e. *K-Y* jelly). Never use an oil-based lubricant because accidental aspiration would cause a severe inflammatory response.

b) Insert the catheter through the nasal cavity to the measured distance marked by the tape.

c) Move it gently into the nare, holding the catheter so that the curvature of the catheter corresponds with the natural curvature of the nasal cavity. If resistance is encountered, rotate the tube by applying gentle pressure. If the catheter cannot be inserted in this nare, try the other nare. Never force the catheter.

d) Check placement by depressing the patient's tongue and using a flashlight to locate the tip of the catheter.

e) After insertion, locate the tip of the catheter and slowly withdraw it until it just disappears behind the uvula. The tip of the properly placed catheter should rest just out of sight behind the uvula.

f) Secure the nasal catheter with nonabrasive tape to the mandible or the bridge of the nose.

## Simple Oxygen Mask (see Fig. 1-5)

This is a dome-shaped, disposable, plastic apparatus that fits over the nose and mouth and is secured by a strap around the back of the head. It is adjusted to the patient's face by a malleable metal nose piece incorporated on the mask. The dome shape of the mask provides an additional 70–100 ml reservoir for oxygen; therefore, it can deliver a moderate range of oxygen concentrations (44–68 percent $O_2$ at 6–10 l/min). The mask requires a snug fit to limit the amount of room air entrained around the edges. It has a series of small holes, or ports, on each side that act as exhalation ports. There are no valves in this mask, so room air is entrained through these ports, thus reducing the delivered oxygen concentration the patient receives.

The following are therapeutic considerations for the use of the simple mask:

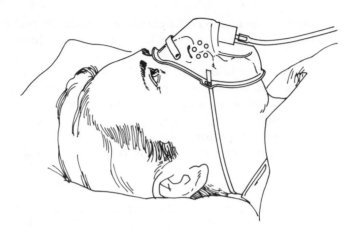

FIG. 1-5. Simple oxygen mask.

1.  The mask can be easily dislodged. This is common with all masks. Its proper position should be understood by the patient and checked frequently. The mask's edges and the elastic bands holding it in place can cause pressure necrosis when the mask is used for extended periods of time.

2.  The minimum flowrate through these masks should never be less than 5 l/min. This flowrate is necessary to force the exhaled gas, which is high in carbon dioxide, out the exhalation ports, thus preventing the rebreathing of exhaled gas.

3.  These masks are contraindicated in patients with levine tubes (nasogastric drain tubes), facial burns, or where proper nursing care requires frequent access to the patient's face. These do not allow for proper fit of the mask and consistent gas delivery.

4.  With vomiting, there is greater hazard of aspiration with a mask because it would inhibit clearance of the vomitus from around the mouth. This hazard is even greater with unconscious and comatose patients. These individuals require close observation when using a simple mask.

Partial Rebreathing Mask (see Fig. 1-6)

This is a simple mask with an attached reservoir bag. It contains no valves. The use of a 500–1000 ml reservoir provides a range of oxygen concentrations from 52–80 percent at 6–10 l/min. The reservoir allows a reserve gas volume to be inhaled from the bag during inspiration. The first one-third of the patient's exhaled volume returns to the bag as the patient exhales and the remaining two-thirds are exhaled through the mask's side ports. The first part of the exhaled volume only reaches the anatomical deadspace of the respiratory tract, and, therefore, has a near-inspired

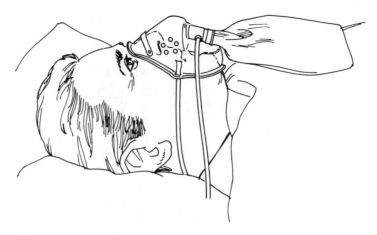

FIG. 1-6. Partial rebreathing mask.

oxygen level and a low carbon-dioxide level. The mask is firmly secured with an elastic band around the back of the head.

The following are therapeutic considerations for the use of a partial rebreathing mask:

1. The flowrate of the source gas should be adjusted so that the reservoir bag does not completely collapse during inhalation. The bag should be about one-third collapsed with each inhalation. This mask conserves oxygen, allowing the part of the exhaled gas volume to be rebreathed during the next inspiration.
2. The mask must be positioned so that the reservoir bag is never kinked, preventing gas to be inhaled from it. If the patient's head position causes the bag to be pinched off, the efficiency of the mask and the delivered oxygen concentration will be reduced to that of a simple mask.

### Nonrebreathing Mask (see Fig. 1-7)

This is a simple mask with a reservoir bag that includes a one-way valve between the bag and the mask and two one-way valves on the mask's exhalation side ports. These valves prevent the entrainment of room air through the exhalation ports and require that the patient receive all the delivered gas from the reservoir bag and mask. Inhaled gas with a properly fitted mask comes only from the bag and the exhaled gas goes only to the room. The gas concentration delivered depends on the concentration of the source gas. This type of mask can be used as a high-gas flow system if the reservoir provides the adequate gas to exceed the patient's inspiratory requirements.

The following are therapeutic considerations for the use of a non-rebreathing mask:

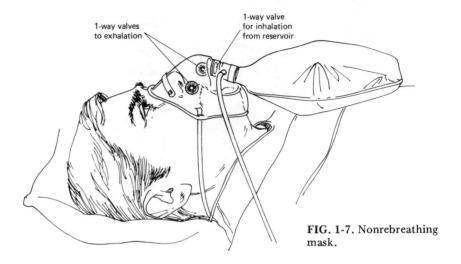

1-way valves
to exhalation

1-way valve
for inhalation
from reservoir

**FIG.** 1-7. Nonrebreathing mask.

1. The ability of the mask to act as a nonrebreathing device requires a high flowrate and a 500–1000 ml reservoir.
2. A snug-fitting nonrebreathing mask is used to deliver oxygen-helium and carbon dioxide-oxygen mixtures. A proper close fit is needed to guarantee delivery of the precise gas concentrations in the mixtures.
3. A safety relief valve is placed between the one-way inhalation valve and the dome of the mask to allow room air to be inhaled by the patient in case the reservoir bag or inhalation valve becomes obstructed or pinched off. This happens if the patient's head is improperly positioned, thus kinking the bag from the mask. This is important since the patient is dependent on the system for his or her total gas volume.
4. An expiratory retard adaptation has been used with this mask to provide positive pressure on expiration. It can be used with patients having pulmonary edema. It can also be used with an adaptor that is a venturi diluter, creating exact oxygen concentrations of 40–95 percent.

## Tent

A tent is a large plastic canopy designed to enclose the patient in a controlled environment. Humidity and/or aerosol and supplemental oxygen may be added to the tent atmosphere. Oxygen concentrations range from 30–50 percent at 10–15 l/min. Oxygen tents for adults cover the upper half of the body, while tents for pediatric patients enclose the entire body. The bottom edges of the tent must be tucked in securely around the base of the bed to allow a build-up of gas concentration to the 30–50 percent range. A minimum flowrate of 10 l/min is recommended to prevent a build-up of exhaled carbon dioxide within the tent. Today, tents are used primarily with pediatric patients.

One modification of the oxygen tent is the *croupette* (see Fig. 1-8). The croupette is specially designed to deliver a cool, high-humidity atmosphere to the pediatric patient. It is used with patients with tracheo-laryngobronchitis (croup), bronchitis, and pneumonia. Pneumatic nebulizers are used to produce an aerosol for evaporation in the tent. If high humidity is desired, a babbington or ultrasonic nebulizer may be used to create a more dense aerosol. Depending on design, the tent may be cooled electrically or by using an ice reservoir. Tents are designed so that all gas flow circulates through the cooling systems prior to entering the patient's environment. The minimum gas flowrate not only removes exhaled carbon dioxide but also circulates cool gas through the tent. A sealed croupette can build up to 30–50 percent gas concentrations at 10–15 l/min.

The following are therapeutic considerations for the use of tents:

1. The edges of the tent must be firmly sealed at the bottom. Tuck the edges under the mattress of the bed. A drawsheet can be used to secure the edge across the patient to prevent leaks. Since oxygen has a greater density than air, the higher gas concentration will be in the bottom of the tent and any leaks would cause a decrease in the delivered gas concentration.

2. The tent should be flushed with oxygen prior to sealing the patient in it. Once the tent is securely tucked in, the oxygen concentration builds up in the tent. Any time the tent is opened, the gas concentration drops and can actually decrease to nearly room-air oxygen levels. Therefore, the

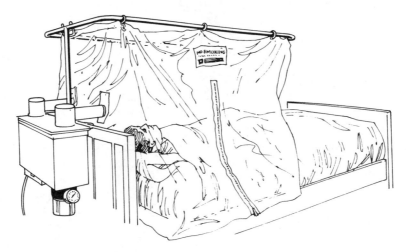

**FIG. 1-8.** Croupette mounted on a pediatric bed.

efficiency of tents is limited if the patient requires frequent nursing care. Oxygen concentrations should be monitored at least every four hours with an oxygen analyzer.

3. Noise pollution is a potential hazard, especially with aerosol delivery into an oxygen hood. High gas flows create sound levels that may affect the patient's hearing and psychological well being. Gas flow and exposure time should be limited to the minimum.

4. A tent is made of a transparent plastic material. Its combustion point is lowered considerably with the increased oxygen levels in the atmosphere. The tent canopy and the patient's room door should be clearly labelled, warning of the hazard of fire and strictly prohibiting smoking. All spark-producing toys or electrical equipment including the nurse call buttons should be kept outside the tent canopy.

The *oxygen hood* is another modification of the tent (see Fig. 1-9). It fits over the patient's head and is primarily used with newborns and infants. Care must be taken that gas flow and aerosol entering the hood do not blow directly onto the patient. Heated aerosol and humidity are recommended. These considerations will help prevent exceptional heat loss by the patient. This is a hazard in newborns because their heads make up approximately one-third of their total bodies. The function of the hood is to provide prescribed gas concentrations and humidity to the infant and newborn. It can be used to provide up to 100 percent oxygen to these small children. Again, caution should be taken to provide only enough oxygen in the atmosphere to maintain a normal range of arterial oxygen tension.

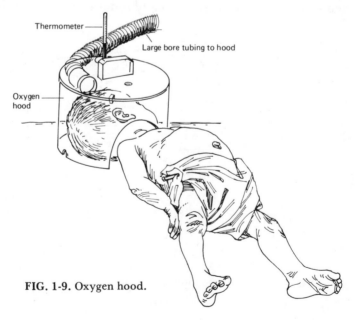

Thermometer

Large bore tubing to hood

Oxygen hood

**FIG. 1-9. Oxygen hood.**

Aerosol Delivery Equipment

Tracheostomy masks, aerosol masks, T-connectors, and face tents are used with large bore tubing to deliver low-flow gas concentrations and aerosols to the patient. Their primary purpose is to deliver humidity and aerosol. The gas concentration delivered from the equipment depends on the source gas concentration and the amount of air being entrained. (Aerosol delivery equipment is described in Chap. 3, Humidity and Therapy.)

## HIGH-FLOW GAS EQUIPMENT

This equipment delivers more than the minimum peak inspiratory flowrate required by the patient, and, therefore, delivers a constant exact gas concentration as described in the operation of high-flow gas systems. The use of high-flow gas systems is a current trend in respiratory care equipment, although these system sometimes require expensive and complex equipment. Table 1-6 shows high-flow gas equipment.

Venturi Mask

This is a simple mask with a venturi device attached to the source gas input port (see Fig. 1-10). The velocity of the source gas flowing through the venturi decreases the lateral wall pressure in the tube of the mask. This draws in room air (20.95 percent) to mix with the 100 percent oxygen source gas to deliver a constant gas concentration to the patient. The entrained room air combined with the source gas maintains a high liter flow of gas through the system. Common available venturi mask gas concentrations are 24 percent, 28 percent, 31 percent, 35 percent, 40 percent.

The following are therapeutic considerations in the use of venturi masks:

1. A venturi mask must fit the face snugly so that no room air can be pulled into the mask when the patient inhales. If this mask is not properly placed on the patient's face, it does not provide the precise oxygen concentration to the patient.
2. Care must be taken to prevent the blocking of the air entrainment ports on the venturi mask. The venturi mask should never be covered with bed sheets, bandages, or surgical drapes. If the venturi is occluded, the efficiency of the venturi mask is reduced to that of a simple mask and the oxygen concentration delivered to the patient will vary.

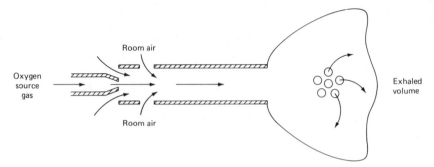

FIG. 1-10. Mask with venturi. The venturi mask functions as a high gas flow device based on Bernoulli's principle that changes in lateral wall pressure are directly related to changes in the velocity of a gas flowing through a tube. At a given gas velocity, a predictable amount of room air will be entrained into the mask, creating a constant gas concentration to be delivered to the patient (see text). The size of the restriction in the diluter determines the velocity of the source gas flowing into the tube. As velocity increases, the amount of air entrained through the ports also increases.

3.   When venturi devices that deliver more than 24 percent are used, the source gas may require humidification. Room air contains some humidity but at higher gas concentrations the amount of room air entrained into the system is limited. The high gas flowrate and the limited amount of room air entrained in these systems may not provide adequate humidity for the gas entering the respiratory tract. This can lead to dehydration and should be closely monitored by observating the patient and looking for thickening secretions. Prolonged continuous use of venturi masks without additional humidity can lead to thickened secretions and mucosal hemorrhage caused by drying. Blood-streaked sputum may appear after two or three days of continuous use of a venturi mask, if the gas contains inadequate humidity.

An aerosol collar adapted to fit the base of the venturi mask is used to attach large bore tubing for aerosol delivery in the entrained air. The nebulizer should be propelled with air so that the delivered oxygen concentration is not increased.

## Mechanical Ventilator-Patient Circuit

This is the tubing assembly that is attached from an artificial mechanical ventilator to the patient via an endotracheal or tracheostomy tube (see Fig. 1-11). It provides the delivery of gas to the patient from the mechanical ventilator and includes an exhalation valve for the removal of exhaled gas. This circuit from the mechanical ventilator provides all the gas required by the patient, and, therefore, can deliver a constant pre-mixed gas concentration. Most continuous mechanical ventilators can

MECHANICAL VENTILATOR-PATIENT CIRCUIT

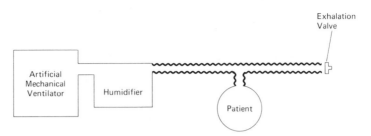

**FIG. 1-11.** Mechanical ventilator-patient circuit.

deliver precise gas concentrations from 21–100 percent. This is described in more detail in Chaps. 8 and 9.

## Intermittent Mandatory Ventilation (IMV)

This is a tubing assembly used in conjunction with mechanical ventilation to provide a constant high-flow system that meets the patient's spontaneous ventilatory demand, as well as delivers periodically required gas volumes to the patient from the mechanical ventilator to assist with the patient's ventilatory needs. This high-flow system allows the patient to continue spontaneous breathing. This is also described in Chaps. 8 and 9.

## Continuous Positive Airway Pressure (CPAP)

This tubing assembly is set up to deliver a high flow of gas to the patient and to continually keep a prescribed level of positive pressure in the respiratory system to prevent the alveoli from collapsing on exhalation. This system is used with patients who are spontaneously breathing. It is also discussed in greater detail in Chaps. 8 and 9.

The following is an important therapeutic consideration of ventilator-patient circuits, IMV circuits, and CPAP circuits:

The patient receiving medical gas administration from these types of equipment assemblies is dependent on the gas delivered in the system to meet his or her inspiratory demands. These assemblies are normally "sealed" into the patient circuits in some manner: with mechanical ventilator patient's circuits, cuffed endotracheal or tracheostomy tubes; IMV circuits are the same; with CPAP circuits, nasal prongs, mask, endotracheal tube, tracheostomy tubes or headbags. Whatever the method, these systems do not always have very efficient fail-safe devices for the patient to breathe through in case gas stops flowing in the system (i.e., with tubing disconnection or power failure). Because the patient is dependent entirely on the system for his gas volume, it is recommended that some type of pressure alarm be incorporated whenever possible and that the equipment be securely fastened when assembled and monitored to assure adequate continuous gas flow to the patient. These systems should be set up only in intensive care units where they can be closely observed, and they should be checked at least once each hour.

## GENERAL PROCEDURES FOR INITIATING MEDICAL GAS ADMINISTRATION

The following is a procedure to follow after an order for medical-gas administration has been received. It does not include the set up of a mechanical ventilation patient circuit, IMV circuit, or CPAP circuit (see Chap. 3, Intensive Respiratory Care).

1. Assemble the needed equipment and check its function in the department. Only pressure-compensated flowmeters should be used.
2. Check the chart for orders. There must be a complete written order by a physician before therapy can be administered. Emergency situations should be described in the department procedure manual and authorized by the medical director. Also, check the chart for the possibility of the patient having a hypoxic ventilatory drive. This may be indicated with chronic emphysema or bronchitis and a compensated respiratory acidosis with reduced arterial oxygen tensions (less than 80 torr).
3. Wash hands. Hospital-acquired nosocomial infections are commonly caused by the transportation of bacteria between patients by health care personnel not using proper cleaning techniques.
4. Introduce yourself to the patient, identify the patient, and explain to him what you are doing and why. Reassure the patient. Explain the no-smoking instructions. With unconscious or comatose patients, explain what you are doing to them as if they were alert and listening. The tone of your voice and your warm, confident touch can be reassuring to them. Also explain the equipment to the patient's relatives that may be staying with him.
5. Attach the pressure-compensated flowmeter to a 50-psig source. Attach humidification equipment filled with sterile water to the flowmeter.
6. Attach the gas-delivery equipment to the humidifier via small bore tubing. Observe proper cleaning techniques while handling the gas delivery equipment and humidifier.
7. Check the safety pop-off valve on the humidification equipment (if present) and set the ordered flowrate.
8. Place the gas delivery equipment in proper position on the patient. Secure the equipment to the patient's face so that it fits snugly, but not tightly enough to obstruct blood circulation.

9.   Place a no-smoking sign on the patient's door.
10.   Wash hands before leaving the patient's room.
11.   Chart the date and time, gas-concentration delivered, type of gas-delivery apparatus, the set flowrate in l/min, and patient reaction to therapy.

Check proper equipment position and function and the patient's condition at least every four hours. With each check, review the patient's chart for new orders and most recent arterial blood gas measurements, and record the status of the equipment (i.e., p.r.n., continuous, h.s.).

## GENERAL CONSIDERATIONS OF MEDICAL GAS THERAPY

### Use of Air/Oxygen Blenders

This type of equipment is used to mix oxygen and air proportionately to provide the prescribed oxygen concentration. A calibrated dial is set on the front of the blender. This is also called an air/oxygen mixer. This equipment requires a constant compressed air and oxygen source to maintain proper blending of the gases. Some equipment has low-pressure alarms to signal if the source gas is below the minimum pressure level. Most units have flowmeter attachments and a 50-psig pressure outlet connection. This equipment provides precise gas concentrations between 21 and 100 percent.

The following are therapeutic considerations with the use of an air/oxygen blender:

1.   The oxygen concentration of the gas delivered by the blender is based on the mixing of air and oxygen in the system. It is not analyzed internally and the control knob for setting the desired oxygen concentration must be kept in proper calibration. Therefore, gas delivered from this system must be periodically analyzed.
2.   Air/oxygen blenders are used to provide source gas for high-flow gas systems. This is often more efficient than blending oxygen and air from two flowmeters. The units available are expensive but do provide a precise, constant gas concentration for the high flow gas systems.

### Use of Cylinders

There are hazards in the storage, handling, and use of any compressed gas cylinders. When use of cylinders is required, the potential of these hazards should be reduced to a minimum. All applicable National Fire Prevention Association standards (NFPA) for the handling and storage of high pressure cylinders should be followed.

## TABLE 1-7

### Conversion Factors for Calculation of Cylinder Flow Duration (l/psig)

|                | D    | E    | G    | H and K |
|----------------|------|------|------|---------|
| Air, $O_2$     | 0.16 | 0.28 | 2.41 | 3.14    |
| $He/O_2$       | 0.20 | 0.35 | 2.94 | 3.84    |
| $O_2/CO_2$     | 0.14 | 0.23 | 1.93 | 2.50    |

Compressed gas cylinders containing 2200 psig pressure should be changed after the pressure of gas in the cylinder reaches 500 psig. This will assure that the cylinder does not empty, interrupting the prescribed gas therapy, and that a cylinder is not completely emptied of gas, allowing moisture or dirt to accumulate in it. Table 1-7 lists the conversion factors for computing the length of time that a cylinder of gas will last at a set flowrate. The following formula is used for calculating the duration of flow and changing the cylinder with 500 psig remaining.

$$\text{Duration of flow} = \frac{(\text{psig} - 500) \times \text{conversion factor for that cylinder size}}{\text{set gas flow rate}}$$

EXAMPLE: If an *H* cylinder has 1500 psig pressure on the regulator and is set up on a patient using a nebulizer set at 10 l/min, it will last the following length of time before requiring to be changed:

$$= \frac{(1500 \text{ psig} - 500 \text{ psig}) \times 3.14 \text{ l/psig}}{10 \text{ l/min}}$$

$$= \frac{1000 \text{ psig} \times 3.14 \text{ l/psig}}{10 \text{ l/min}} = \frac{3140 \text{ liters/psig}}{10 \text{ l/min}}$$

314 min = 5 hrs 14 min

## REFERENCES

Bendixen, H.H., *et al.*, *Respiratory Care*, C.V. Mosby, St. Louis, 1965.

Brunner, L.S., Suddarth, D.S., *Lippincott Manual of Nursing Practice*, Lippincott, Philadelphia, 1974.

Bushnell, S.S., *Respiratory Intensive Care Nursing*, Little, Brown, Boston, 1973.

Egan, F. *Fundamentals of Respiratory Therapy*, 3rd edition, C.V. Mosby, St. Louis, 1977.

Grenard, S., *et al.*, *Advanced Study in Respiratory Therapy*, Glenn Educational Medical Services, New York, 1971.

Hedley-White, J., *et. al.*, *Applied Physiology of Respiratory Care*, Little, Brown, Boston, 1976.

Johnson, R.F., *Pulmonary Care*, Grune and Stratton, New York, 1973.

McPherson, S.P., *Respiratory Therapy Equipment*, C.V. Mosby, St. Louis, 1977.

Rau, J.C. and M.Y. Rau, *Fundamental Respiratory Therapy Equipment*, Glenn Educational Medical Services, New York, 1977.

Safar, P., *Respiratory Therapy*, F.A. Davis, Philadelphia, 1965.

Shapiro, B.A., *et. al.*, *Clinical Application of Respiratory Care*, 2nd edition, Year Book Medical Publishers, Chicago, 1979.

Slonim, N.B. and Hamilton, L.H., *Respiratory Physiology*, 2nd edition, C.V. Mosby, St. Louis, 1978.

Taylor, J.P., *Manual of Respiratory Therapy*, 2nd edition, C.V. Mosby, St. Louis, 1978.

Wade, J.F., *Respiratory Nursing Care*, 3rd edition, C.V. Mosby, St. Louis, 1977.

West, J.B., *Ventilation/Blood Flow and Gas Exchange*, 2nd edition, Blackwell Scientific Publications, Oxford, 1970.

Young, J.A. and Crocker, D., *Principles and Practices of Respiratory Therapy*, 2nd edition, Year Book Medical Publishers, Chicago, 1976.

# CHAPTER

# 2

# Oxygen Analyzers

Oxygen is a potent drug. The physician prescribes it in specific concentrations for clinical use. The use of oxygen requires precise measurement and periodic checking of administration equipment. Advances and improvements have been made in oxygen-delivery equipment, oxygen-monitoring and alarm systems, and oxygen-analysis equipment to provide continual delivery of accurate oxygen concentrations. It is important to know how much oxygen is being delivered to the patient. Delivering inadequate or excessive amounts of oxygen can result in pulmonary and systemic complications; for example, retrolental fibroplasia in neonates and pulmonary and systemic oxygen toxicity in adults. Delivering inadequate amounts can lead to cardiac arrest, central nervous-system lesions, and cerebral damage.

## PRINCIPLES OF OPERATION

Oxygen analyzers are classified on the basis of their principle operation. Those most often used in the clinical practice of respiratory therapy fall under one of four basic principles:

1. the paramagnetic principle (Pauling's principle)
2. thermal conductivity (the Wheatstone Bridge)
3. the Galvanic Cell (Fuel cell)
4. the Polarographic Electrode (Clark Electrode, Amperometer)

The safe, effective use of oxygen-analyzing equipment mandates that the therapist have a fundamental understanding of how each type of analyzer operates.

## PARAMAGNETIC PRINCIPLE

Oxygen is unique among gases because it is paramagnetic; that is, it is affected by a magnetic field. When a gas containing oxygen is exposed to a magnetic field, the oxygen molecules are attracted to the magnetic field and align themselves within the field. Most other gases are diamagnetic, which means that they are either repelled or unaffected in a magnetic field. Oxygen, in essence, becomes "magnetized" and the force of this effect is dependent on the amount of oxygen present in the gas. Figure 2-1 shows a schematic representation of the paramagnetic effect within such an oxygen analyzer. The Beckman D2 Oxygen Analyzer operates on the paramagnetic principle. This analyzer consists of a set of hollow glass dumbbells whose spheres are filled with nitrogen and suspended by two quartz fibers between the poles of two permanent magnets within the sampling chamber. The nitrogen within the spheres is not affected by the magnetic field. The glass and quartz are used because they also are unaffected within the same field. This sets up a density gradient

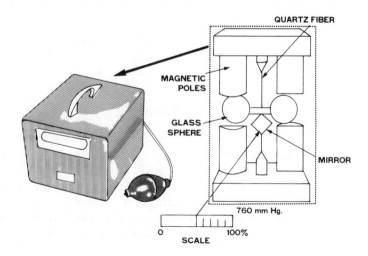

**FIG. 2-1.** Paramagnetic principle.

which applies a force to the glass sphere which is, in turn, proportional to the partial pressure of the oxygen in the sample. The dumbbell is displaced away from the poles. Situated on the bar of the dumbbell, directly between the bells, is a small mirror, onto which a lamp shines a beam of light. As the dumbbell turns, the mirror is turned and the light beam is displaced up or down on a scale depending on whether the gas sample is higher or lower in $O_2$ concentration. Only a small rotation of the dumbbell is necessary to cause a large deflection on the scale. The position of the light beam on the scale indicates the oxygen content of the sample and is calibrated in percent of $O_2$ concentration on the bottom part of the scale and in partial pressure of oxygen on the upper portion of the scale.

Paramagnetic analyzers are affected by barometric pressure because they measure the partial pressure of oxygen within the gas sample. They read out in both millimeters (mm) of mercury and percent concentration (Beckman D2). Even though the percent of oxygen in the air is the same regardless of altitude, the partial pressure varies with changes in altitude. The oxygen-concentration reading of this analyzer represents a percentage of the barometric pressure at that elevation. The unit must be factory calibrated for the altitude at which the analyzer will be used. For example, for an oxygen analyzer that has been calibrated at sea level (760 mm of mercury), and an ambient temperature range, the scale should read 20.9 percent $O_2$ and 158.8 mm Hg pressure. Oxygen analyzers using the paramagnetic principle will read inaccurately with varying altitudes and extreme temperatures. If this same analyzer were taken to an area with a barometric pressure of 600 mm Hg, the scale would also read inaccurately. The partial pressure of oxygen would be 125.4 mm Hg and the scale would read 16.5 percent $O_2$. This is corrected by using the following equation:

$$\frac{\text{Indicated } O_2\% \times 760 \text{ mm Hg}}{\text{Actual Pb}} = \text{Actual } O_2\%$$

Using above data:

$$\frac{16.5 \times 760 \text{ mm Hg}}{600 \text{ mm Hg}} = \text{approx. } 20.9\% \, O_2$$

The Beckman D2 uses silica gel to take moisture from the sample. The silica gel turns pink when the gel is saturated with water. The Beckman D2 Analyzer does not require daily calibration; however, the unit should be tested prior to use to see that it is functioning correctly. This can be done by either an air or 100 percent $O_2$ reference. If the analyzer is not functioning accurately, the unit should be returned to the factory to be recalibrated.

## THERMAL CONDUCTIVITY
## (WHEATSTONE BRIDGE)

The thermal conductivity of a gas describes the way in which it conducts heat. Oxygen conducts heat at different rates than does nitrogen, the major balancing gas in room air. Oxygen analyzers using this principle of thermal conductivity measure the concentration of oxygen in a gas sample by observing the changes in electrical resistance within the analyzer. Oxygen removes heat from an óbject more rapidly than other gases. The speed at which this conduction occurs is a function of the oxygen concentration; therefore, the higher the concentration, the faster the rate of conduction and thus the faster the rate of cooling. In analyzers using this cooling principle, an electric current is carried through a wire with a given resistance. The oxygen changes the resistance in that wire because of its ability to absorb heat. As the wire cools, the electrical resistance is reduced. This current reaches a bifurcation in the wire and splits equally if the resistance in both branches is equal (see Fig. 2-2). The current then passes through each pair of resistors in each wire, which forms the Wheatstone Bridge. Given that $R_1$, $R_2$, $R_3$, and $R_4$ are individual resistances and a galvonometer is connected between this parallel electrical circuit, the potential difference which can be created between these two circuits can be measured. In such an electrical circuit, if the ratio of $R_1/R_2 = R_3/R_4$, the galvonometer should read zero; that is, no potential difference. In

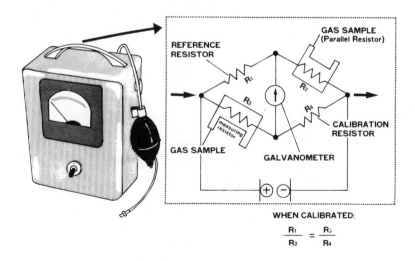

FIG. 2-2. Wheatstone bridge (thermal conductivity).

analyzers using the thermal conductivity principle, when this equation is balanced, the galvonometer is adjusted to read 21 percent. The sample gas is passed across one side of the Wheatstone Bridge ($R_3$, see Fig. 2-2). Remembering that resistance is a function of the amount of heat, the equation given above will be disrupted and the galvonometer will register a greater current through the side of the Bridge exposed to the sample gas. Since the opposite side is kept constant as a reference with room air, this potential difference is a function of the amount of oxygen available. The galvanometer is actually reading potential difference; however, it is calibrated in percent oxygen since the amount of oxygen is proportional to the electrical flow.

In oxygen analyzers using the thermal conductivity principle, the amount of carbon dioxide in the sample gas is important because carbon dioxide, like oxygen, has the property of thermal conductivity. The Mira and OEM oxygen analyzers are common examples of thermal conductivity units. The Mira unit uses a wet gas in its measurement of oxygen, and, therefore, silica gel is used to add moisture to the sample gas. The OEM unit, on the other hand, uses a dry gas measurement, and it uses silica gel to remove moisture from the sample. Units operating on the thermal conductivity principle are unaffected by changes in altitude and temperature. Because the thermal conductivity analyzers have the measuring resistor or circuit exposed to the gas sample and because an electrical current is running through this exposed wire, these units should not be used in an explosive atmosphere and not in an operating room nor with an anesthesia circuit.

Oxygen analyzers using the paramagnetic principle and the principle of thermal conductivity are used for intermittent oxygen analysis (static sampling) and both use a hand aspirator process.

## ELECTROCHEMICAL (AMPEROMETRIC) PRINCIPLE

There are two types of oxygen analyzers that use the electrochemical principle: the galvanic fuel cell and the polarographic electrode (Clark electrode). The primary difference between these two is that the galvanic fuel-cell polarizing principle is generated by the fuel cell itself, and the polarographic electrode sensor is generated by an external power source. In each of these units, a current flow (amperage) is set up that is related to the amount of oxygen available in the sample gas. In both analyzers, oxygen diffuses through a semipermeable membrane ($PO_2$ membrane) and an electrolyte solution. The membranes are usually made of Teflon or a polypropylene. Oxygen diffuses across the membrane because of the partial pressure gradient between the sample gas and the $PO_2$ in the liquid phase of the electrolyte. The oxygen molecules congregate at the cathode of the cell and in the presence of the electrolyte solution, an oxidation-reduction reaction occurs. For example,

$$4e^- + 2H_2O + O_2 \rightarrow 4OH^-$$

In essence, the oxygen is consumed. This generates an electrical current proportional to the rate of diffusion of oxygen across the membrane. The current is proportional to the number of oxygen molecules, and, therefore, to the partial pressure of oxygen. The rate of diffusion is directly proportional to the partial pressure of oxygen. The rate of diffusion is directly proportional to the partial pressure of oxygen in the gas phase. The anode of the elecfrode serves as the reference and supplies the electrons necessary for the oxidation-reduction of oxygen.

$$2OH^- + Pb \rightarrow PbO_2 + 2H_2O + 2e^-$$

This reaction is limited only by the amount of oxygen that is available at the anode and the amount of electrons produced. The electrons that establish the current are produced at the anode and used in the redox reaction at the cathode. The current is calibrated on the scale as oxygen percentage. Oxygen analyzers operating by this amperometric principle must do so at a constant temperature, since temperature changes would affect the rate of reaction; therefore, a thermistor is incorporated in these electrodes to maintain the constant temperature.

Gases under positive pressure cause an increase in the density or number of molecules per unit, and thus will increase the current. This increase in current will be read as an elevated oxygen percentage even though the actual oxygen percentage may be unchanged.

Figure 2-3 is a schematic of oxygen analyzers using the fuel cell. The Biomarine, Teledyne, Airshields and Hudson models of oxygen analyzers all use this principle. The Clark electrode operates basically in the same manner as does the galvanic fuel cell (see Fig. 2-4). Oxygen diffuses across the membrane, and is reduced at the cathode by the external voltage provided to the unit. This sets up the electrical current between the cathode and anode, thereby enabling the oxygen concentration to be measured. The Clark electrode responds to partial pressure in a manner similar to the galvanic fuel cell. Both the galvanic fuel cell and the Clark electrode are affected by humidity and moisture that may condensate on the measuring electrode, thus creating an inaccurate reading.

The difference between the galvanic fuel cell and the Clark electrode is that the galvanic fuel cell, being able to generate its own voltage at the anode, has a specific life span. On the other hand, by utilizing an external power source, the Clark electrode can last indefinitely under proper care. The polarographic unit will require changes in electrolyte solutions and in the oxygen membrane. The galvanic fuel cell will not. Analyzers that use

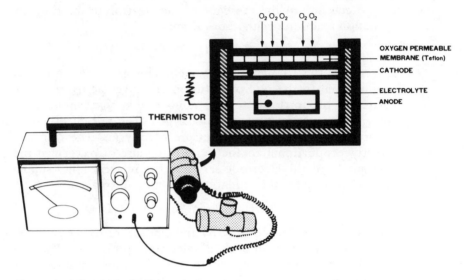

**FIG. 2-3.** Galvanic fuel cell.

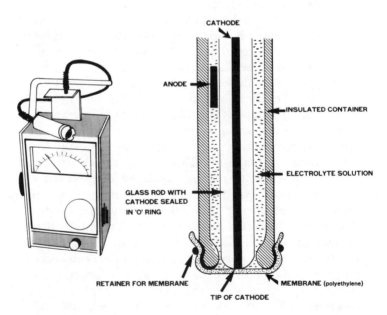

**FIG. 2-4.** Polarographic.

40

the polarographic or Clark electrode principle include the IL401, the Ohio, the Beckman OM10, the IMI and the Foregger analyzers. Tables 2-1, 2-2, and 2-3 provide a summary of the basic analyzers, their characteristics, and the factors that will cause inaccuracies.

TABLE 2-1

**List of Various Analyzers and Their Respective Principles and Modes of Sampling**

| Oxygen Analyzer | Principle of Operation | Sampling Function |
|---|---|---|
| Beckman D$_2$ | Paramagnetic | Intermittent |
| Mira | Thermal Conductivity | Intermittent |
| OEM | Thermal Conductivity | Intermittent |
| Beckman OM10, OM11 | Polarographic | Continuous |
| IL 402, 404, 406, 407 | Polarographic | Continuous |
| Ohio 200, 400, 600 | Polarographic | Continuous |
| IMI 3300, 3700 | Polarographic | Continuous |
| Foregger 7–029–005 | Polarographic | Continuous |
| Biomarine 0A202, 0A233, 0A288 | Galvanic Fuel Cell | Continuous |
| Teledyne 3300, 330F, 334 | Galvanic Fuel Cell | Continuous |
| Harlake Sentry I & II | Galvanic Fuel Cell | Continuous |

TABLE 2-2

**List of Analyzer Principles and Their Respective Calibration Procedure**

| Principle of Operation | Calibration |
|---|---|
| Paramagnetic | Does not require calibration. They are factory calibrated. Should be checked for accuracy with known O$_2$ concentration. Return to factory if re-calibration is necessary |
| Thermal Conductivity | These units require a two-point calibration (21% and 100%) |
| Galvanic Fuel Cell | Normally requires only a single point calibration (21%); however, if desired, can use a two-point calibration (21% and 100%) |
| Polarographic (Clark Electrode) | Normally requires only a single point calibration (21%); however, if desired, can use a two-point calibration (21% and 100%) |

**TABLE 2-3**

**List of Various Factors on Operation of Oxygen Analyzers**

| Principle of Operation | Pressure | Factors Humidity | Temperature |
|---|---|---|---|
| Paramagnetic (Beckman $D_2$) | Accuracy affected by ambient pressure | Read dry gases | Not affected by ambient temperature |
| Thermal Conductivity | Generally unaffected by ambient pressure ranges | Can read wet or dry gas depending on the unit. | Compensated through the calibration process |
| Polarographic | Will read higher % under increasing pressure | Unaffected by humidity unless condensate forms on electrodes | Electronically compensated |
| Galvanic Fuel Cell | Will read higher % under increasing pressure | Unaffected by humidity unless condensate forms on electrodes | Electronically compensated |

# CHAPTER

# 3

# Humidity and Aerosol Therapy

Humidity and aerosol therapy are basic modalities used in the treatment of respiratory disease. To provide effective therapy, one must clearly understand humidity and aerosol, the goals of each therapy, the equipment used, and the therapeutic considerations of such treatments.

## HUMIDITY

Water can exist in a gaseous atmosphere in two forms, as humidity and as aerosol. Though related, they are two separate forms of matter having individual characteristics (see Table 3-1). Humidity (also called water vapor) exists as individual water molecules and enters the air as a gas. The amount of water that the air can hold is directly related to the air temperature and atmospheric pressure. The maximum amounts of water that the air can hold as a gas at a given temperature is called the *maximum humidity*. As the temperature and/or pressure of the air increases, the capacity of the air for water vapor increases, therefore increasing the maximum

TABLE 3-1

Separate Characteristics of Humidity and Aerosol

|  | *Humidity* | *Aerosol* |
|---|---|---|
| Physical State: | Gas | Liquid |
| Partial Pressure (B.T.P.S.): | 47 torr | 0 torr |
| Produced by: | Evaporation | Atomization, nebulization |
| Unit of measure: | mg/l or g/m$^3$ (density) | Micron (diameter) |
| Stability factors: | Temperature Atmospheric pressure | Particle concentration Particle size Relative humidity |
| Possibility of transporting bacteria: | None | Can be transported on aerosol particles |

humidity (see Table 3-2). The transformation of water from a liquid to a gas is caused by the movement of gas molecules from the liquid surface into the surrounding atmosphere. This process is called *evaporation*. Evaporation requires a specific amount of energy called the *heat of vaporization*. The heat of vaporization is the number of calories required to convert one gram of liquid to a vapor without a change in temperature. The amount of humidity in the atmosphere in measured with a hygrometer.

Humidity is described in relationship to temperature in the following terms:

1. *Absolute humidity* is the actual amount of water vapor measured in the air at a given temperature. It is the amount of humidity that is present. (Example: The amount of humidity in the air at 28°C is measured and is 9.5 mg/l. Then 9.5 mg/l is the absolute humidity at 28°C.)

2. *Maximum humidity* is the greatest amount of water vapor that can be held in the air at a given temperature. It is the potential capacity of the air to contain water vapor at that specific temperature. Air containing maximum humidity would be described as being 100 percent saturated. (Example: At 28°C the absolute humidity was 9.5 mg/l, but the most it could be if 100 percent saturated at 28°C is 27.2 mg/l. Therefore, 27.2 mg/l would be the maximum humidity of the air at 28°C.) (See Table 3-2.)

3. *Relative humidity* is a comparison of the absolute humidity in the air and the maximum humidity the air could hold. It is expressed as a percent and is determined by the following formula.

$$\frac{\text{absolute humidity} \times 100}{\text{maximum humidity}} = \text{relative humidity (\%)}$$

Table 3-2

**Relationship Between Temperature and Maximum Humidity**

| Temperature (°C) | Temperature (°F) | Maximum Humidity (mg/l) |
|---|---|---|
| 37 | 98.6 | 43.9 |
| 35 | 95 | 39.6 |
| 30 | 86 | 30.4 |
| 27 | 80.6 | 25.8 |
| 25 | 77 | 23.0 |
| 20 | 68 | 17.3 |
| 17 | 62.6 | 14.5 |
| 15 | 59 | 12.8 |
| 10 | 50 | 9.4 |

The capacity of the air to be saturated by water vapor is directly related to the air temperature. This chart lists the maximum humidity that can exist at the specific temperatures (measurements at sea level, 760 torr).

(Example: The absolute humidity of the air is measured. At 28°C the absolute humidity was measured and is 9.5 mg/l. The maximum humidity of the air at 28°C equals 27.2 mg/l. Therefore, the relative humidity would equal:

$$\frac{9.5 \times 100}{27.2} = 35\%$$

The relative humidity equals 35 percent.)
4. *Body humidity* is the water content of the humidity in the lungs at 37°C. (98.6°F). It amounts to 44 mg of water per liter of air and exerts a partial pressure of 47 torr.

## AEROSOL

An *aerosol* is a colloidal suspension of liquid or solid particles in a gas. It is synonymous with a mist or fog. The mechanical breaking up of the liquid or solid into these particles is done by atomization or nebulization. An aerosol may be natural or man-made. Most naturally occurring aerosol particles are $50\mu$ (microns) or less in size.

An example of a natural aerosol would be the spray coming off the ocean or a sneeze. A man-made aerosol could be the spray from a pressurized deodorant can or a paint sprayer. The stability of an aerosol depends on particle size, particle concentration, and relative humidity. If the absolute humidity of the air is low, then the aerosol particle will evaporate to add water to the air until the maximum humidity is reached. The greater the particle concentration and the more optimal the particle size, the more stable the aerosol will be.

Many of the most common examples of aerosol exist as air pollutants in our environment. Coal dust and cotton dust, which can cause pneumoconiosis, are particle suspensions. Also the condensate nuclei of sulfur dioxide and ozone, which make up the smog that shrouds many of our metropolitan areas, are examples of common artificial aerosols. Aerosol can be effective therapeutically when produced and delivered to the patient in a controlled procedure.

## HUMIDITY THERAPY

The primary purpose of humidity therapy is to increase the amount of humidity (water vapor) in the gas being inhaled by a patient. The additional humidity is used to reduce the patient's physiological humidity deficit. The *humidity deficit* is the difference between the absolute humidity in the inhaled gas and the maximum humidity at 37°C that is required for the normal functioning of the lower respiratory system. The normal functioning of the respiratory mucosa and the gas exchange in the alveoli require gas that is 100 percent saturated with water vapor at 37°C. The maximum humidity at 37°C equals 43.9 mg/l.

For example: If a patient is breathing room air at an average room temperature of 68°F which normally has a relative humidity (R.H.) of approximately 50 percent, then the patient's inhaled air would contain 50 percent of the maximum humidity of 17.3 mg/l. 68°F., or 8.6 mg/l. To reach the maximum humidity of 43.9 mg/l at 98.6°F, 35.3 mg/l of water must be added. The humidity deficit of this patient would equal 35.3 mg/l.

The temperature control and humidification of the inhaled air is the natural function of the upper respiratory tract. This system normally adds all the needed additional humidity. The highly vascular nasal cavity provides gas to the lung containing 43.9 mg/l at 98.6°F.

Humidity therapy provides more water vapor in the inhaled air, increasing its relative humidity and reducing the amount that must be supplied by the upper respiratory tract.

### PHYSIOLOGICAL EFFECTS

Adequate humidity levels in the patient's atmosphere are an important consideration for normal lung functioning. In the normal healthy individual, about 700 g of water from the body are used each day to evaporate into the air in the respiratory tract. Humidity therapy provides an artificial humidity source. The effects of humidity therapy are:

1.  Reduces the humidity deficit. The addition of humidity to inspired gas decreases the physiological demand on the patient. The absolute humidity of the air is increased, decreasing the amount that the body needs to completely saturate the air at $37^\circ C$ (body humidity). This may reduce the water lost through the respiratory system.

2.  Prevents drying of the respiratory mucosa. The brushlike cilia and mucus and serous layers that line the respiratory system must function normally to remove foreign particles and microorganisms and to keep the lower respiratory tract sterile. Their mucosal layer must be moist and the secretions must have a low viscosity to be efficiently removed. The addition of humidity to the inspired air helps prevent the excessive water loss from this layer that may occur when providing the normal humidity requirements of an ill patient.

## THERAPEUTIC CONSIDERATIONS

1.  The patient may need additional humidity in the inspired air to reduce the amount that his or her body would have to provide. Any disease that inhibits the normal air "conditioning" by the nasal cavity may cause drying and damage to the lower airway mucosa, leading to the pooling of secretions, increased airway resistance, and a greater chance of infection. Added humidity also is needed with the dehydrated patients. The production of very thick secretions or a dry nonproductive cough can be indications of the need for additional humidity.

2.  All patients that have a tracheostomy tube or endotracheal tube should be provided with increased humidity. Since the upper airway is being bypassed, the normal means of humidification by the respiratory system are limited. Warming the air should also be considered since the nasal cavity also normally provides that air-conditioning process, and warming will increase the maximum humidity. Weak and debilitated patients who breathe primarily through their mouths should be observed and provided with artificial humidification if necessary.

3.  When a medical gas is delivered to a patient, it should have humidity added. Medical gas contains minimal water vapor (6 ppm) and may cause an increased physiological demand on the patient's respiratory system. (See Chap. 1.)

4.  A potential hazard of humidity therapy is overhydration. This is more likely to occur when the delivered gas is 100 percent saturated with water vapor at near body temperature when inhaled by the patient. This may

inhibit the normal use of body water in the respiratory system as well as add water through condensation. This should be closely monitored in patients who are confined to bed, are receiving I.V. therapy, and/or have reduced renal output. An increase in daily weight of greater than 1 percent or an increase in blood pressure may indicate the development of overhydration. This is a greater potential problem in newborns and patients with congestive heart failure.

5.  Humidity is used in the treatment of disease and should be considered a drug. It is also applied topically to the respiratory system, which is a sterile area; therefore, the water used in the humidity production should be sterile. It should be handled as a drug and its containers dated when opened and discarded at least every 24 hours to prevent contamination.

## HUMIDITY-PRODUCING EQUIPMENT

Humidity and aerosol-therapy equipment produce both humidity and aerosol. They are distinguished by their primary functions. Devices that primarily produce humidity are called humidifiers. Humidifiers are designed around one or both of the following physical principles:

1.  Gas must be in direct contact with a liquid for evaporation to take place. Therefore, the greater the surface area of the liquid that is in contact with the gas, the more evaporation that can take place. This is similar to the relationship of a pond to the sky above it. This relationship is described as a *gas-liquid interface*. Humidity-producing equipment increases the area of contact between the liquid and the gas delivered to the patients.

2.  As described earlier, the amount of humidity a gas can hold is dependent on *temperature and pressure*. On a daily basis, atmospheric pressure remains relatively constant but the temperature does vary. The higher the temperature, the greater the maximum humidity of the gas. Some humidifiers are designed with a heating mechanism incorporated within them, or that may be added, to increase the potential maximum humidity.

### PRINCIPLES OF OPERATION

Humidifiers are described in four categories based on the physical design of the equipment to increase the gas-liquid interface.

### Diffusion Head Humidifier

This type of device increases the gas-liquid interface by directing all the gas flow to the patient through a porous filter at the base of a water-filled container. The porous object fragments the gas flow, allowing it to

FIG. 3-1. Diffusion head humidifier. Gas flow enters the humidifier at (A) and travels down a capillary tube (B) to the base of the reservoir. A porous diffusing surface (C) separates the gas into parts allowing the gas to escape into the reservoir in small bubbles. Evaporation takes place as the gas flow passes through the reservoir and at the surface of the water (C and D). Humidified gas flows from the humidifier to the patient at outlet (E).

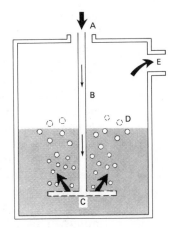

spread and emerge as multiple bubbles moving to the surface of the water at the top of the jar (see Fig. 3-1). This porous filter creates an amount of diffusing bubbles dependent on the number and size of the holes within it. Such porous materials as stone, plastic, and fabric are used as diffusing heads. The greater the number of bubbles and the smaller the bubbles, the more the gas surface area that will be exposed to the liquid. Evaporation also will occur at the surface of the water in the reservoir. The greater the gas-liquid interface, the more evaporation that can take place. This diffusion head design is commonly incorporated in humidifiers that are used in low-flow oxygen administration. These humidifiers are available in many designs.

## THERAPEUTIC CONSIDERATIONS

The following are therapeutic considerations of diffusion head humidifiers:

1.  This type of humidifier is most often used when the primary purpose is to increase the amount of humidity in a medical gas that is being delivered to a patient. It produces a low concentration of humidity. These humidifiers provide approximately 40–50 percent relative humidity at room temperature, which is only about 20–30 percent at body temperature. Therefore, their effectiveness is limited. It will decrease some of the water loss from the respiratory system, but it will not prevent all loss. The patient having thick secretions may require greater humidity than this humidifier will provide.

2.  A diffusion head humidifier is attached directly to a pressure-compensated flowmeter in the wall outlet or on the cylinder regulator. As the flowrate delivered to the patient increases, the temperature in the water

reservoir decreases caused by the heat loss into the flow gas. Another factor that influences the water temperature is the heat loss from evaporation, which was described earlier as the heat of vaporization. This temperature decrease will decrease the humidity carrying-capacity of the gas. The temperature decrease from the flowrate and evaporation is noted by the coldness to the touch of the water reservoir and by the observation of the formation of condensate on the outside of the jar. This heat loss may be compensated by heating the water in the humidifier. Heating equipment will be discussed later in this chapter.

3. The humidifier should have a pressure-relief valve in the reservoir to prevent pressure build-up that may occur if the delivery tubing becomes kinked or occluded between the humidifier and the patient, such as when a patient is lying on the tubing or when the tubing becomes plugged with mucus. This pressure build-up can cause cracking or explosion of the water reservoir. The pressure-relief valve presently in use in some humidifiers relieves pressures at 2 psig and at 40 torr. When it is set up, proper functioning of the pop-off should be checked by occluding the humidifier outlet until the valve pops off.

4. Diffusion head humidifiers are built as disposable and nondisposable units. Some of these are prefilled with sterile water for convenience and to prevent contamination. When in operation, humidifiers should be checked for proper functioning and refilled every four hours. As the water level in the humidifier reservoir decreases, the evaporation of water in the gas decreases; therefore to be most efficient the humidifiers should be kept filled. Sterile water should be used to refill humidifiers and the humidifier should be emptied and rinsed before being refilled.

5. Many disposable humidifiers that are prefilled with sterile water contain a bacteriostatic solution such as methyl paraben to inhibit bacterial contamination. They can be set up for use on a standby basis. These are convenient for emergency and recovery-room use and may be changed weekly or bimonthly if not used. They should be dated to assure that they are disposed of at the scheduled time.

## Spinning Disc Humidifier

This humidifier uses the action of centrifugal force to expand the gas-liquid interface (the Shiger principle). A single stemmed plate is attached to a small motor that turns the plate and conical stem at a high number of revolutions per minute (see Fig. 3-2). The stem extends into a reservoir of water. As it revolves, the water is drawn up the stem and onto the plate by centrifugal force and the principle of a screw. As the plate revolves the water is thrown against a comb-teeth baffle located around the dome of the humidifier. Striking the comblike structure, the water is fragmented, thus increasing the surface area exposed to the air. This increases the air-water interface and evaporation. The motor also drives a fan that creates

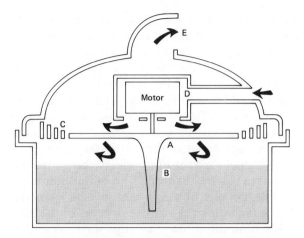

**FIG. 3-2.** Spinning disc humidifier. Room air enters inlet ports (D). Air is drawn by a fan attached to an electrical motor that also propels humidifed air out (E). Gas entering the humidifier passes through a water reservoir (B) where a large air-water interface enhances evaporation. A disc with a conical stem (A) is rapidly spun by the motor. As it revolves, water is drawn up the stem from the reservoir (B) and thrown from the disc onto a set of comb-shaped baffles that line the inside of the reservoir (C). Evaporation can take place along the surface of the reservoir and from the fragmented particles of water at the buffles.

air flow through the system and carries the humidified air out into the room. Evaporation occurs at the air-liquid interface of the fragmented water and the surface of the water in the reservoir. The water particles are aerosol, produced to evaporate and increase the absolute humidity in the air. The large water particles drop back into the reservoir while the smaller particles act as aerosol and are carried out with the air flow to evaporate in the room. This design is typical in room humidifiers commonly used at home and in hospital care.

## THERAPEUTIC CONSIDERATIONS

The following are therapeutic considerations of spinning disc humidifiers:

1. The spinning disc is used in humidifiers that are manufactured to increase general room humidity. These humidifers are not directly connected to the patient. The room humidifier should be placed near the

patient, preferably on a stand next to the bed. The output port should not be placed so that the expelled air blows directly on the patient, but rather in the patient's general direction. The draftlike effect is not usually well tolerated by the patient. These humidifiers also may be used with tent therapy by attaching a large bore tube from the humidifier port to the tent to add humidity to the enclosed environment.

2. These humidifiers have limited use in the hospital. They are most effective in small, closed rooms. The humidified air they deliver disseminates rapidly into the surrounding room air. There is no control over the actual amount of humidity the patient receives, unless the patient is restricted to the bed and the humidifier is properly positioned. Clinically, the therapeutic value can only be estimated by the patient's verbal feedback regarding the relative dryness of the air he or she is inhaling.

3. This humidifier uses a large water reservoir that normally requires filling every eight hours. Due to the possible bacterial growth in this warm, aqueous medium, the water reservoir and dome should be wiped off with a disinfectant and rinsed each time it is refilled. Use of sterile water for rinsing and refilling may be used to delay bacterial growth. Proper functioning of the humidifier and the water level should be checked at least every four hours.

4. All spinning disc humidifiers used for hospital patient care should be replaced or completely decontaminated after each seven days of use to further prevent bacterial contamination of the units. Some units available today allow complete disassembly for more accessible decontamination.

## Pass-over Humidifier

This type of humidifier has a very basic structure. Gas is exposed to a body of water by being blown across the surface of the liquid. Evaporation occurs as the gas flows through the water-filled reservoir (see Fig. 3-3). This design alone has limited use today in humidity-producing equipment. It has been the standard humidifier used on the Emerson

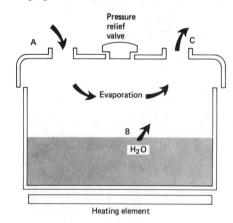

FIG. 3-3. Pass-over humidifier. This sketch describes a blower humidifier in which all gas flow passes over the surface of the heated reservoir of water (B) allowing evaporation of water to take place. Evaporation is enhanced by the heating of the water reservoir. (A) Inlet port of gas flow. (B) Point of evaporation. (C) Output port for humidified gas.

volume ventilator and the physical pass-over design is incorporated with other designs in all humidity producing equipment.

## THERAPEUTIC CONSIDERATIONS

The following are therapeutic considerations of pass-over humidifiers:

**1.** As the gas flowrate across the surface of the water in a reservoir increases, the temperature of the water falls, decreasing the capacity of the gas to hold humidity. This may be reduced by heating the water. The pass-over humidifier on the Emerson adult ventilator sits on a heating plate that can increase the water temperature considerably. Therefore, potentially the unit can deliver saturated gas equivalent to body humidity and temperature to the patient.

**2.** These humidifiers should be sterilized at least every 24 hours and only sterile water should be used to prevent bacterial contamination.

**3.** The water added to these units should be preheated to reduce the temperature drop that would occur if cold water were added when the unit needed to be filled. It is recommended that the unit not be "topped off" but, if possible, emptied and refilled each time it requires refilling. With the pass-over humidifier used in the Emerson, this requires disconnecting the unit from the patient circuit to refill it (see Chap. 9).

### Cascade Humidifier

This humidifier combines the diffusion head and pass-over principles to increase the gas-liquid interface. Gas entering the humidifier is directed to the bottom of the humidifier and forced up through a fine grid. The incoming gas flow pushes water and gas through the perforated grid, increasing the water fragments and gas bubbles to enhance maximum evaporation. Once leaving the grid, the gas flow is directed across the surface of the water in the reservoir. Most cascade humidifiers in use today have heating elements incorporated in their design (see Fig. 3-4). As the gas flows through the Cascade humidifiers, it can be warmed to above

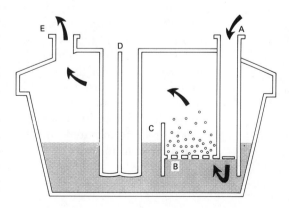

**FIG. 3-4. Cascade humidifier.** This humidifier combines a heated reservoir with a blow over and diffusion head design. Flow enters the humidifier at (A) and is pushed through a plastic grid (B) creating fine bubbles to increase evaporation. The gas flow passes across the surface of the water as water molecules continue to move into it (C). The gas flow exits at (E) to be delivered to the patient. (D) is housing for a double heating device which warms the reservoir.

body temperature and it comes in contact with enough water to saturate it to 100 percent body humidity. Cascade humidifiers are commonly used with artificial methanical ventilation systems to provide optimal patient humidity. The Cascade humidifier is also used with CPAP and IPPB equipment to deliver gas saturated at body temperature to the patient receiving these types of therapy.

## THERAPEUTIC CONSIDERATIONS

The following are therapeutic considerations of Cascade humidifiers:

1.  For the effective delivery of humidity to the gas system, the water in the Cascade humidifiers must be maintained above the minimum water-level mark. When the water level in this humidifier falls below that level, the patient will receive an absolute humidity close to that of the surrounding room air.

2.  It is recommended that the Cascade humidifier be sterilized at least every 24 hours and that the water level and equipment function be checked at least every four hours in general patient care and every two hours when used in critical care.

These are very efficient, high-output humidifiers that use a large amount of water. As described above, it may be hazardous to the patient for improper water levels to go unchanged. Only sterile water should be used in the system. Also, inappropriate heater settings increase body temperatures and may cause respiratory tract burns.

3.  Nondisposable Cascade humidifiers are made up of a large number of parts. Following disinfection or sterilization, great care should be taken to properly reassemble the equipment, assuring tight fits and replacing any worn parts. Improper reassembly can create a dangerous leak in the closed high-flow gas system when used in critical care.

4.  These humidifiers also can be useful in treating patients such as severely burned patients, in wound and skin isolation. Humidity, being a molecular form of water, does not transport bacteria, and, therefore, limits the possibility of patient contamination through inhalation or skin exposure to the humidified gas.

5.  Large bore tubing should be used with heated Cascade humidifiers because of the very high humidity output. As the temperature drops along the tubing, the humidity condenses and this condensation could block a small bore tube with water. When checking equipment functioning, the tubing should not be drained back into the Cascade humidifiers because it may be contaminated with bacteria from the patient, which would contaminate the humidifier's water reservoir.

# AEROSOL THERAPY

Aerosol therapy is the therapeutic use of a suspension of particles in a gas to deposit a significant amount of the medication in the respiratory tract. Clinical evaluation of this therapy is based on observation and measurement of the patient's reaction to the medications delivered. Aerosol therapy is administered to deliver medications directly to the surface of the respiratory tract.

## PHYSIOLOGICAL EFFECTS

The effects of aerosol therapy for the treatment of patients with respiratory disease are:

1. *Reduction of body humidity deficit.* An aerosol of sterile water or isotonic solution (0.9 percent NaCl) may be used to add moisture directly to the lungs in the form of a liquid and a gas. As an aerosol particle exists in the gas, it is affected by evaporation. As it evaporates it adds to the absolute humidity of the gas as well as delivers particles of water on the respiratory mucosa. Therefore, an aerosol of water or normal saline also can be delivered to provide humidity, reduce the body humidity deficit, and add liquid to mucosal secretions.

2. *Topical application of medications.* Epithelial inflammation, smooth muscle bronchospasm, thickened mucosal secretions, and pulmonary infections can be treated through the direct application of medication to the affected site. Specific drugs can be prescribed for delivery as an aerosol to treat the individual respiratory conditions.

3. *Sputum induction.* Aerosols of hypertonic (greater than 0.9 percent NaCl) can induce coughing and add moisture to mucosal secretions to aid in removal of secretions for collection as sputum samples.

4. *Local anesthesia.* Localized areas of the respiratory tract can be anesthetized using an aerosol of 1–2 percent lidocaine, or other agent, prior to a bronchoscopy, tracheostomy, or intubation procedure.

## HAZARDS OF AEROSOL THERAPY

1. *Bronchospasms.* The delivery of a high density of fine aerosol particles onto the lower respiratory-tract mucosa may actually irritate the airway lining, causing bronchospasms. If this occurs, a decreased concentration of aerosol particles may be required, or if the lower density cannot be tolerated, then such high-density aerosol therapy should be discontinued. This occurs most often with nebulizers that produce high concen-

trations of particles between 0.5 to 10$\mu$ in size, such as the ultrasonic or babbington nebulizers. This may occur more frequently with patients with asthma, emphysema, or chronic bronchitis. The initiation of or an increase in wheezing and/or coughing indicates that this is occurring. Therapy should be evaluated and modified or discontinued.

2. *Overhydration.* Overhydration also may be a hazard of continuous aerosol therapy. Patients receiving large volume fluid replacement or having renal dysfunction and also receiving long-term continuous aerosol therapy should be carefully monitored. Overhydration can occur as early as two to four hours from the start of therapy. The acute development of rales in the lower lobes of the lung may indicate pulmonary edema from fluid overload. Aerosol therapy, unlike humidity therapy, adds particulate water to the respiratory tract, creating an even greater hazard of overhydration. It is a consideration to be aware of, especially in nebulizers that put out 3 ml/min or more. Daily weight and electrolytes should be monitored. Gradual weight increases, acute pulmonary congestion, increased blood pressure and/or reduced electrolytes may indicate overhydration.

3. *Transport of microorganisms.* Since an aerosol is actually particulate matter, it is capable of carrying microorganisms. Bacterial contamination of a nebulizer reservoir or delivery system can be transported to the patient via the aerosol. Hence care must be taken during aerosol therapy to prevent bacterial contamination of the equipment. Nebulizers and aerosol delivery systems should be completely changed and disinfected at least every 48 hours. Also, it is recommended that only sterile solutions be used in all nebulizers.


## THERAPEUTIC CONSIDERATIONS

1. When aerosol therapy is prescribed to deliver a medication into the lower respiratory tract, the patient should be instructed to breathe in through his mouth so that the normal filtration taking place in the nose will be bypassed. The patient also should be instructed and encouraged to take slow, deep breaths and to pause momentarily before exhaling to allow for greater aerosol deposition in the lower respiratory system. This will improve gas distribution and aerosol deposition. Exhalation should be slow and relaxed.

2. The patient should be positioned in a semi-Fowler's or sitting position to allow maximum chest expansion for deep breathing and to provide a more effective position in which the patient may cough.

3. Patients receiving aerosol should be encouraged to cough during and

following treatment. Effective coughing is vital to clearing secretions and providing effective aerosol therapy. Postural drainage and chest percussion should also be incorporated with aerosol therapy when the patient has very thick, tenacious secretions. Given prior to the postural drainage, secretion removal can be enhanced by the increased moisture and medication delivered to the airways.

## AEROSOL-PRODUCING EQUIPMENT

Aerosol-producing equipment mechanically breaks liquid into small, fine particles. Equipment that produces liquid particles of indiscriminate size and concentration is described as an *atomizer*. A *nebulizer* (*nebula* means cloud) is basically an atomizer that uses a baffle or series of baffles to refine the aerosol to create a more uniform, evenly distributed therapeutic size (0.5–3 $\mu$) (see Table 3-3). Gas flow containing the produced aerosol is directed toward the baffles of the nebulizer, with inertia causing larger particles to collide with the baffle, while smaller, more stable particles are diverted around the baffle with the gas flow. Liquid drops smashing into the baffle will be further fragmented and the aerosol that cannot be carried by the gas flow will drop back into the water reservoir or tubing of the nebulizer (see Fig. 3-5). Most nebulizers use specific baffles such as spheres or plates but the 90° angle in the elbow of a tube or side of the aerosol delivery tubing can also act as a baffle to eliminate large, less stable particles from the gas flow. A baffle is simply a method of changing the direction or deflecting a flow of gas. The nebulizer is most frequently used in the delivery of aerosol therapy because its aerosol particles are more consistent, stable, and refined than that of the atomizer.

TABLE 3-3

**Therapeutic Aerosol Deposition**

| Area of Deposition | Aerosol Particle Size |
|---|---|
| Too large to enter respiratory tract | 50 $\mu$ |
| Mouth, nose, pharynx | 10–50 $\mu$ |
| Larynx, trachea, bronchi | 3–10 $\mu$ |
| Bronchiole, alveolar ducts, sacs | 0.5–3 $\mu$ |
| May be removed with the exhaled gas, act as molecules | < 0.5 $\mu$ |

These are predicted areas of aerosol deposition based on aerosol size and the patient breathing through his mouth (1 micron ($\mu$) equals 1/25,000 in).

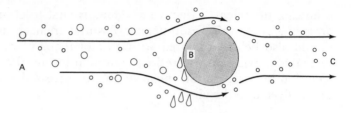

FIG. 3-5. A baffle. The circular structures (B) cause the laminar gas flow to be deflected from its path. Aerosol particles traveling in the gas flow (A) that are small enough will be deflected with the gas flow, while large particles will impact against the ball baffle (B) and fall back into the reservoir. The remaining gas flow of more stable, uniform particles (C) travel on to be delivered to the patient. Any part of the equipment may act as a baffle if it deflects the flow of gas from its straight laminar flow.

## PRINCIPLES OF OPERATION

Nebulizers are divided into three categories based on the physical design of the equipment to disperse a liquid into a fine aerosol.

### Venturi Nebulizers

This type of nebulizer uses a venturi to create an aerosol. This is the most common design incorporated in nebulizers. A venturi device is a function of the Bernoulli principle. This principle states that as the velocity of a gas through a tube increases, the lateral wall pressure decreases (see Fig. 3-6). In a nebulizer the venturi draws the medication out of a reservoir through a capillary tube. As the fluid enters the high velocity gas flow, it breaks down into a vast array of aerosol particles. This primary particle spray is directed into a baffle that creates a more stable, refined secondary spray of aerosol, which is directed to the patient through an aerosol delivery system (see Fig. 3-7). The amount of aerosol produced depends on the velocity of the gas through the venturi jet and on the ratio of gas through the venturi jet and the ratio of gas and liquid flow.

### PHYSICAL CONSIDERATIONS

The venturi nebulizer can be distinguished by three forms in which the venturi is set into the nebulizer in relation to the main gas flow (see Fig. 3-8). The following are physical considerations of venturi nebulizers:

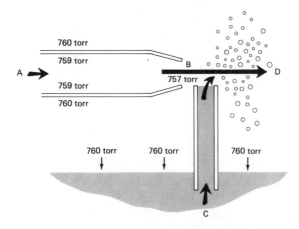

FIG. 3-6. A venturi device. The Bernoulli effect is combined with a gas flow through a restriction in a tube (A) and an entrainment tube (B) placed in a lateral position at an angle to the gas flow to form a venturi device. Using the above numerical examples, as the gas flows through the horizontal tube (A) the pressure along the inside wall of the tube is 759 torr due to the velocity of the flowing gas. At (B) where the horizontal and vertical tubes are in close proximity there is sharp narrowing of tube (A). This restriction causes an increase in the gas velocity and this results in a decrease in the lateral pressure to 757 torr. Due to the pressure difference between point (B) and point (C), liquid is pushed up the tube into the gas flow by the atmospheric pressure being exerted upon it. In this manner, the venturi device utilizes the Bernoulli principle to draw liquids or additional gas into the original gas flow to produce a combined flow at (D).

FIG. 3-7. A venturi nebulizer with baffle. This nebulizer is pneumatically powered by a gas source (A) with a venturi (B) used to entrain a medication through the capillary tube from the reservoir at (E). (C) is a ball baffle used to reduce particle size and the liquid in the reservoir at (D) would also act as a baffle. The final aerosol concentration would exit at the output port (F).

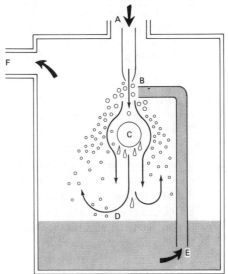

59

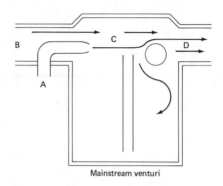

Mainstream venturi

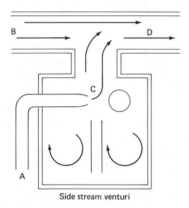

Side stream venturi

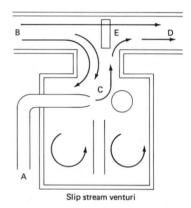

Slip stream venturi

**FIG. 3-8.** Physical design of venturi nebulizers. Mainstream, side stream, slip stream nebulizers. (A), gas source to the venturi jet. (B), main flow of gas to the patient. (C), the venturi and baffle within the nebulizer. (D), the flow of gas and aerosol combined after passing the nebulizer. (E), a baffle to divert part of the mainstream gas flow into a slip stream nebulizer.

1. *Main-stream venturi.* In this nebulizer the venturi is located in the midstream of the gas flow to the patient. Therefore, all the gas delivered to the patient goes through the nebulizer. Clinically, this will increase the density of the aerosol leaving the nebulizer and the amount of medication delivered per minute. It also may increase the mean particle size resulting from less baffling within the nebulizer. This main-stream nebulizer would deliver a denser aerosol than the following other two nebulizer designs. The main-stream construction is the most common pattern of venturi nebulizers used for aerosol therapy. It is incorporated in most large reservoir venturi nebulizers and in many small reservoir treatment nebulizers.
2. *Side-stream venturi.* With the side-stream design, the venturi is separate from the main gas flow to the patient. As the main gas flow passes the nebulizer, the gas flow from the venturi jet propels the aerosol into the

main gas stream. None of the central gas flow to the patient passes through the nebulizer. This design will provide a less dense aerosol and it will decrease the amount of medication delivered per minute. Because of increased baffling prior to the aerosol entering the main gas flow, the particle size should be more uniform and stable as it leaves the nebulizer. Use of this venturi nebulizer style would prolong the aerosol treatment and deliver a finer, drier, aerosol to the patient. Many IPPB-treatment nebulizers use this design.

3. *Slip-stream venturi.* In this nebulizer, the venturi is also separated from the main gas flow path. A baffle is placed in the central gas stream superior to the nebulizer input port. As gas flows by the nebulizer, the baffle deflects part of the flow into it. Therefore, though the venturi and main gas flow are physically separated, part of the main flow does pass through the nebulizer and combines with the flow from the venturi jet to carry aerosol out of the nebulizer. The quality of the aerosol produced by the slip-stream venturi nebulizer would be between that produced by the other two nebulizer designs. This construction is incorporated in some IPPB-treatment nebulizers manufactured today. It is the *least* common of the three designs.

## THERAPEUTIC CONSIDERATIONS

The following are therapeutic considerations of venturi nebulizers:

1. Most respiratory therapy equipment is calibrated for use with a 50 psig gas source. The venturi nebulizer is also such a pneumatically powered device. A pressure compensated flowmeter can be used to connect the venturi nebulizer to a gas cylinder regulator or piped-in gas outlet to provide calibrated flowrates up to 15 l through the nebulizer.

2. Large and small reservoir nebulizers deliver varying amounts of water outputs. Large reservoir venturi nebulizers deliver approximately 1–3 ml/min while the small reservoir treatment nebulizers deliver approximately 0.5–0.75 ml/min. This total water output includes humidity plus aerosol and would increase with increasing gas flowrates and heating of the nebulizer reservoir.

3. A minimum flowrate of 10 l/min should be used in operating a large reservoir nebulizer. These minimum flowrates will assure proper operation of the venturi and baffling of the aerosol produced. Many large reservoir nebulizers use a venturi to entrain air into the nebulizer to create varying oxygen concentrations that can be delivered to the patient. The air-entrainment ratios are listed in Chap. 1. The minimum flowrates also ensure the appropriate entrainment of room air at the prescribed setting on the nebulizer.

4.  Large bore tubing should be used with all nebulizers. The large bore tubing provides a large passageway for aerosol to the patient and is not easily occluded by any aerosol "rain out" that occurs. The tubing on equipment providing long-term continuous aerosol therapy should be checked at least every four hours to prevent the build-up of water from particle deposition in the tubing. Aerosol "rain out" collects in the low point of tubing and can affect nebulizer function. Any water in the tubing should be emptied into a sink, bucket, or plastic-lined basket, and not placed back into the nebulizer reservoir. This precaution will decrease the possibility of bacterial contamination of the nebulizer.

5.  Proper functioning of the nebulizer should be checked at least every four hours during continuous aerosol therapy, and the nebulizer should be refilled with sterile water. With each refill, the nebulizer should be emptied, completely rinsed, and then refilled. All nebulizer equipment should be changed at least every 48 hours and sterilized if nondisposable or discarded if disposable.

6.  Nondisposable nebulizers require periodic maintenance. The venturi jets and capillary tubes must be cleared regularly and any mineral deposits that form around the jet should be removed. This may be done every three months, depending on amount of use. Care also must be taken in reassembling the nebulizer to ensure proper functioning.

7.  All transport of soiled equipment should be done in plastic bags when moving it from the patient's room to the decontamination unit.

8.  Nondisposable venturi nebulizers should have a pressure relief valve to prevent the build-up of excessive pressure resulting from equipment malfunction or accidental occlusion of the tubing. Valves commonly used today have pop-off pressures of either 2 psig or 40 torr. This safety feature prevents cracking or explosion of the reservoir.

9.  Nebulizers are affected by the same cooling that occurs with humidifiers. The nebulizers may be heated to increase the maximum humidity and prevent cooling of the delivered gas, thus creating more stable particles by eliminating the need for evaporation that takes place as the aerosol enters the warm respiratory tract. The nebulizer reservoir can be heated to above body temperature to deliver a warm, saturated gas filled with aerosol. The extent of heating depends on the type of equipment used. This will be described at the end of this section on nebulizers. These also require more frequent checks for build-up of condensate in the patient delivery tubing and refill of water.

## Ultrasonic Nebulizers

This nebulizer uses high-frequency sound waves to produce an aerosol. A power unit converts a 60 cycle, 100-V (volt) electrical current to a radio frequency of 1.3 to 1.4 MHz (megahertz), depending on the commercial model. This frequency is transferred to a piezoelectric transducer

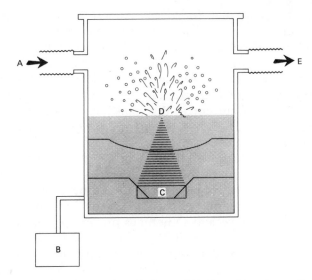

**FIG. 3-9.** Ultrasonic nebulizer. (A) flow from a small blower fan evacuates aerosol from the nebulizer through port (E) to be delivered to the patient. A power unit (B) converts standard current to high frequency and by having the energy focused through a piezoelectric transducer (C) the vibrational energy is used to physically break down liquid to aerosol (D).

within a nebulizing unit (see Fig. 3-9). The piezoelectric quality means that a ceramic disc within the transducer will uniformly vibrate and change height and width when energy is applied to it. The transducer creates a sound energy that is directed into the nebulizer reservoir. The sound vibrations are aimed at a central focal point in the reservoir at which all liquid is physically broken into a large volume of fine aerosol particles. The sound frequency of ultrasonic nebulizers is regulated by the Federal Communications Commission. Ultrasonic nebulizers have a power and nebulizer unit. There are several commercial designs available.

## THERAPEUTIC CONSIDERATIONS

The following are therapeutic considerations of ultrasonic nebulizers:

1. The nebulizer is electrically powered and does not require an external gas source to carry the aerosol to the patient because a blower fan is incorporated into its power unit. The fan also cools the power unit. The fan filter in the power unit should be cleaned at least every seven days.

2. Ultrasonic nebulizers deliver a maximum of 3–6 ml/min total water content depending on the model. The majority of the particles are 1–3 $\mu$,

which is optimal for deep respiratory tract deposition. Because the nebulizer is very efficient, a very stable particle concentration is generated and the delivered air is nearly 100 percent saturated.

3.  The on-off switch on an ultrasonic nebulizer controls the electric current flow to the power unit of the nebulizer. The frequency is preset internally and remains constant. A dial on the nebulizer console adjusts the amplitude of current to the transducer. An increase in the amplitude will increase the density of the aerosol produced by the nebulizer. A decrease will decrease the density.

4.  All nebulizer equipment that comes in contact with the aerosol delivered to the patient should be changed every 24 hours. When cleaning the transducer or diaphragm, care should be taken to prevent any oil residue from remaining on the parts. Even touching these parts can leave body oil on their surface and sometimes prevent proper nebulization from taking place. Vinegar or alcohol can be placed on the transducer at least every seven days and nebulized to remove any build-up of mineral or oil residue.

5.  Ultrasonic nebulization is a process of transforming electrical energy to sound energy, which is then converted to mechanical energy. The Occupational Safety and Health Administration (O.S.H.A.) requires a minimal leakage of less than 100 $\mu$A (microamperes) from all hospital electrical equipment coming in contact with a patient. The electrical leakage of the ultrasonic nebulizer should be checked periodically and the equipment should only be used with a three-prong electrical plug for proper electrical grounding.

6.  Ultrasonic nebulizers have available single-use disposable cups for intermittent aerosol therapy, and they have available large reservoir feed systems for continuous therapy. These cups allow convenient delivery of bronchodilators and mucolytic solutions to the patients. Large bore tubing and sterile water should be used with this as with other nebulizers.

7.  Supplemental oxygen may be given to the patient by using an external gas source rather than the blower fan to carry the aerosol to the patient. A venturi or air-oxygen blender may be used to deliver exact oxygen concentrations. This may be connected to the nebulizer at the input for the hose from the blower fan. Use of a venturi requires an unrestricted gas flow from the venturi device.

8.  Patients receiving long-term high-density aerosol therapy with an ultrasonic nebulizer have a greater chance of overhydration or bronchospasm. The total water content delivered to the patient is high and the small particle size provides more opportunity for peripheral lung deposition. An aerosol of normal saline may become hypertonic because of evaporation during inhalation and may irritate the lower respiratory mucosa, causing coughing and wheezing. In some chronic lung-disease patients, a dense aerosol of just sterile water via an ultrasonic nebulizer may cause severe bronchospasms. Caution must be taken and the patient must be closely

observed for coughing spasms or wheezing when this high density aerosol therapy is initiated.

9. When an ultrasonic nebulizer is used for continuous therapy, the water level and equipment function should be checked at least every four hours. If the water covering the transducer dries up, the equipment can overheat and be permanently damaged. Some ultrasonic nebulizers have automatic shut-off switches to protect the electrical components, but if the nebulizer shuts off, the patient will no longer receive an aerosol concentration.

10. The high water content produced by ultrasonic nebulizers is very useful in the treatment of severely dehydrated patients with dry, inflamed, respiratory mucosa and patients with thick, tenacious secretions such as severe bronchitis or cystic fibrosis patients. The dense aerosol will add both humidity and aerosol to the respiratory tract and provide particles for deposition in the peripheral lung areas.

## Babbington Nebulizers

The Babbington nebulizer incorporates a hollow glass sphere of compressed gas and a fine film of sterile water to create an aerosol. The Babbington principle creates an aerosol by directing a high-velocity compressed gas source through a film of water and into a baffle. The sphere containing compressed gas is continually covered with a thin layer of water from a reservoir above it. A small hole in the sphere allows the compressed gas to escape at a supersonic velocity. As this high-velocity gas strikes the film of water, the liquid is broken into a dense aerosol that is immediately driven into a small ball baffle (impactor) to create a minute, uniform particle concentration (see Fig. 3-10).

### THERAPEUTIC CONSIDERATIONS

The following are therapeutic considerations of Babbington nebulizers:

1. This nebulizer is pneumatically powered. It requires no electronics or moving parts. It will operate with a supply source of 10–50 psi. The supply source may be compressed air or oxygen.

2. This Babbington nebulizer produces a uniform aerosol of which 97 percent are less than 10 $\mu$ in size and the median mass diameter is 3–4 $\mu$. It delivers 3–6 ml per minute total water content using a 3-ft long bore aerosol tubing. This fine mist can be used in aerosol therapy to provide both aerosol and humidity to the patient. The delivered gas is 100 percent saturated with water.

3. The nebulizer has an air entrainment port that allows delivery of a wide range of oxygen concentrations. It can deliver between 30–100 percent oxygen depending on the model and the setting of the air entrain-

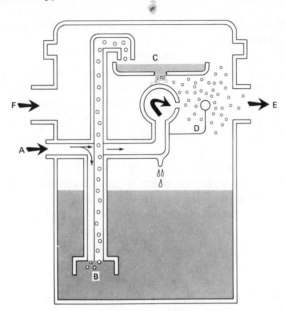

FIG. 3-10. Babbington nebulizer. (A) Compressed gas enters the nebulizer and part is directed through a pneumatic column (B) which acts as a pump to carry water to the reservoir (C), while part is directed to a pressurized hollow sphere at (D). High velocity gas from the sphere (D) breaks through a thin film of water covering the outside of the sphere from reservoir (C) creating a fine dense aerosol. This is driven against a baffle directly in front of the orifice in the hollow sphere (D). The gas flow from the sphere and that which is entrained at inlet (F) carries with the aerosol out of the nebulizer at port (E).

ment device. The air entrainment is caused by the Bernoulli effect of the gas flow through the nebulizer. Gas flows of up to 135 l/min can be delivered with some models.

4. This nebulizer may be connected directly to a 50 psig gas source or be operated from a pressure compensated flowmeter. A chart accompanies most nebulizers which can be used to calculate oxygen concentrations delivered. It is based on flowrate, the number of spheres, and the occlusion of the air entrainment port.

5. This equipment should be checked at least every four hours for proper functioning and water level. If the water level falls below the minimum operating level, no aerosol will be produced by the nebulizer. A continuous feed system may be used with some models. The total nebulizer and delivery system should be changed and sterilized every 24 hours.

6. The design of this pneumatic system requires that all parts must be properly assembled for any aerosol to be produced. All seals and gaskets

must be in place and have a tight fit for the pneumatic pump system to continually cover the spheres with a thin layer of water.

7. Since this nebulizer design requires no electrical input, there is no electrical hazard to the patient. This eliminates some basic maintenance problems. Care must be taken in handling, though, because several key parts (i.e., spheres, some reservoirs) are presently made of glass, making them breakable.

8. The large reservoir on these units does not allow convenient delivery of any aerosol medication other than saline solutions or sterile water, since exact measured doses of bronchodilator or mucolytic solutions cannot be completely nebulized from the reservoir.

9. The Babbington nebulizer delivers an aerosol concentration and water content comparable to high-output ultrasonic nebulizers; therefore, it may be used with the same favored therapeutic results to treat dehydrated patients and patients with thick, tenacious secretions.

## HEATING EQUIPMENT

There are multiple designs used in heating elements for humidifiers and nebulizers. These include probe-type heating elements, wrap-around heaters (see Fig. 3-11), and hot-plate devices. The purpose of heating equipment is to increase the temperature of the water in the nebulizer or humidifier reservoir. Through convection, the heat of the water will be transferred to the gas flowing through the equipment, and, therefore, the maximum humidity that the gas can hold will be increased.

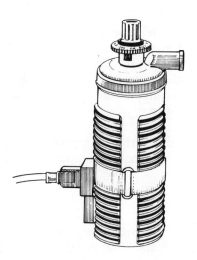

FIG. 3-11. Wraparound heater on nebulizer.

## THERAPEUTIC CONSIDERATIONS

The following are therapeutic considerations of heating elements:

1.  Many types of respiratory therapy equipment have a heating device already designed into them, such as the Cascade humidifier. The use of heating elements can increase the water content of the delivered gas to above body humidity depending on their efficiency. This is most beneficial in the critically ill patient.

2.  When mucosal inflammation and swelling is the problem, such as with croup or epiglottitis, then a cool aerosol can reduce swelling and a heating device is not desirable.

3.  If a heating device does not function properly, it can be very dangerous. One extreme is that if the device does not work at all, the gas temperature delivered to the patient can actually be 5–10°F below room temperature because of heat loss with evaporation. This will decrease the maximum humidity the gas can hold, and, therefore, reduce the efficiency of the equipment to produce humidity. Second is the problem of over-heating caused by dysfunction or lack of calibration of the device. If the heating element increases the temperature of the gas delivered to the patient in excess of body temperature, the gas may cause mucosal drying and pulmonary burns. Heating equipment should be inspected with the other equipment at least every 4 hours.

4.  The temperature of the inspired gas should be monitored to maintain it below body temperature. A gas temperature of 85–95°F at the patient provides a safe range at near body temperature for delivery of heated, saturated gas to the patient. If the gas temperature is not measured at the patient, then it should be remembered that the temperature will drop approximately 1°C for each foot of tubing it travels through to the patient.

5.  When a heating element is used, the rapid cooling of the gas along the delivery tube will increase condensation and liquid will pool more rapidly because of the increase in the efficiency of the equipment to produce humidity. With continuous use, the equipment will require refilling at least every four hours. With this equipment a continuous feed system may be advantageous.

6.  Warm solutions provide a good medium for bacterial growth. Therefore, people handling this equipment should follow proper cleaning procedures and should change equipment on a routine basis.

## HUMIDITY AND AEROSOL DELIVERY EQUIPMENT

The following equipment is primarily used with nebulizers. Its function and design are aimed at delivering humidity and aerosol, although nebulizers are commonly prescribed with an increased oxygen concentration to be delivered to the patient.

1. *Aerosol mask.* This is a cone-shaped shell, similar to a simple oxygen mask. It fits over the nose and mouth of the patient. Unlike the simple oxygen mask, it has large, round, open exhalation ports and a connection fitting for the large bore tubing used with nebulization equipment. The shell of the mask acts as a 100–150 ml reservoir for the aerosol. The large exhalation ports vent excessive carrier gas from the nebulizer. (See Fig. 3-12.)

2. *Tracheostomy mask.* This mask is held around the neck of the patient by an elastic band and fits directly over the stoma of the tracheotomy, or the tracheostomy tube. There is a round opening in the top of the mask for exhalation and a large bore tubing connection. The tubing connection should swivel to allow adjustment with the patient's position. (See Fig. 3-13.)

3. *Face mask (face tent).* This is an enclosure that covers the lower half of the face and fits snugly under the chin to provide aerosol to the patient's nose and mouth. It is open at the top at about the level of the patient's eyes. Exhaled gas flows out of the top of the mask as incoming gas enters through a large bore tubing connection in the base of the shield. The face tent can be used when an aerosol mask cannot be tolerated by the patient. (See Fig. 3-14.)

4. *Briggs adaptor (T tube).* This connection attaches the large bore tubing from the nebulizer directly to an endotracheal or tracheostomy tube. The three way connector contains a 15 mm opening that will fit the endotracheal tube adaptor. Exhaled gas leaves the system from the third opening. If a large bore tube is not placed on the exhalation port of the Briggs adaptor, the patient may inhale 30–50 percent of his tidal volume from the room air, diluting the delivered aerosol concentration and the oxygen concentration. (See Fig. 3-15.)

5. *Tent.* This was described in Chap. 1. The enclosure is primarily used to deliver humidity and aerosol to pediatric patients.

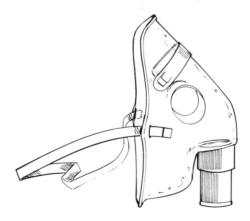

**FIG. 3-12.** Aerosol mask.

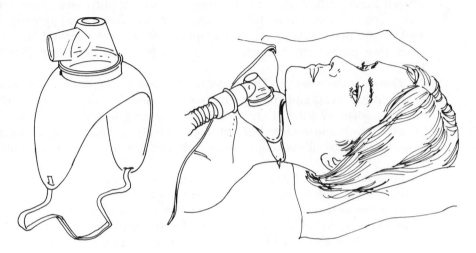

**FIG. 3-13.** A. Tracheostomy mask. B. Mask on patient.

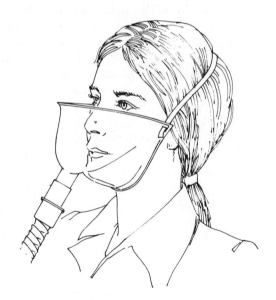

**FIG. 3-14.** Face mask on patient.

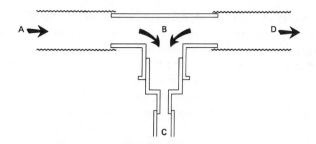

**FIG. 3-15.** Briggs Adaptor ("T" piece). This fitting allows direct connections to the patient with an endotracheal or tracheostomy tube (C). Large bore tubing carries humidity and aerosol to the patient connector (A). On inhalation, the patient draws gas in from the system (B). A length of aerosol tubing can be attached to the exhalation side (D) to act as a gas reservoir so that on inhalation the patient will not dilute the oxygen concentration he is receiving by drawing in room air.

## THERAPEUTIC CONSIDERATIONS

The following are therapeutic considerations of humidity and aerosol delivery equipment.

1. It is important to remember that this equipment is primarily designed to deliver humidity and aerosol. The large exhalation ports in aerosol delivery equipment allow the dilution of the oxygen concentration delivered by the nebulizer. Air is entrained by the patient during inhalation so that the oxygen concentration will be less than that set on the nebulizer oxygen control. For example, if the oxygen control on a venturi nebulizer is set on 60 percent oxygen, then the *nebulizer* will deliver 60 percent oxygen from its output port. When the patient inhales, some air from the room enters through the exhalation ports so that the actual oxygen concentration received into the patient's lungs will be less than 60 percent. How much less will depend on the patient's respiratory rate, tidal volume, and peak inspiratory flowrate. Without an additional reservoir the oxygen concentration could be at least 20 percent less than the oxygen concentration setting on the nebulizer.

2. When using a Briggs adaptor an exact oxygen concentration can be delivered if a large bore reservoir tube is placed on the exhalation side. Aerosol must be visible throughout inhalation and exhalation for the exact oxygen concentration to be delivered. The length of tube required will depend on the flowrate through the nebulizer system (which should be as high as possible) and the ventilatory demands of the patient. When-

ever a reservoir tube is used if aerosol is not visible during exhalation, the patient may be rebreathing his exhaled gas leading to carbon-dioxide build-up; so it is critical that during end exhalation aerosol is flowing from the exhalation port. If not, the reservoir tubing length should be decreased immediately. A 50-100 ml reservoir tube can usually be used safely to decrease the amount of room air entrained.

3. Any dependent (hanging) large bore tubing will collect water from condensation and aerosol deposition. It should be checked and drained at least every four hours with equipment functioning checks. It should never be drained back into the humidifier or nebulizer for this can lead to bacterial contamination. Also, any blockage of the tube will decrease the aerosol concentration delivered to the patient and will cause an increase in the oxygen concentration delivered. Blockage would cause the normal air entrainment ratio of the nebulizer's venturi dilution control device to decrease, leading to a higher delivered oxygen concentration.

4. Patients receiving aerosol therapy via a face-fitting aerosol mask or tent may complain of a feeling of "suffocating." This is common with high-density aerosol therapy. This may be resolved by reassuring the patient and, if an ultrasonic nebulizer is used, by decreasing the amplitude. Aerosol may also deposit on the patient's face, and so require periodic face care.

5. Effective delivery of the aerosol and oxygen concentration requires a properly fitted mask. Mask placement should be checked with proper nebulizer function at least every four hours and should be replaced at least every 48 hours or when soiled. The patient, nurse, and therapist should be aware of proper fitting so that the mask is properly placed all the time with continuous therapy.

6. Aerosol tubing or any respiratory therapy equipment should be positioned so that it fits snugly to the patient but does not "pull" on the patient at the point of attachment in any way. The large bore aerosol tubing should never be allowed to hang in such a position so that it "pulls" on the patient. This is of vital importance especially in the attachment of large bore tubing to endotracheal and tracheostomy tubes. If tubing is in any position to put pressure by pulling or pushing on the tube, it will cause damage to the patient's trachea. It is also uncomfortable and may lead to pressure necrosis at the point of stress.

# BIBLIOGRAPHY

Brunner, L.S., and D.S. Suddarth, *Lippincott Manual of Nursing Practice*, J.B. Lippincott, Philadelphia, 1974.

Bushnell, S.S., *Respiratory Intensive Care Nursing*, Little, Brown, Boston, 1973.

Comroe, J.H., *et al.*, *The Lung*, 2nd edition, Year Book Medical Publishers, Chicago, 1962.

Cotes, C.E., *Lung Function: Assessment and Application in Medicine*, 2nd edition, F.A. Davis, Philadelphia, 1979.

Garrett, D.F., *et al.*, *Physical Principles of Respiratory Therapy Equipment*, Ohio Medical Products, Madison, Wisconsin, 1975.

Guenter, C.A. and M.H. Welch, *Pulmonary Medicine*, J.B. Lippincott, Philadelphia, 1977.

Hedley-White, J., *et al.*, *Applied Physiology of Respiratory Care*, Little, Brown, Boston, 1976.

Hunsinger, D.L., *et al.*, *Respiratory Technology: A Procedure Manual*, 2nd edition, Reston, Reston, Virginia, 1976.

Johnson, R.F., *Pulmonary Care*, Grune and Stratton, New York, 1973.

McPherson, S.P., *Respiratory Therapy Equipment*, 2nd edition, C.V. Mosby, St. Louis, 1977.

Petty, T.L., *Pulmonary Diagnostic Techniques*, Lea and Febiger, Philadelphia, 1975.

Rau, J.C. and M.Y. Rau, *Fundamental Respiratory Therapy Equipment*, Glenn Educational Medical Services, Sarasota, 1977.

Ruppell, Greg, *Manual of Pulmonary Function Testing*, 2nd edition, C.V. Mosby, St. Louis, 1978.

Shapiro, B.A., *et al.*, *Clinical Application of Respiratory Care*, 2nd edition, Year Book Medical Publishers, Chicago, 1979.

Slonim, N.B. and L.H. Hamilton, *Respiratory Physiology*, 2nd edition, C.V. Mosby, St. Louis, 1971.

West, J.B., *Ventilation/Blood Flow and Gas Exchange*, 2nd edition, Blackwell Scientific Publications, Oxford, 1970.

Young, J.A. and D. Crocker, *Principles and Practices of Respiratory Therapy*, 2nd edition, Year Book Medical Publishers, Chicago, 1976.

# CHAPTER

# 4

# RESPIRATORY PHARMACOLOGY

Pharmacology is the study of drugs and their effect upon the body. Cells are made up of chemical compounds and water, whose structure and interaction within the living cell provide the foundation for our understanding of pharmacodynamics. For the health practitioner, pharmacology stresses the basic properties of drugs, their effects upon the body, their interaction with other drugs, and the general condition of the patient as a result of drug therapy. Respiratory care personnel must be able to use information about respiratory drugs and those drugs that pertain to the cardiopulmonary care of a patient.

## DEFINITION OF TERMS

Drugs are chemical compounds that alter the function of living cells. They are used not only in the treatment of diseases and alleviation of pain, but also in the prevention and diagnosis of diseases.

*Drug*                        Originally, the word drug meant a dry herb (French derivation). More specifically, a drug is a chemical compound or a mixture of compounds used in the treatment, prevention, and diagnosis of diseases. In the United States these compounds must meet the rigid standards of the United States Pharmacopeia (USP) and the National Formulary (NF). The federal standards for drugs are under control of the Food and Drug Administration (FDA) of the Department of Health and Human Services (formerly HEW).

*Pharmacology*

Pharmacology is the study of the properties of drugs, including their chemical interactions, and their effect on living organisms. Pharmacology uses the sciences of biology, chemistry, biochemistry, and physiology in research efforts.

*Pharmacy*

Pharmacy is an area of pharmacology that deals primarily with the properties and dosages of drugs. The pharmacist is responsible for the preparation and dispensing of drugs. Many of the drugs available to the general public have a restricted use and are available only by the written order (prescription) of a licensed physician.

*Generic name*

The generic name of a drug is the name given by the laboratory, company, or manufacturer who developed the drug. Generally, this name is some modification of the true chemical name. For example, isoproterenol hydrochloride is a generic name.

*Chemical name*

The chemical name is actually a description of the chemical structure of the drug. The chemical name for isoproterenol hydrochloride is 3,4-dihydroxy-[isopropylamino]-benzyl alcohol hydrochloride.

*Trade name*

The trade name of a drug is the brand name given by the manufacturer. For example, a trade name for isoproterenol hydrochloride is Isuprel (Winthrop) or Norisodrine (Abbott).

*Official name*

This is the name registered with the U.S.P. for the drug. Oftentimes, this is the same as the generic name.

# DRUG INTERACTIONS

With the increased use of drugs in medicine, the likelihood that a patient will be receiving two or more drugs simultaneously increases. In such situations, one of two general possibilities will exist: (1) the actions of each drug will be independent; that is, the action of one drug will have no observable effect on the other drug; or (2) the combined effect of two or more of the drugs will be different from that normally observed when each drug is used alone.

*Antagonistic*

Antagonism of two or more drugs occurs when the action of one drug is opposed by the action of another drug. The result will be either: (1) no observable effect by either drug; or (2) the effect of each drug will be greatly reduced. For example, if equal physiologic amounts of a central nervous system stimulant and depressant are given, the net result may be no appreciable change in central nervous system activity. If two or more drugs compete for the same receptor site, these drugs are said to be competitive. The action of a histamine and antihistamine is competitive.

*Additive*

When the net effect of two drugs is equal to the sum of the effects of each drug independently, the effect is said to be additive. This is also called summation. Isoproterenol and isoetharine are additive when used together.

*Synergism*

When one drug increases the effect of another drug, the effect is said to be synergistic. This definition suggests that only one of the two drugs has a greater than normal effect. For example, if drug A and drug B are given, and because of the presence of drug A, drug B has a greater than normal effect, then the interaction is said to be synergistic. In synergism, only one of the two drugs has the desired action.

*Potentiation*

When the combined effect of two or more drugs is greater than the additive effect, then the drugs are said to potentiate one another. This definition suggests that each drug has a greater than normal effect when used together. For example, if drug A and drug B are given, and because of the presence of these two drugs together, drug A has a greater than normal effect and drug B also has a greater than normal effect, then the interaction is said to be potentiated. In clinical practice, there is really no difference between these two (potentiation and synergism). The differentiation is primarily of pharmacological interest.

Two additional terms need to be defined at this point. They do not represent drug interaction, but rather the effect that may occur within the patient.

| | |
|---|---|
| *Cumulation* | Drugs all have a range of action. That is, they will be effective for a given period of time after being administered. If a drug is given in successively short periods of time so that the body has not had time to remove previous doses, the effect is said to be cumulative, and in some instances may be toxic. In situations where cumulation becomes toxic, the therapeutic or maintenance dosage levels have been exceeded. When giving theophylline, the patient dosage and sequence are important to prevent cumulation of the drug. |
| *Tolerance* | When a drug is administered over a period of time and increasing amounts of the drug are needed to achieve the same therapeutic effect, the patient is said to be developing a tolerance for the drug. Repeated use of narcotics will cause the patient to develop a tolerance. |

## ROUTE OF ADMINISTRATION

Many drugs currently in use have specific variations in their make-up or concentration that permit them to be given through different routes of administration. The action of a drug often will be dependent upon the route of administration. The effect may be quite different, and unwanted, if a drug designed for intramuscular use is given intravenously or through inhalation. For this reason, when giving a patient a drug, it is absolutely necessary that the preparation being used is correct for the intended route of administration. For example, epinephrine can be administered intravenously, or subcutaneously, or through inhalation. The preparations and concentrations of the drug are not the same for all routes. It could prove harmful to the patient if the incorrect form of the drug is used.

Drugs may initially be classified by the type of effect desired. Drugs are either administered for a local effect or they are given for a desired systemic effect.

## LOCAL EFFECTS

Drugs that are administered for their local (topical) effect are most often applied directly to the skin or mucous membrane. The skin does not readily absorb drugs unless the epidermal layer is broken. A large number of drugs that are applied to the skin have either an antibacterial or an antiseptic action. Generally, topical drugs are not of primary importance in respiratory therapy.

## SYSTEMIC EFFECTS

Drugs that relate to the respiratory and cardiopulmonary systems are given for their systemic effects. Any route of administration has the potential to produce a systemic effect; however, it should be noted that all routes are not equally effective in producing the desired change.

1. *Oral administration.* Oral administration is the most common route because such a large number of drugs are easily absorbed through the digestive system. The main disadvantage of the oral route is that it takes a longer period of time before the drug will begin to produce its effect. For this reason, oral administration is not used in emergency situations. Drugs taken orally are in the form of pills, capsules, tablets, and liquids. Because pills, tablets, etc. must be in solution before they are absorbed through the digestive tract, they should be taken with water or some other liquid. Obviously, oral administration is contraindicated in nauseated, vomiting patients. Likewise oral drugs cannot be given to unconscious patients. Oral bronchodilators are helpful for patients on a home bronchodilator therapy program, (Alupent, Bricanyl).

2. *Sublingual administration.* Sublingual administration uses the mucous membranes beneath the tongue for a drug route. Relatively few drugs are used in this fashion. Notable exceptions include nitroglycerine and oxytocin.

3. *Rectal administration.* Drugs that are given rectally or in an enema are generally limited to children or adults who are unable to take drugs orally. Suppositories are the most often used form of drugs given rectally. Aminophylline can be given via a rectal suppository.

4. *Inhalation administration.* At one time, drugs given through inhalation consisted primarily of anesthetic gases. Today, however, an increasing number of drugs are given through inhalation for their systemic and local effects. Such drugs include bronchodilators, mucolytic agents, proteolytic enzymes, wetting agents, and asthma inhibitors.

5. *Parenteral administration.* Parenteral administration includes those drugs given by injection. Routes of injection are subcutaneous, intradermal, intramuscular, intravenous, and intra-arterial (some anticancer drugs). Drugs given parenterally are quickly absorbed and distributed in the body. Generally, such drugs are less concentrated and more soluble than those drugs given through other routes of administration. Aminophylline is generally given through the intravenous route.

## GUIDELINES FOR DRUG ADMINISTRATION

Initially, only physicians administered medications. As the demands on the physician increased, he delegated this function to supportive personnel, historically the nurse. Today, individuals from various health care disciplines are responsible for drug administration. The important word here is responsibility. When a therapist is administering a drug, he or she is responsible for the well being of the patient. Certain guidelines should govern the administration of a drug by a therapist:

1. Do not administer any medication without a prescription, preferably written. Verbal orders should only be carried out when written by a nurse or given directly by the physician.
2. Read the label on the drug bottle. Make sure that you have the correct drug, that the drug is in the form acceptable for the intended route of administration, and that you have the correct concentration of the drug. Never give a drug that does not have a label on the bottle.
3. Dispense the appropriate amount of medication. At this time check the physical characteristics for unusual color, odor, or consistency. For example, Bronkosol may show a red tinge of color when outdated. Never use discolored or outdated medications.
4. If you draw up the drug, then give the treatment yourself. Do not give a treatment with a drug dispensed by another individual unless you watched that person draw up the medication, or, the container has been properly labeled and signed. Remember, if you give the treatment with the drug, then you are responsible.
5. Stay with the patient during the drug administration (treatment). Watch for unwanted side effects. Know the drugs and their potential side effects. Always discontinue the drug when side effects occur.
6. Using the charting procedure accepted in your institution, be sure to chart all pertinent information concerning the procedure.

## ABSORPTION AND DISTRIBUTION OF DRUGS

Absorption is the process whereby the drug enters the body for systemic circulation. How readily absorption occurs depends upon the route of administration and the physical properties of the drug. The patient's physiologic status may also have an effect upon the rate of absorption. However, the concentration of a drug and its physical properties have the greatest effect on absorption. Absorption may take place from the gastrointestinal tract, the alveolar-capillary surface area, and, if the drug is given parenterally, the muscle tissue, blood tissue, or dermal tissues. When drugs are administered parenterally, blood flow through the tissues is the prime factor in absorption.

In the absorption of drugs, the drug must pass across body membranes. The types of transfer across membranes can be classified as passive or active transport. Examples of passive transport are diffusion and filtration. In diffusion, a concentration gradient exists that causes the drug to be absorbed. Both diffusion and filtration are passive because no energy (ATP) is used in the transport of the drug. Bronchodilator absorption is an example of diffusion. The second classification is active transport. Included in active transport are pinocytosis and facilitated transfer. In active transport, certain carriers or substrates are needed to transfer the drug across cell membranes. All forms of active transport must use energy in order for absorption to occur.

Once a drug has passed into the circulatory system and reaches the plasma (by either passive or active transport), the compound must be distributed to the various receptor sites (sites of drug action). It is important to repeat here that drugs are not always distributed equally throughout the body. For example, the blood-brain barrier prevents many compounds from easily penetrating the cerebral spinal fluid. This selective permeability of cell membranes partially accounts for the specific action of many drugs. It is important to note that inflammation can also change the permeability of various cell membranes and thus alter the normal distribution of a drug.

## METABOLISM AND ELIMINATION OF DRUGS

The body does not rely solely upon the excretory system as a method of drug elimination. Many drug-metabolizing enzymes are found in the liver and play an important role in drug elimination. In addition, the kidney aids in the elimination of drugs from the body. Most drugs or metabolized substrates of drugs are excreted in the urine. Not to be overlooked, the lung plays a major role in the elimination of anesthetic gases.

## REVIEW OF THE CENTRAL NERVOUS SYSTEM (CNS)

In order to understand even the fundamental actions of drugs used in anesthesia and respiratory therapy, a basic foundation in the CNS is necessary. The following discussion of one division of the CNS, the autonomic nervous system, is not intended to be exhaustive. Its purpose is to provide working knowledge of autonomic agents. The autonomic nervous system automatically controls a large number of physiologic functions in the body. These functions are necessary to maintain a constant internal environment (homeostasis). There are several centers within the central nervous system that function to integrate all autonomic nervous system activities. Table 4-1 provides a breakdown of the central nervous system and its divisions. We will be concerned with the autonomic division.

The autonomic nervous system is composed of two systems of nerves: the sympathetic and the parasympathetic. The actions of these two systems are physiologically opposed in what is called a *balanced antagonism*. Autonomic drugs are those that either oppose or mimic the autonomic nervous system (see definitions below).

| | |
|---|---|
| *Parasympathomimetic (Cholinergic)* | An agent causing stimulation of the parasympathetic nervous system sites. |
| *Parasympatholytic (Anticholinergic)* | An agent blocking or inhibiting effects of the parasympathetic nervous system. |
| *Sympathomimetic (Adrenergic)* | An agent causing stimulation of the sympathetic nervous system sites. Such agents are alpha-stimulants (Phenylephrine), beta-stimulants (Isoproterenol), beta-two stimulants (Isoetharine) or alpha and beta stimulants (Epinephrine). |
| *Sympatholytic (Anti-adrenergic)* | An agent blocking or inhibiting the effect of the sympathetic nervous system. |

Generally speaking, the parasympathetic nervous system is the stabilizing force in the body. The related functions are conservative, constructive, repairative, and vegetative. The parasympathetic system deals with the maintenance of body functions. The effects are predominant in times of rest and are very specific. The sympathetic nervous system deals with the body's protective system. It is designed for a mass response and uses a

Table 4-1

**Division of the Central and Peripheral Nervous System**

A. *Central*
   1. Brain
   2. Spinal cord
B. *Peripheral*
   1. Sensory (afferent)
   2. Motor (efferent)
   3. Autonomic
     a. Parasympathetic—controls bladder, peristalsis, bronchial glands, heart rate, pupil size, sweat glands, etc.
     b. Sympathetic—controls many of the above mentioned glands and smooth muscles, including heart contractile force, bronchial smooth muscles and circulation.
       (1) alpha-sympathetic: peripheral vasoconstriction, bronchoconstriction
       (2) beta-one sympathetic: cardiac excitation
       (3) beta-two sympathetic: bronchodilation, skeletal muscle vasodilation

great deal of energy. The sympathetic system provides for the body "fight or flight" mechanism (see Table 4-2).

The autonomic system is an efferent system. That is, it conducts messages from the CNS to the periphery. The efferent connections of the autonomic nervous system are composed of a two neuron system:

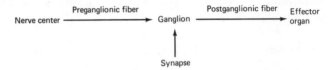

The transmission of the impulse takes place at a junction or synapse. The peripheral synapses are located in ganglia. The neuron that conducts the impulse from the CNS to the ganglion is called the *preganglionic fiber.* This fiber is longer in the parasympathetic system. The neuron carrying the impulse from the ganglion to the target or effector organ is called the *postganglionic fiber.* This fiber is longer in the sympathetic system. The transmission of a nerve impulse from one fiber to another or from a nerve fiber to a target site is possible because of a chemical mediator found at the synapses. This mediator is called *acetylcholine.* Acetylcholine aids in nerve impulse transmission in both the sympathetic and the parasympathetic nervous systems. Acetylcholine is inactivated at the synapse by enzymes called *cholinesterases.* Cholinergic drugs (parasympathomimetic) bring about effects similar to acetylcholine.

In certain nerve synapses in the sympathetic nervous system, the chemical transmitter is norepinephrine. This occurs where the postganglionic fiber meets the target site (see Figure 4-1). Drugs that produce effects similar to norepinephrine are called *adrenergic* drugs (sympatho-

Table 4-2

**Parasympathetic and Sympathetic Responses**

| Organ | Parasympathetic System | Sympathetic System |
|---|---|---|
| Pupil | Constrict | Dilate |
| Lung | Bronchoconstriction | Bronchodilation |
| Stomach | ↑ Tone and motility | ↓ Tone and motility |
| Intestines | ↑ Tone and motility | ↓ Tone and motility |
| Heart | ↓ Rate | ↑ Rate |
| Atrial musculature | ↓ Force of contraction | ↑ Force of contraction |
| Glands (salivary, bronchial, etc.) | ↑ Secretions | ↓ Secretions (generally) |
| Urinary bladder | Sphincter relaxation | Sphincter contraction |
| Blood vessels | Vasodilatation | Vasoconstriction (generally) |
| Ventricle | No effect | ↑ Force of contraction |

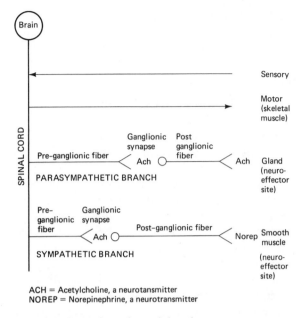

FIG. 4-1. Central and peripheral nervous sytem. (From Rau, J.L.: Respiratory Care 22:263, 1977, with permission.)

mimetic). Autonomic drugs are divided into four main classes based on the two chemical mediators in the autonomic nervous system, and on the action of the drugs:

1. *Adrenergic drugs:* effects similar to those produced by epinephrine and norepinephrine.
2. *Cholinergic drugs:* effects similar to those produced by acetylcholine.
3. *Adrenergic blocking agents:* block the effect of norepinephrine at the myoneural junction.
4. *Cholinergic blocking agents:* block the effect of acetylcholine.

## RECEPTORS

The therapeutic action of a drug may be explained by the concept of receptors. Adrenergic drugs are those drugs that have effects similar to epinephrine or norepinephrine (catecholamines); that is, they affect the sympathetic nervous system. It is postulated that two basic types of adrenergic receptors exist.

1. *Alpha receptors (α):* Alpha receptors constrict arterioles by causing the smooth muscle to contract. Alpha stimulation will cause an eleva-

tion of arterial blood pressure through its vasopressor action. An alpha-stimulating drug will also cause decongestion through the same mechanism.

2. *Beta receptors (β):* Beta receptors in general cause vasodilation, increased cardiac rate, and bronchial dilatation. The classification of receptors can be further delineated as:

β-1: Stimulation of β-1 receptors results in an increase in heart rate and force of contraction.

β-2: Stimulation of β-2 receptors results in relaxation of the smooth muscle and, therefore, bronchial dilatation.

α, β-1 and β-2 receptors are found throughout the cardiovascular and respiratory systems; however, each receptor seems to be predominant in given areas. For example, α activity is greatest in the cardiac musculature, while β-2 activity is greatest in the smooth muscle of bronchioles. Figure 4-2 demonstrates the balance of the sympathetic and parasympathetic activity in the lung.

The action of the β receptors in the lung is of primary importance to the respiratory therapist. Figure 4-3 presents a scheme for the function of a β receptor in the lung. Adenyl cyclase is an enzyme found in the cell membrane of the smooth muscle of the bronchiole. Normally, adenyl cyclase in the presence of ATP (energy form) will form cyclic AMP. The presence of cyclic AMP within the cell will cause bronchodilatation and also will reduce the release of histamine. When an adrenergic bronchodilator is given, this will stimulate the adenyl cyclase to form increased amounts of cyclic AMP and thus, the bronchodilator effect. The cyclic AMP is then broken down into 5-AMP by the enzyme phosphodiesterase. The 5-AMP is inactive and has no effect on the bronchial smooth muscle. From this, one can see that bronchodilatation can bring about one of two results.

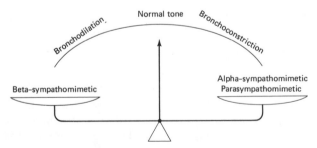

FIG. 4-2. Autonomic control equilibrium in the lung. (From Rau, J.L.: Respiratory Care 22:263, 1977, with permission.)

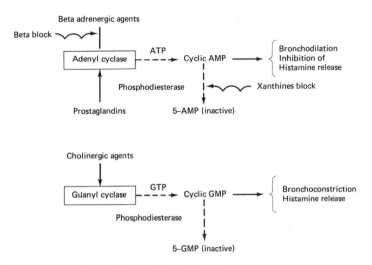

**FIG. 4-3.** Metabolic activity of bronchoactive drugs in the lung. (From Rau, J.L.: Respiratory Therapy Pharmacology, Year Book Medical Publishers, Chicago, 1978.)

1. It can stimulate the adenyl cyclase to produce more cyclic AMP;
2. It can inhibit the breakdown in cyclic AMP by blocking the action of phosphodiesterase.

Many adrenergic drugs such as isoproterenol hydrochloride are $\beta$ stimulants and produce cyclic AMP, while drugs such as aminophylline interfere with the breakdown of cyclic AMP. In both situations, the net result is bronchodilatation.

A similar scheme can be noted in Fig. 4-3 for the cholinergic drugs. Guanyl cyclase is the initial enzyme of this scheme. Note that the production of cyclic GMP will result in histamine release and bronchoconstriction. This scheme plays an important role in the asthma patient.

Some drugs have the ability to block the action of an adrenergic agent or drug on a $\beta$ receptor. Such a drug is often simply called a $\beta$ blocker. The effects of a $\beta$ blocker would include:

1. Decreased heart rate
2. Decreased force of contractions
3. Bronchoconstriction.

$\beta$ blockers generally are given for their antiarrhythmic effects. Propanolol is an often used $\beta$ blocker.

## BRONCHODILATORS

The adrenergic drugs, or sympathomimetics, stimulate the receptor sites, thus producing effects similar to the sympathetic nervous system. The β-sympathomimetics are strong bronchodilators. Their function is to increase the lumen of the bronchioles by relaxing the smooth muscle in the bronchiole wall. As a class of drugs, the bronchodilators are used in the symptomatic treatment of asthma, emphysema, bronchitis, and other disorders where bronchospasm is a problem.

### Isoproterenol Hydrochloride

**Mode of Action:**  The primary action is that of β-1 and β-2 adrenergic stimulation; therefore, action is primarily in the heart and bronchiole smooth muscle.

**Indications:**  Isoproterenol is also available for nebulization and in mistometers. Nebulized isoproterenol is used in the treatment of bronchospasm complicating asthma, bronchitis, emphysema, bronchiectasis, and pneumonoconiosis. Parenteral isoproterenol (for injection) is used in the treatment of shock and cardiac arrest.

**Precautions:**  Isoproterenol hydrochloride is contraindicated or should be used with extreme caution in patients with cardiac disease, hypertension, diabetes, cardiac arrhythmias, and hyperthyroidism.

**Adverse Reactions:**  Tachycardia, palpitations, anxiety, and nausea may occur with the use of isoproterenol. If such symptoms occur, the treatment should be discontinued. Such reactions usually will subside when the treatment is stopped. As a general rule, during a treatment, the cardiac rate should not be permitted to increase greater than 10–15 percent over the resting level.

**Dosage:**

1.  Parenteral isoproterenol hydrochloride is a 1:5000 solution. Generally, it is diluted in 500 cc of I.V. solution. The rate of administration is determined by the patient's status.

2.  Isoproterenol for nebulization is available in two concentrations: 1:100 solution. 10 mg/cc (1 percent). The usual dose is 0.25 ml diluted in 2ml to 4ml of sterile water or normal saline and nebulized for approximately 15 min. 1:200 solution. 5 mg/cc (0.5 percent). The usual dose is 0.25 ml up to 0.50 ml diluted in 2ml to 4ml of sterile water or normal saline. Treatment time is generally 15 min.

**Brand Names:**

Isuprel
Norisodrine
Isuprel Mistometer

## Metaproterenol Sulfate

**Mode of Action:** The primary action is that of a $\beta$ ($\beta$-1 and $\beta$-2) adrenergic stimulator. The action of metaproterenol is of longer duration than isoproterenol hydrochloride; however, the bronchodilator activity is considerably less.

**Indications:** Metaproterenol sulfate is used as a bronchodilator for asthma, bronchitis, and emphysema where bronchospasm is reversible.

**Precautions:** Because of the nonspecific $\beta$ activity, the drug is contraindicated or should be used with extreme caution in patients with cardiac disease where tachycardia and cardiac arrhythmias are evident.

**Adverse Reactions:** Excessive use may cause paradoxical bronchospasm. Tachycardia palpitations, anxiety, and nausea may occur. Safety in pregnancy has not been established.

**Dosage:** Metaproterenol is available in 20-mg tablets and in a metered dose inhaler.

**Oral:** 20 mg taken three or four times daily for adults.

**Inhalation:** Two or three inhalations, not to be repeated more than every three to four hours. The total dosage should not exceed 12 inhalations per day. Each inhalation delivers approximately 0.65 mg of metaproterenol sulfate.

**Brand Names:**

> Alupent
> Alupent Metered Dose Inhaler
> Metaprel Tablets

## Isoetharine Hydrochloride

**Mode of Action:** The primary action of isoetharine hydrochloride is a sympathomimetic $\beta$ stimulation with predominance of $\beta$-2 activity.

**Indications:** Isoetharine hydrochloride is used for its bronchodilator effect in bronchial asthma, chronic bronchitis, and emphysema where bronchospasm is reversible. Isoetharine in Bronkosol is useful with congested or swollen mucosa, for example in post-intubation edema, where the phenylephrine additive reduces swelling caused by vascular engorgement.

**Precautions:** Isoetharine hydrochloride is contraindicated or should be used with extreme caution in patients with cardiac disease, hypertension, diabetes, cardiac arrhythmias, and hyperthyroidism.

**Adverse Reactions:** Tachycardia, palpitations, anxiety, nausea, headache, tension, dizziness, and tremor may result if used too often. Such reactions are common with all sympathomimetic amines.

**Dosage:**   Oral Inhalation:

1. Hand nebulizer: 3–7 inhalations (average 4) undiluted
2. Oxygen aerosolization: 0.25–0.50 ml diluted 1:3 with sterile water or normal saline.
3. IPPB nebulization: 0.25–1.0 ml diluted 1:3 with sterile water or normal saline.

**Brand Names:**

Dilabron
Bronkosol[1]

## Epinephrine

**Mode of Action:**   Epinephrine has the action of $\alpha$, $\beta$-1, and $\beta$-2 stimulation.

**Indications:**   Epinephrine is available in numerous forms where the $\alpha$ and $\beta$ effects are desired. Epinephrine is indicated where elevation of blood pressure is desired such as in acute anaphylactic reactions, and/or where bronchodilation is desired such as in acute asthma attacks, bronchitis, and emphysema where bronchospasm is reversible. Compounds containing epinephrine are also effective in reducing mucosal edema.

Because of the significant cardiac effects of epinephrine, it is generally not used in oral inhalation or nebulization. A synthetic form called racemic epinephrine is less potent as a cardiac stimulant and vasopressor and yet remains an effective bronchodilator. This form of epinephrine is used in respiratory care. In the area of respiratory therapy, racemic epinephrine is used in the treatment of croup, COPD, bronchial asthma, and related airway diseases where bronchospasm is reversible.

**Precautions:**   Compounds containing racemic epinephrine should be used with extreme caution in patients with cardiac disease, hypertension, diabetes, cardiac arrhythmias, and hyperthyroidism.

**Adverse Reactions:**   Tachycardia, palpitations, nausea, and vomiting may be observed with too frequent use. Heart rate should be watched carefully and the treatment given accordingly.

**Dosage:**   The usual dosage of racemic epinephrine is inhalation of a 1:1000 nebulized solution. A 1:500 solution can also be used if necessary for adequate response. For microNefrin this range may be achieved by 4–8 drops of

---

[1]Bronkosol is isoetharine hydrochloride 1 percent and phenylephrine hydrochloride 0.25 percent. Phenylephrine is an $\alpha$ stimulator and thus adds the action of vasoconstriction of mucosal membranes.

solution diluted with 4.6–4.8 ml of sterile water. This produces approximately 5 ml of solution for administration.

**Brand Names:**

> microNefrin
> Vaponefrin Solution (OTC)[2]
> Adrenalin (for parenteral use only)

## Phenylephrine Hydrochloride

**Mode of Action:** The action of phenylephrine hydrochloride is that of α adrenergic stimulation. Phenylephrine is a synthetic sympathomimetic.

**Indications:** Since phenylephrine is an α stimulant, no significant bronchodilator effect exists when used alone. Phenylephrine is available in many forms: tablets, injection, ophthalmic solution, elixir, and intranasal solution (decongestant). In respiratory care, phenylephrine is generally used either as a vasopressor (systemic effect) or as a decongestant (local effect). As a vasopressor phenylephrine is used to treat hypotension related to anesthesia, shock, and circulatory collapse. Phenylephrine slows the heart rate and increases stroke volume. When used topically, phenylephrine is a decongestive, and is useful in the symptomatic relief from colds, sinus congestion, and edema associated with asthma, bronchitis, and allergies.

**Precautions:** Phenylephrine should be used with caution in patients with hypertension, heart disease, diabetes, or hyperthyroidism.

**Adverse Reactions:** Excessive use of phenylephrine hydrochloride may result in ventricular arrhythmias in patients with coronary heart disease.

**Dosage[3] (local decongestant):**

> Nasal spray: 0.25% solution (children)
> 0.50% solution (adults)
> Nasal drops: 0.125% solution (infants and small children)
> 0.25% solution (children)
> 0.50% solution (adults)
> 1.00% solution (extra strength)

**Brand Name:** Neosynephrine
Phenylephrine hydrochloride is also supplied in combination with a bronchodilator: Bronkosol–2 (isoetharine).

---

[2]over-the-counter
[3]Use as directed for each solution strength.

## Cyclopentamine and Isoproterenol Hydrochloride

**Mode of Action:**  Cyclopentamine as well as isoproterenol are sympathomimetic and result in $\alpha$ and $\beta$ stimulation.

**Indications:**  Cyclopentamine and isoproterenol are used in the treatment of bronchospasm associated with bronchial asthma, emphysema, and bronchitis where bronchospasm is reversible.

**Precautions:**  This combination compound is contraindicated or should be used with extreme caution in patients with hypertension, cardiac disease and associated arrhythmias, hyperthyroidism, or a known sensitivity to cyclopentamine or isoproterenol.

**Adverse Reactions:**  Palpitations, insomnia, anxiety, vertigo, and tachycardia may occur.

**Dosage:**  Cyclopentamine and isoproterenol compound is designed for inhalation only:

1. Oral inhalation: 4–10 inhalations using a hand nebulizer
2. Oxygen aerosolization and IPPB: 0.25–0.50 ml of drug diluted in 1–4 ml of sterile water or saline.

**Brand Name:**  Aerolone Compound

## Terbutaline Sulfate

**Mode of Action:**  Terbutaline sulfate is a sympathomimetic $\beta$ stimulator with preferential $\beta$-2 stimulation.

**Indications:**  Terbutaline sulfate is used for its bronchodilator action in bronchial asthma, chronic bronchitis, and emphysema where bronchospasm is reversible.

**Precautions:**  As with other sympathomimetic drugs, terbutaline sulfate is contraindicated or should be used with extreme caution in patients with hypertension, cardiac disease, diabetes, cardiac arrhythmias, and hyperthyroidism. The safety of terbutaline sulfate during pregnancy has not been established.

**Adverse Reactions:**  Increased cardiac rate, palpitations, anxiety, tremor, and dizziness have been observed. Excessive dosages may cause nausea, vomiting, and headache.

**Dosage:**  Terbutaline sulfate is available for subcutaneous injection. The normal dose is 0.25 mg. If clinical improvement does not occur within 30 minutes, a second dose may be given. Dosage should not exceed 0.50 mg within a 4 hour period.

**Brand Name:** Bricanyl

## Theophylline

**Mode of Action:** Theophylline is classified as a xanthine drug. Xathines are found in many types of plants and are found in many commercial beverages: coffee (caffeine), tea (caffeine and theophylline), cola (caffeine), and cocoa (caffeine and theophylline). Xanthines stimulate the central nervous system and produce a variety of other effects including diuresis, cardiac stimulation, bronchodilatation, and coronary vasodilatation.

Our primary interest in theophylline is its bronchodilator effect. Aminophylline is a commercial form of theophylline and is a widely used intravenous bronchodilator. The action of xanthines is to inhibit the phosphodiesterase and thus increase levels of cyclic AMP in the cell (see Fig. 4-3). This produces the relaxation of bronchial smooth muscle.

**Indications:** Theophylline is used most widely in the control and prevention of bronchospasms related to asthma.

**Precautions:** Compounds containing theophylline should not be used concurrently with sympathomimetics. The use of theophylline is contraindicated or should be used with extreme caution in patients with cardiac disease where stimulation may be harmful. Theophylline blood levels should be measured daily to prevent toxicity.

**Adverse Reactions:** Headache, nausea, vomiting, anxiety, palpitations, tachycardia, and dizziness may be observed.

**Dosage:** Because of the large number of drug combinations using theophylline, dosage depends on the type of product used. Products containing theophylline are available in tablets, elixirs, injections, syrups, enemas, suppositories, and capsules.

**Brand Names:** (representative list):

> Elixophylline—KI
> Theoglycinate
> Isuprel Compound Elixir
> Bronkolixir
> Bronkotabs
> Fleet Theophylline
> Tedral
> Quibron
> Aminophylline (pure theophylline)

## *MUCOLYTIC AGENTS*

Quite often expectorants and mucolytic agents are jointly classified. Primarily this is due to the fact that both types of agents promote the removal of secretions from the respiratory tract. Generally expectorants are found in cough medicines and are taken orally; whereas, mucolytics are administered through inhalation.

Mucolytic agents alter the viscosity of the sputum through direct chemical action on the bonds of the mucoprotein component.

### Acetylcysteine

**Mode of Action:**   The primary action of acetylcysteine is through the breakdown of the disulfide bonds in mucus. Figure 4-4 demonstrates this action. This reaction reduces the viscosity and thus promotes removal. Acetylcysteine also reduces the viscosity of purulent sputum. The maximum effectiveness is pH related and has greatest activity in an alkaline range of approximately pH 7–8.

**Indications:**   Acetylcysteine is used as a mucolytic agent for chronic bronchopulmonary diseases, pneumonia, cystic fibrosis, airway care, mucus obstruction, acute bronchopulmonary diseases, and related conditions where viscid mucus is a complicating factor.

**Precautions:**   Acetylcysteine may be irritating to some patients and produce irritation, coughing, and bronchospasm. Asthmatic patients should be closely watched when using acetylcysteine.

**Adverse Reactions:**   Moderate to severe bronchospasm, hemoptysis, vomiting, and nausea may occur with use. It has been suggested that the use of bronchodilators with acetylcysteine may reduce the possibility of bronchospasm.

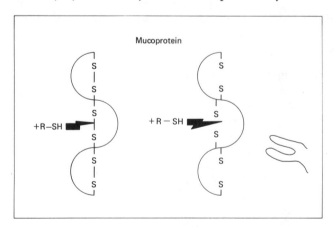

**FIG. 4-4.** Mode of action for acetylcysteine.

**Dosage:**   3–5 ml of the 20 percent solution of acetylcysteine
6–10 ml of the 10 percent solution

**Brand Names:**

Mucomyst (20 percent acetylcysteine)
Mucomyst–10 (10 percent acetylcysteine)

## PROTEOLYTIC AGENTS

Proteolytic agents break down the DNA structures found in pus and thus result in a decrease in viscosity. Specifically, the deoxyribonucleo-protein of purulent sputum is the target of the drug action.

Pancreatic Dornase

**Mode of Action:**   The action of pancreatic dornase is the hydrolysis of the deoxyri-bonucleoprotein of purulent sputum and cellular debris (nonliving). Pancreatic dornase is a natural enzyme prepared from beef pancreas and the action is specific for DNA-containing material; therefore, pancreatic dornase would not be expected to act on mucus.

**Indications:**   Pancreatic dornase is used as a mucolytic agent in bronchiectasis, pulmonary abscess, pneumonia, chronic bronchitis, and related disorders where purulent mucus is a complicating factor.

**Precautions:**   Irritation and bronchospasm have been observed with use. Because pancreatic dornase is a derivative of animal pancreas, sensitivity (allergic) reactions can be observed in some patients.

**Adverse Reactions:**   Airway irritation and anaphylactic reactions may occur with use in hypersensitive patients.

**Dosage:**   50,000–100,000 units, 1–2 times daily.

> NOTE: Pancreatic dornase is unstable at room temperature and thus, once reconstituted, should be used immediately. In addition, pancreatic dornase is very expensive and its high cost should be a consideration.

**Brand Name:**   Dornavac

Trypsin

**Mode of Action:**   The primary action of trypsin is the breakdown of proteins, respiratory and intestinal mucin, fibrin, and protein products. It is a naturally occurring enzyme.

**Indications:** Used as mucolytic agent in the breakdown of mucoproteins associated with purulent sputum. Helpful when fibrin is present in the sputum.

**Adverse Reactions:** Hoarseness and vomiting have been observed after oral inhalation. Anaphylaxis is a danger when this enzyme is used. Trypsin has been found to be very irritating to the bronchial tract and hypersensitivity is common.

**Dosage (oral inhalation):** 125,000 units dissolved in 3–4 ml of normal saline one or two times daily.

**Brand Names:** Tryptar

> NOTE: Because of the hypersensitivity and irritating side effects, the use of trypsin in respiratory care is cautioned.

## Streptokinase-Streptodornase

**Mode of Action:** Streptokinase-Streptodornase is an enzyme mixture used as a proteolytic agent for purulent secretions; materials where blood, fibrin, and pus are present. In respiratory care, the mixture is used for the removal of purulent bronchial secretions. The streptokinase is used to dissolve blood clots and blood-thickened secretions, while streptodornase liquifies nucleoprotein secretions. The mixture is a derivative of the streptococcus bacterium.

**Indications:** Streptokinase-streptodornase is used to remove blood clots, fibrin, and purulent secretions materials.

**Precautions:** Streptokinase-streptodornase may reopen closed bronchopleural fistulae, especially with active tuberculosis. Allergic reactions are rare.

**Dosage (oral inhalation/instillation):** 125,000 units in 10–20cc sterile water or normal saline.

**Brand Name:** Varidase

## WETTING AGENTS

Under the category of wetting agents, two primary classes of drugs or agents exist:

1. Humidifying agents
2. Surface-active agents

The humidifying agents aid in the clearance of bronchial secretions by reducing their viscosity. Normal saline is probably the most widely used humidifying agent. It is used to hydrate secretions, as a vehicle for other drugs, and as a diluent for many bronchodilators. Normal or physiological saline is in the concentration of 0.9 percent. Half strength (0.45 percent saline) and quarter strength (0.25 percent saline) are also used. Saline is less irritating to the bronchial mucosa than water, which explains its popularity. The use of saline as a respiratory medication should be taken into account with patients on a sodium-restricted therapy.

Sterile distilled water has the same hydrating effect on bronchial secretions as saline. The disadvantage of water is that the mist can be irritating to the bronchial mucosa and can cause excessive coughing. Because of the danger of overhydration of the circulatory as well as the respiratory system, excessive use of aerosols is cautioned against. This is particularly true in infants and small children.

**Dosage:**   The dosage for saline and water may vary with the use. When used for hydration purposes, 2–4 cc are aerosolized as directed. When used as a diluent for bronchodilators, the amount will vary according to the desired concentration to be delivered.

> NOTE: *Bacteriostatic* water or saline is not recommended because of the irritating effect of the preservative on the bronchial mucosa.

## Ethyl Alcohol

**Mode of Action:**   The action of ethyl alcohol is to reduce the surface tension of the bubbles, thus causing the bubbles to break and liquefy.

**Indications:**   Ethyl alcohol is used almost exclusively in the treatment of pulmonary edema where frothing secretions are a complicating factor.

**Precautions:**   Ethyl alcohol should be used with extreme caution on patients who may be sensitive to alcohol.

**Adverse Reactions:**   Excessive use or concentrations may irritate the airways.

**Dosage:**   3–5cc of a 30 percent concentration via nebulizer.

**Brand Name:**   Sold under the generic name Ethyl Alcohol ($C_2H_5OH$).

## ADRENOCORTICOSTEROIDS

The group of drugs commonly called steroids may be classified by their primary mode of action:

1. *Glucocorticosteroids* cause the conversion of proteins into fats. This form of steroid possesses the anti-inflammatory action and thus is of concern to those providing respiratory care.

2. *Mineralocorticosteroids* regulate the sodium and potassium metabo-

lism. Aldosterone is the primary mineralocorticoid produced by the adrenal cortex. Deoxycorticosterone is available and causes sodium and water retention while promoting the loss of potassium. No therapeutic use is made of this preparation related to respiratory therapy.

3.  *Androgens* affect male sex hormone activity.

The uses of glucocorticosteroids are varied. They are used to treat endocrine disorders, rheumatic diseases, collagen diseases, dermatologic disorders, respiratory diseases, and numerous other clinical situations. In general, they cause significant metabolic changes and modify the body's immune response. They may cause a reduction in the body's resistance to infection.

In the area of respiratory care, glucocorticosteroids have been valuable in the treatment of asthma and pulmonary emphysema where edema and bronchospasm were complicating factors.

The adverse reactions of the corticosteroids include fluid and electrolyte disturbance, menstrual irregularities, musculoskeletal disorders, hypertension, osteoporosis, convulsions, impaired wound healing, edema, gastrointestinal disturbances, and development of a Cushingoid state (including "moon-face," and "buffalo hump"). The type and severity of adverse reactions vary and are related to dosage and length of therapy.

## Dexamethasone

**Mode of Action:**  The action of dexamethasone is that of an anti-inflammatory agent with modification of the body's immune response. It reduces the swelling associated with inflammation.

**Indications:**  Dexamethasone is used in the treatment of adrenocortical insufficiency, rheumatic disorders, systemic lupus, control of allergic reaction, pulmonary emphysema, and diffuse interstitial pulmonary fibrosis.

**Precautions:**  Dexamethasone, like all corticosteroids, may cause adrenal insufficiency, sodium and water retention (mild), and potassium and nitrogen loss, as well as the adverse reactions listed previously.

**Brand Names:**

| | |
|---|---|
| Decadron | (various forms) |
| Dexameth | |
| Deronil | |
| Gommacorten | |
| Hexadrol | |
| Vanceril | Inhaler (for oral inhalation only) |

NOTE: Other often used glucocorticosteroids include Hydrocortisone, and Methylprednisolone.

## ANTIBIOTICS

An antibiotic is a compound that is produced by a microorganism that is detrimental to or has an inhibitory effect on other microorganisms. The term has been generalized to include synthetic compounds.

Antibiotics are complex compounds. The presence of one antibiotic in the system may have an effect on the action of another. For this reason, antibiotics are often classified as Type I or Type II antibiotics. The Type I group consists of the penicillins, the streptomycins, neomycin, and the polymyxins. The Type II group consists of the tetracyclines, erythromycin, the sulfonamides, chloramphenicol, and novobiocin. The antibiotics in Type I are additive and may, in fact, show a degree of synergism, while those in Type II are thought to be simply additive in their effect. Also, antagonism may occur between Type I and Type II antibiotics when given together.

The antibiotics also can be classified on the basis of the type of bacteria they act against. For example, some antibiotics act primarily against gram-negative microorganisms, while others have their action primarily against gram-positive bacteria. Antibiotics also can affect other types of organisms such as fungi and viruses. Antibiotics that affect many types or classes of microorganisms are called *broad spectrum* antibiotics.

Antibiotics are either bacteriocidal (lethal) or bacteriostatic (inhibitory) on microorganisms. Often, their effect depends on the concentration of antibiotic and the type of organism present, and on the susceptibility of the organism to the particular agent used.

Since the introduction of antibiotics into medical practice, many strains of microorganisms have become resistant to specific antibiotics. Fortunately, however, many new drugs have become available to use in such situations. Aside from any particular side effects that may result from using a specific agent, one should always realize that an allergic reaction is a real possibility when administering antibiotics.

The aerosolization of antibiotics is not uniformly accepted in the practice of pulmonary medicine. Antibiotics are administered through oral inhalation for the following reasons:

1. The topical treatment of local colonizing bacterial growth may be more effective, in some instances, than systemic treatment.
2. The use of an antibiotic in conjunction with a mucolytic agent may help reduce the secretions in order to expose the local bacteria to the antibiotic.
3. The aerosolization of a bronchodilator with an antibiotic may serve two purposes:

    a) It may reduce bronchospasm which may accompany the antibiotic.
    b) It may allow for greater penetration.

## PENICILLINS

The penicillins are produced by the penicillium strain of mold, which explains their name. Different types or varieties of penicillin are produced by changing the culture media in which the molds are grown.

Penicillin is both bacteriostatic and bacteriocidal, depending on the dosage concentration. Penicillin remains the most widely used antibiotic, in part, because the drug lacks many of the toxic side effects, and so people can tolerate large doses with few side effects. The antibacterial activity is due to the fact that the penicillins inhibit the bacteria from synthesizing an adequate cell wall. Thus, the bacteria are easily killed by body defense mechanisms.

The primary disadvantage of the penicillins is the incidence of allergic reactions. Such reactions generally appear with repeated doses. Perhaps 10-15 percent of the population may be hypersensitized to one or more of the penicillins.

Potassium Penicillin G

**Mode of Action:**  Penicillin G is bacteriocidal against penicillin-sensitive organisms. Action is through inhibition of the biosynthesis of cell-wall mucopeptides, allowing the bacteria to be destroyed by normal blood defensive components.

**Indications:**  Penicillin G is used in the treatment of infections resulting from penicillin G-sensitive microorganisms.

**Precautions:**  Penicillin should be used with caution in individuals with histories of significant allergies and/or asthma.

**Adverse Reactions:**  Hypersensitivity reactions may occur with use. Because of the low toxicity, other reactions such as hemolytic anemia and leukopenia are rare.

**Brand Names:**  Potassium Penicillin G for Injection, U.S.P. (Squibb)
Brand names of other penicillin-containing drugs include:

> Bicillin
> Duracillin
> Polycillin
> Wycillin

## STREPTOMYCINS

The streptomycin antibiotic is of historical importance to those providing respiratory care because of its effectiveness in the treatment of pulmonary tuberculosis. Generally, streptomycin is used in combination with other drugs for maximum effectiveness.

Streptomycin is not absorbed through the digestive tract and thus is generally given by intramuscular injection. The primary toxic side effect is the loss of hearing (progressive and irreversible) that can occur with prolonged use.

## Streptomycin Sulfate

**Mode of Action:**   Streptomycin sulfate is both bacteriostatic and bacteriocidal. The action is thought to be inhibition of protein synthesis in the microorganism.

**Indications:**   Streptomycin is used in the treatment of a variety of infections, particularly those of acid-fast and gram-negative bacteria. It is useful against the mycobacterium tuberculosis.

**Precautions:**   Streptomycin should be used with caution in treating patients with hypersensitivity to the streptomycins.

**Adverse Reactions:**   Hypersensitivity reactions may occur with use. Damage to the vestibular nerve can occur with prolonged use.

## TETRACYCLINES

The group known as tetracyclines are broad spectrum antibiotics that are effective against both the gram-negative and gram-positive bacteria. The tetracyclines are generally bacteriostatic but show bacteriocidal properties in high doses. The tetracyclines are less toxic than the streptomycins.

The use of tetracyclines may cause nausea, vomiting, and irritation of the gastrointestinal tract.

## Tetracycline Hydrochloride

**Mode of Action:**   Tetracycline hydrochloride inhibits protein synthesis by the bacteria. The general action is bacteriostatic.

**Indications:**   Tetracycline hydrochloride is used in a variety of infections, including respiratory tract infections, surgical infections, and urinary tract infections.

**Precautions:**   Tetracycline should not be given to patients with known hypersensitivity to any tetracycline group.

**Adverse Reactions:**   Nausea, vomiting, diarrhea, and gastrointestinal disturbances may occur with the use of tetracyclines.

**Brand Names:**

Achromycin
Panmycin
Robitet

### DIURETICS

Diuretics are agents that increase urine flow through the kidney. In doing this, they reduce the amount of water in the body. Two general mechanisms within the kidney produce diuresis: (1) increased glomerular filtration rate, and (2) decreased reabsorption. The second is the primary action of most diuretics. The most effective diuretics primarily influence the excretion of sodium or other ions, rather than water itself. The mechanism of such diuretics is an increased sodium excretion and with it, an osmotic equivalent of water. In order for normal electrolyte balance to exist, the concentration of cations ($Na^+$, $K^+$, etc.) must be equal to the concentration of anions ($Cl^-$, $HCO_3^-$, etc.). Water is obligated to the sodium ion in the body. If the sodium concentration increases, so will the water content. Likewise, if sodium decreases, the body will lose water.

## Osmotic Diuretics

**Mode of Action:**   The presence of osmotic diuretics in the glomerular filtrate will be poorly absorbed by the kidney, and, therefore, its osmotic equivalent of water will be lost to the urine.

**Indications:**   Osmotic diuretics are useful in the treatment of cerebral edema and in the reduction of intraocular pressure.

**Precautions:**   Rapid intravenous solution of osmotic diuretics may cause hemolysis. Osmotic diuretics should be used with caution in patients with renal disease.

**Adverse Reactions:**   Headaches, nausea, and vomiting may occur with use.

**Brand Names:**

> Mannitol I.V.
> Sucrose and glucose I.V. solutions also show diuretic properties

## Xanthines

**Mode of Action:**   Xanthines interfere with the reabsorption of sodium and chloride in the proximal tubules.

**Indications:**   Generally, the xanthines have been replaced by newer agents for use as diuretics. Their primary use today is for the bronchodilator action.

**Precautions:**   Xanthines should be used with caution in patients with hyperthyroidism, myocardial damage, or renal disease.

**Adverse Reactions**: Nausea, vomiting, palpitations, dizziness, and nervousness may occur with use.

**Brand Names**:

> Neothylline
> Fleet Theophylline

## Mercurial Diuretics

**Mode of Action**: Mercury inhibits the enzyme actions involved in the reabsorption of sodium throughout the nephron. Sodium excretion thus occurs with the obligatory water. The mercurial agents are extremely potent diuretics. Mercurial diuretics are given by injection.

**Indications**: Mercurial diuretics are used for the treatment of edema secondary to congestive heart failure and nephrotic syndrome.

**Precautions**: Caution must be taken to prevent deficient sodium levels.

**Brand Name**: Thiomerin

## Carbonic Anhydrase Inhibitors

**Mode of Action**: Inhibition of carbonic anhydrase stops the formation of $H^+$, since $H_2CO_3$ is not synthesized from $CO_2$ and $H_2O$. In normal renal function, $H^+$ enters the lumen while $Na^+$ is absorbed in its place and the $Na^+$ returns to the blood (with $HCO_3^-$). If $H_2CO_3$ is not formed, then no $H^+$ are produced, and $Na^+$ is lost in the urine, carrying with it obligatory water.

**Indications**: For the most part the carbonic anhydrase inhibitors have been replaced by the thiazide diuretic agents. They are used, however, for the treatment of glaucoma.

**Precautions**: Carbonic anhydrase inhibitors should be used with caution in patients with reduced sodium and/or potassium levels, liver disease, and hypochloremic acidosis.

**Brand Names**:

> Diamox
> Cardase

## Hormone Antagonist

**Mode of Action**: Hormone antagonists cause increased $Na^+$ excretion resulting from the action of aldosterone in the distal tubules of the kidney.

**Indications:**  Hormone antagonists are used for the treatment of edema resulting from congestive heart failure. They also are used in the treatment of essential hypertension.

**Precautions:**  Hyperkalemia may occur when renal impairment exists.

**Adverse Reactions:**  Drowsiness, lethargy, headache, and gastrointestinal disturbance may occur with use.

**Brand Name:**  Aldactone

## Thiazide Compounds

The thiazide group of diuretics is a large class of sulfonamide or sulfonamide derivatives. Their action in the kidney tubules is inhibition of sodium reabsorption.

This class of diuretics is a very potent group used in edema secondary to congestive heart failure, renal disease, and liver disease.

Precautions and adverse reactions vary with dosage, duration of treatment, and specific diuretic used. Examples include:

> Diuril
> Hydrodiuril
> Edecrin
> Lasix
> Renese
> Nagua
> Hydromox
> Enduron
> Exna

## NEUROMUSCULAR BLOCKING AGENTS

The neuromuscular blocking agents have the ability to increase the degree of muscular relaxation in skeletal (striated) muscles. Historically, these drugs have been used during surgery to allow for the use of a lighter degree of anesthesia and to reduce the amount of muscle spasm that otherwise might be encountered during the surgical procedure. Of particular interest to respiratory therapists is the fact that the skeletal muscle relaxants or neuromuscular blocking agents have been of considerable value in controlling patients on continuous ventilation. In addition, these drugs have been helpful in orthopedic procedures where muscle relaxation is essential, and they have been used to prevent trauma during electroshock therapy.

The neuromuscular blocking agents are generally divided into two main groups; the *depolarizing agents* and the *nondepolarizing agents*. The nondepolarizing agents are competitive blocking agents in that they inhibit neuromuscular transmission by competing with acetylcholine for the endplate. Examples of nondepolarizing or competitive blocking agents are D-tubocurarine and pancuronium. The depolarizing agents produce end-plate depolarization at the myoneural junction, which is followed by a refractory state during which subsequent impulses will not be transmitted. Examples of such depolarizing agents are from the succinylcholine group: Anectine, Quelicin, and Sucostrin Chloride. Depolarizing agents often cause muscular twitching or contraction prior to the state of total muscle relaxation.

It is very important that the clinical practitioner be aware of the drug interactions that can occur with many of the nondepolarizing agents (curare). For example, anesthetics such as ether, halothane, and cyclopropane increase the action of the nondepolarizing agents. Therefore, the level of dosage is generally reduced. Many of the antibiotics such as neomycin, streptomycin, and kanamycin potentiate the action of the neuromuscular agents. In addition, the nondepolarizing neuromuscular agents may cause adverse reactions in the patient such as bronchospasm, hypotension, and extended periods of apnea.

Neuromuscular blocking agents affect all skeletal muscles. The diaphragm and other accessory muscles of respiration are skeletal muscles, and, consequently, are affected by the neuromuscular blocking agents. When any of these drugs are given, the ventilatory action of the patient will be weakened and in some cases may even stop, depending on the dosage. Whenever skeletal relaxants are being used, the patient must be watched very carefully for he or she is in an extremely compromised position.

## Nondepolarizing Agents

**Mode of Action:**  The action of nondepolarizing agents is to block neuromuscular transmission to the skeletal muscle by competing with acetylcholine for the endplate.

**Indications:**  The nondepolarizing agents are used to provide muscle relaxation during anesthesia, during electroshock therapy, and during other situations where a significant degree of relaxation is necessary for adequate patient therapy.

**Precautions:**  Because the use of neuromuscular blocking agents can produce depression of respirations and even respiratory paralysis, close observation must be made of patients receiving such agents.

**Adverse Reactions:**  Bronchospasm and hypotension have been observed in patients receiving curare. This is apparently due to the histamine release.

**Brand Names:**

>  Pavulon
>  Tubarine
>  Metubine

Depolarizing Agents

**Mode of Action:**  The depolarizing agents produce depolarization at the myoneural junction followed by a refractory state at the endplate. This produces the skeletal muscle relaxation.

**Indications:**  Depolarizing agents have a relatively short-term effect and therefore are only useful for brief procedures including endotracheal intubation, bronchoscopy, cardioversion, and preventing the convulsions of electro-shock therapy.

**Precautions:**  Depolarizing agents should be used with caution in patients with impaired cholinesterase activity and patients with liver disease, malnutrition, and anemia.

**Adverse Reactions:**  Cardiac arrhythmias, prolonged respiratory depression, and cardiac arrest have been reported with use.

**Brand Names:**

>  Anectine
>  Quelicin

## CARDIAC DRUGS

The use of cardiac agents has proven invaluable in the treatment of patients with congenital or acquired cardiac diseases in which an effective cardiac output is no longer maintained. When this occurs, clinical signs and symptoms of heart failure result. The cardiac drugs can be divided into classes depending on their action on the heart. One such class of drugs is called *cardiotonic agents* because they increase the force of cardiac contraction and thereby increase the cardiac output. The cardiac glycosides (digitalis preparations) and the sympathomimetic amines are representative samples. A second class of cardiac drugs is anti-arrhythmic drugs. Propanolol and Diphenylhydantoin (Dilantin) are examples of drugs used to correct cardiac arrhythmias. The third class of cardiac drugs is those that serve as *coronary vasodilators*. Nitroglycerin is an example of such a drug.

## Cardiotonic Agents

The cardiac glycosides improve the function of the heart by increasing the force and efficiency of the cardiac contraction. This corresponds also to an increase in oxygen consumption by the heart. The result of such action includes increased cardiac output, slower rate via the vagus, lower venous pressure, diuresis secondary to an improved renal circulation, and improved ventilation.

**Mode of Action:** The cardiac glycosides are represented by the various digitalis preparations. The action is to increase the contractile force of the myocardium.

**Indications:** The digitalis preparation agents should be used in cases of congestive heart failure, atrial fibrillation, supraventricular tachycardia, and premature ventricular beats.

**Precautions:** The digitalis preparation agents should be used with extreme caution in patients with potassium depletion secondary to diuretic therapy.

**Adverse Reactions:** Nausea, vomiting, headache, depression, confusion, and reduction of pulse rate have been observed with the use of digitalis preparations.

**Brand Names:**

> Lanoxin (Digoxin, USP)
> Digitaline Nativelle (Digitoxin, USP)
> Digitalis

### SYMPATHOMIMETIC AMINES

The sympathomimetic amines are generally used in emergency situations to increase the cardiac muscle's contractility. The action is for very short periods of time. Because of their side effects, sympathomimetic drugs have no clinical use for long-term therapy in the treatment of cardiac patients.

### ANTIARRHYTHMIC AGENTS

## Xylocaine Hydrochloride

Xylocaine hydrochloride is one of the most common antiarrhythmic agents used in the practice of medicine.

**Mode of Action:** Xylocaine hydrochloride exerts its effect by increasing the electrical threshold of the ventricles during diastole.

**Indications:** Xylocaine may be administered in several forms such as intravenous, suppository, and viscous solution. The intravenous route is used in treatment of cardiac arrhythmias.

**Precautions:** The use of Xylocaine is contraindicated or should be used with extreme caution in the presence of severe liver or renal disease and with patients in shock or with sinus bradycardia.

**Adverse Reactions:** Hypotension, cardiovascular collapse, and bradycardia have occurred with the use of intravenous Xylocaine.

**Brand Name:** Xylocaine

## CORONARY VASODILATORS

Nitroglycerin

The third group of cardiac agents consists of the coronary vasodilators. Nitroglycerin and its various combination agents serve to represent this group.

**Mode of Action:** Nitroglycerin relaxes smooth muscles, especially those in the smaller blood vessels, and thus causes vasodilatation of the arterioles. The result is an increase in the blood supply to the myocardium and thus, relief of myocardial ischemia.

**Indications:** Nitroglycerin is used for the treatment of acute anginal attack and the management of angina pectoris resulting from coronary insufficiency.

**Precautions:** The use of nitroglycerin is contraindicated in patients suffering from a recent myocardiac infarction, glaucoma, an increase in intracranial pressure, and hypotension.

**Adverse Reactions:** Headache, flushing, and tachycardia have been observed with the use of nitroglycerin products.

**Brand Names:**

Nitro-Stat
Nitro-Bid
Nitroglyn

## CENTRAL NERVOUS SYSTEM DRUGS

Several different types or classes of drugs have a primary effect on the central nervous system. To a large extent, the pharmacologic effect depends on where the agent modifies in the central nervous system. For example, some drugs depress the motor areas of the brain while others have their primary action on higher brain centers. The types of agents that cause central nervous system depression include general anesthetics, the sedatives and hypnotics, the tranquilizers, and the analgesics. The barbiturates are examples of the sedatives and hypnotics. Morphine, codeine, and demerol are examples of the narcotic type of analgesics. This section will deal only with barbiturates and narcotics because of their frequent use with patients receiving respiratory therapy.

## Barbiturates

A sedative is a drug that is used to calm a patient or individual by mildly depressing the higher brain centers. Barbiturates, which are the primary type of sedative used, do not relieve pain. If anxiety, restlessness, or wakefulness is a result of pain, then barbiturates used alone would not be a method of treatment.

Quite often the barbiturates are administered as preoperative sedatives to relieve anxiety and calm the patient, thus facilitating general anesthesia induction. In addition, the barbiturates have been useful in the treatment of psychiatric patients; one of the primary barbiturates used, Amytal, has been termed "truth serum." It should be kept in mind, however, that this is a misnomer and information given by patients under the effect of such barbiturates may not actually be the truth.

The normal dosage of barbiturates does not have a major effect on respiration. However, large doses may significantly depress the respiratory center. The barbiturates have a minimal effect upon the cardiovascular and muscular systems.

**Mode of Action:**   The primary action of the barbiturates is that of central nervous-system depression. In larger doses they are used as a hypnotic to produce sleep.

**Indications:**   The barbiturates are used for sedation, sleep, anxiety, and the control of acute seizures.

**Precautions:**   The use of barbiturates is contraindicated in patients with known sensitivity to barbiturates, with a history of porphyria, and with significant liver dysfunction. The use of barbiturates would be cautioned in patients with severe respiratory and cardiac disease.

**Adverse Reactions:**   Dizziness, headache, nausea, and diarrhea may occur with the use of barbiturates.

**Brand Names:**

> Seconal (Secobarbital Sodium)
> Amytal (Amobarbital Sodium)
> Nembutal (Pentobarbital Sodium)

## Narcotics

The narcotic drugs are analgesics that are used primarily in the control of moderate to severe pain. They may be derived either from natural sources such as opium or cocaine or they may be prepared synthetically with structures functionally similar to that of the opiates. As a group of drugs, the narcotics are central nervous-system depressants. In many individuals, the use of narcotics produces euphoria and thus has a potential for drug abuse.

**Mode of Action:** The narcotics produce analgesia and sedation by interfering with pain conduction or the response of the central nervous system to pain. The exact mechanism is unknown.

**Indications:** The narcotics are used for the relief of moderate to severe pain, as a preoperative sedative, and as a supplement to anesthesia.

**Precautions:** The narcotics can produce addiction in patients and, therefore, their use should be monitored carefully. Narcotics also have a particular depressive effect on the cough mechanism and, therefore, may interfere with the removal of secretions by patients. Because of the respiratory and circulatory depression that may occur with use, careful monitoring of patients using moderate to large dosages of narcotics is recommended.

**Adverse Reactions:** Light-headedness, nausea, vomiting, sweating, and extreme restlessness or nervousness may occur with the use of narcotics.

**Brand Names:**

Morphine Sulfate
Demerol (Meperidine Hydrochloride)
Codeine Sulfate

### ASTHMA INHIBITORS

## Cromolyn Sodium

Cromolyn Sodium has been shown to inhibit the degranulation of mast cells in animal studies. The Cromolyn Sodium inhibits the release of histamines and the slow-reacting substance of anaphylaxis (SRS-A). The drug Cromolyn Sodium has no therapeutic effect during the bronchial asthma attack, and it must be stressed that this drug has only a prophylactic value.

**Mode of Action:** Cromolyn Sodium inhibits the release of histamines and the slow-reacting substance of anaphylaxis.

**Indications:** Cromolyn Sodium is used as a prophylactic measure in the management of patients with asthma induced by the inhalation of specific antigens.

**Precautions:**  The use of Cromolyn Sodium is contraindicated in patients who have been proven to be hypersensitive to the agent.

**Adverse Reactions:**  Urticaria, cough, and bronchospasm may occur with the use of Cromolyn Sodium.

**Dosage:**  Each capsule contains 5 mg of Cromolyn Sodium powder. The dosage for adults and children five years and older is the contents of one capsule inhaled four times daily at regular intervals. Each capsule contains 20 mg of the Cromolyn Sodium agent. Oral inhalation devices are supplied with medication.

**Brand Names:**

>  Intal
>  Aarane

## CALCULATIONS

### Percentage Preparations

Often the respiratory therapist needs to administer solutions of a certain percentage strength. Percentage means parts of the active ingredient in a preparation that are contained in one hundred parts of the total preparation. Generally, there are three types of percentage preparations: (1) weight-to-weight solutions, (2) weight-to-volume solutions, and (3) volume-to-volume solutions.

For weight-to-weight preparations, percentage means parts by weight of a drug and parts by weight of a mixture. This is true because solids are more easily weighed. The weight-to-weight type of preparation denotes the number of grams of a drug or an active ingredient in one hundred grams of the mixture.

For preparations where solids are dissolved in a liquid, percentage means parts by weight of the drug or active ingredient in one hundred parts by volume of the mixture. This is true because solids are more easily weighed than measured and at the same time the total amount of the mixture is more easily measured than weighed. Weight-to-volume mixtures express the number of grams of the drug or active ingredient in one hundred milliliters of the total mixture.

For preparations where liquids constitute the total mixture, percentage means parts by volume of a drug or active ingredient in one hundred parts by volume of the total mixture. Again, this is true because liquids are more easily measured than weighed. In volume-to-volume mixtures or solutions, the percentage is expressed as the number of milliliters of the drug or active ingredient in one hundred milliliters of the total mixture.

Often, when diluting a medication for use in an aerosol or an IPPB treatment, a ratio is given, e.g. Isoproterenol 1:200 or Bronkosol 1:8. In the Isoproterenol example, the percentage strength is indicated as such: 1 g/200 ml of solution equals 0.5 percent strength. For Epinephrine 1:100 equals a 1 percent strength and likewise Epinephrine 1:1000 equals 0.1 percent strength. Ratio solutions are expressed by simple parts. For example, a solution of Bronkosol 1:8 simply means 1 part of medication (Bronkosol) to 8 parts of solvent (sterile water or saline). In a medication IPPB order of 1 part to 8 parts or any similar type of ratio, it is generally expected that this means 1 cc to 8 cc ratio, which is the same as a 1/4 cc (0.25cc) to 2 cc ratio. When such a ratio order is given the IPPB treatment and is expected to be carried out over a specific time interval, it is acceptable to set up the ratio to provide the amount of volume that will be necessary to complete the treatment.

When solving percentage problems, always convert measurements to metric units. The following equation can be used to solve percentage problems that occur generally in the practice of respiratory therapy:

$$\text{Percent} = \frac{\text{g of active ingredient (solute)}}{\text{g/ml of total amount (solute and solvent)}}$$

Set up your known, and solve for the unknown. This may require some algebraic rearrangement.

An alternate form of setting up a problem is to use a proportional expression:

$$\frac{\text{amount of solute}}{\text{total amount}} = \frac{\text{amount of solute}}{\text{100 parts (g or ml)}}$$

EXAMPLE:

Isuprel 1/200 equals what percentage strength?

$$\text{Percent strength} = \frac{\text{g of active ingredient}}{\text{g/or ml to total amount}}$$

$$= \frac{1}{200}$$

Percent strength = 0.5%

# BIBLIOGRAPHY

Abbott Laboratories, *Parenteral Administration*, Chicago, 1970.

American Pharmaceutical Association, *National Formulary*, 14th edition, Mack Printing Company, Easton, Pennsylvania, 1974.

Asperheim, Mary, K. and Laurel A. Eisenhauer, *The Pharmacologic Basis of Patient Care*, 2nd edition, Saunders, Philadelphia, 1973.

Aviado, Domingo, M., *Pharmacologic Principles of Medical Practice*, 8th edition, Williams and Wilkins, Baltimore, 1972.

Dekornfeld, Thomas J., *Pharmacology for Respiratory Therapy*, Glenn Educational Medical Services, Sarasota, Florida, 1976.

Fields, Lawrence, J., Williams, Thomas, J., and Mary M. Garavoglia, *Pharmacologic Review for Intensive Cardiopulmonary Therapy*, Glenn Educational Medical Services, Sarasota, 1975.

Garb, Solomon, Aim, Betty Jean, and Garf, Thomas, *Pharmacology and Patient Care*, 3rd edition, Springer, New York, 1970.

Goodman, Louis S. and Alfred Gilman, *The Pharmacological Basis of Therapeutics*, 4th edition, Macmillan, New York, 1970.

Goth, Andres, *Medical Pharmacology*, 7th edition, C.V. Mosby, St. Louis, 1974.

*Physicians Desk Reference*, 29th edition, Medical Economics Company, Oradell, New Jersey, 1975.

Rau, J.L., "Autonomic Airway Pharmacology," *Respiratory Care*, Vol. 22, No. 5, March, 1977.

Rau, J.L., *Respiratory Therapy Pharmacology*, Year Book Medical Publishers, Chicago, 1978.

# CHAPTER
# 5

# CHEST PHYSICAL
# EXAMINATION

## INTRODUCTION

At one time, the examination of a patient, whether in a hospital setting or
a doctor's office, was the sole responsibility of the physician. Because of
changes in health-care delivery, more and more nonphysician personnel
are now involved in examining patients. Because of the emphasis placed
on the respiratory system, respiratory therapy personnel are becoming
increasingly involved in performing physical examinations of the chest.
This is due to the large amount of time the respiratory therapist spends
with patients during IPPB, mechanical ventilation, aerosol and humidity
therapy, and seeing patients in pulmonary rehabilitation programs.

The chest physical examination involves four features:

1. Inspection, which is the visual observation of the patient. During inspection special attention is paid to ventilation patterns, structure of the
chest, patient color, apparent work of breathing, and any abnormalities of
ventilation or symmetry.

2.   Palpation, which is touching the patient with the hand for the purpose of determining any abnormalities of the chest, the consistency of surface chest tissues, and any abnormalities of structure that are not visually evident.

3.   Percussion, which is the process of striking the chest wall, and often the upper abdomen, for the purpose of determining the nature of the underlying structures relative to air or solid material. Furthermore, percussion is helpful in determining the position and boundaries of organs within the thorax as well as areas of the lung.

4.   Auscultation, which is the process of listening to the chest sounds. Chest auscultation can be either direct, by placing one's ear against the chest wall, or indirect, by the use of a stethoscope. Auscultation using a stethoscope is the procedure of choice.

The physical examination of the chest should be performed in an orderly manner. First perform inspection. This will provide an overview of the anatomical aspects of the patient and make the examiner aware of visual abnormalities at an early stage of the examination. Then palpate the chest for abnormalities. Third, perform percussion, which involves setting up vibrations in the chest wall that can provide information concerning lung functions. Finally, perform auscultation of breath sounds with a stethoscope. Following this procedure allows the examiner to identify suspected abnormalities that can be significant in the patient's therapy program.

## INSPECTION

During inspection, the therapist should be particularly observant of three aspects of the chest: (1) the configuration of the chest; (2) the rate and pattern of respiration, and (3) the movement of the chest during ventilation. When performing inspection of the chest, it is best to be in a warm, quiet environment. The patient should be stripped to the waist and draped accordingly. During inspection, the examiner will be facing the patient and also inspecting from the side and behind the patient. For this reason, the examiner should have ample room to move about so that the patient does not have to change positions. When looking at the configuration of the chest, the patient should be sitting unaided in an upright position. If the patient is unable to remain in a sitting position without help, have the patient lie in bed in a semi-upright position (approximately at a 45°-angle). When looking at the configuration of the chest, the therapist should pay particular attention to symmetry both of structure and movement. Examine the posterior chest first, then the anterior chest. While at the patient's back, observe the movement of the chest with special attention to symmetry. Compare one side of the chest with the other and perform the examination from top to bottom. With the patient in an upright position, observe the entire thorax as a single unit and pay particular attention to the movement of the chest during ventilation. First, observe whether or not both sides of the chest show the same movement during inspiration and expiration. Look to see that excursion of the chest wall is qualitatively the same. Look to see whether or not the shoulders are level and if the thorax is wider from side to side (transverse) than from front to back (anterior-posterior). Check to see if there is restriction of the chest wall on either side during maximal inspiration. In the normal pa-

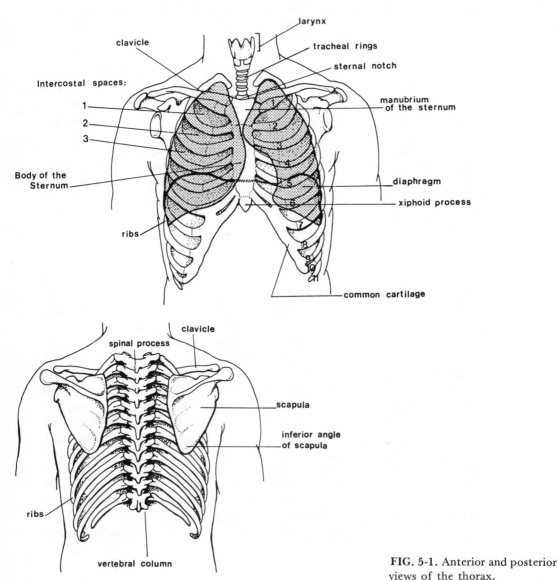

FIG. 5-1. Anterior and posterior views of the thorax.

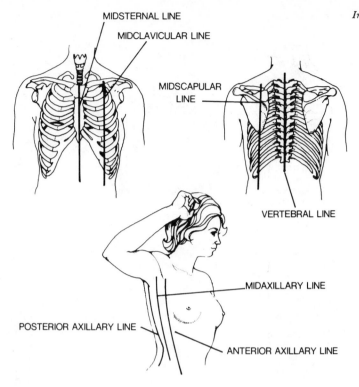

MIDSTERNAL LINE

MIDCLAVICULAR LINE

MIDSCAPULAR LINE

VERTEBRAL LINE

MIDAXILLARY LINE

POSTERIOR AXILLARY LINE

ANTERIOR AXILLARY LINE

**FIG.** 5-2. Anatomical reference areas.

tient, both sides of the chest should be symmetrical, no tissue bulges should be present, the spine should be straight, and the scapulae level in relation to each other.

Figures 5-1 and 5-2 provide basic anatomical information concerning the anatomy of the chest. Familiarize yourself with these before continuing this chapter.

Many variations from the normal can occur that have no major ill-effect or compromise upon the patient (see Fig. 5-3). Such variations include pectus excavatum, a funnel shaped depression of the lower part of the sternum; kyphosis, an exaggeration of the spine convexity; scoliosis, an abnormal deviation of the spine laterally; and kyphoscoliosis, the combination of kyphosis and scoliosis; pectus carinatum, an abnormal projection of the sternum beyond the frontal plane; and barrel chest, an increase in the anterior-posterior diameter. In and of themselves, these are minor variations; however, some of them, such as barrel chest, may be indicative of an underlying pathology, for example, chronic obstructive pulmonary disease. Others, such as kyphoscoliosis, may prevent or impair normal ventilation when severe.

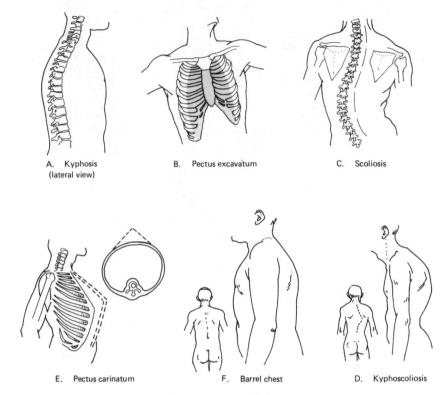

A. Kyphosis
(lateral view)

B. Pectus excavatum

C. Scoliosis

E. Pectus carinatum

F. Barrel chest

D. Kyphoscoliosis

**FIG. 5-3.** Skeletal abnormalities.

While the patient is breathing, the examiner should look at the ribs themselves and the excursion of the chest wall. Women generally breathe with their costal cage and therefore thoracic expansion is obvious. Most males, on the other hand, are diaphragmatic breathers and bulging of the abdomen during inspiration is typical.

During inspiration the entire rib cage moves upward and laterally in a rising motion. It is at this point that right and left symmetry can most easily be noticed. If the excursion of the thorax is difficult to observe during ventilation, it is helpful to place the hands on the patient's chest wall during the ventilatory maneuver and watch the excursion of the hands (see Fig. 5-4). Attention should also be paid to the intercostal spaces during inspiration. Normally the ribs will not react or bulge during an inspiratory maneuver. When retraction is seen in adults, this is often a sign of an increased work of breathing. During inspection, the therapist should be talking with the patient, making him or her feel more comfortable and at the same time gathering additional information. The therapist should be observing whether or not the patient appears to be in pain, whether any respiratory distress is observed, whether or not respiratory noises are heard without the aid of a stethoscope, and the general status of the patient. Also, in out-patient clinic facilities it may be helpful to observe the state of the patient's nutrition, whether or not the patient appears to be in a state of dehydration (which often occurs in chronic obstructive pulmonary patients), and the presence of any vascular pulsations. Observe the patient for increased ventilatory effort, use of accessory muscles, and signs of airway obstruction. This might include difficulty exhaling, pursed lip breathing, nasal flaring, retraction of upper sternum, and splinting secondary to pain.

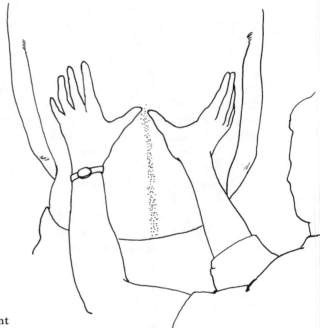

**FIG. 5-4.** Hand placement for chest wall excursion.

## RESPIRATORY PATTERN

The rate and pattern of respiration are very important when doing a chest examination. The rate of respiration may vary among the normal population. However, normally the rate will be between 12 and 16 breaths per minute (eupnea). When the respiratory rate increases to greater than 20 breaths per minute, the term *tachypnea* is generally used. Tachypnea may be nothing more than a sign of patient anxiety caused by being in the hospital, clinical facility, or even by the examination itself. The individual performing the chest examination must be able to evaluate the situation and determine whether or not an elevated respiratory rate appears to be the result of patient nervousness or an underlying disease pathology. Children and infants have a much faster than normal respiratory rate. And quite often, obese individuals will show a slightly faster rate. In order to get an accurate respiratory rate for that particular patient, the individual performing the examination should not be obvious in counting the rate. He or she should attempt to distract the patient or be very subtle and count the rate while performing the physical examination. In doing this, the patient's rate will not increase simply because he or she is aware of being counted. Diseases or disorders that are responsible for tachypnea include: both acute and chronic lung diseases, cardiac diseases, obesity, fever, anemia, and psychotic and neurotic disorders.

Bradypnea is a reduction or slowing of the respiratory rate, usually to less than 10 breaths per minute. In most instances, a severe reduction in respiratory rate is significant of an underlying disease or disorder. Those diseases associated with bradypnea include damage to the central nervous system, drug overdose, metabolic disorders, alcoholism, and diseases involving neuromuscular transmission to the respiratory muscles.

The pattern of respiration can be very helpful during the physical examination in identifying disease processes. The three most common types of abnormal respiratory patterns include (see Fig. 5-5):

a. Cheyne-Stokes respiration
b. Biot's respiration
c. Kussmaul respiration

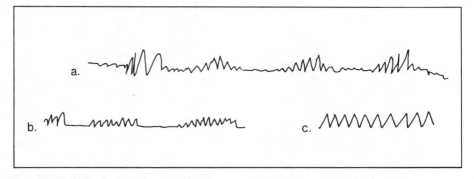

FIG. 5-5. Ventilatory patterns.

Cheyne-Stokes respiration is a periodic form of breathing characterized by alternate phases of increasing and decreasing depths of respiration with periods of apnea. The typical type of pattern seen with Cheyne-Stokes respiration is when the depth of respiration progressively becomes deeper until some maximum depth is reached, and then the subsequent breaths become more and more shallow until a period of apnea occurs, after which progressively deeper respirations begin again and the process is repeated. Cheyne-Stokes respiration is seen in patients with congestive heart failure, damage to the cerebrum, elevated cerebral spinal fluid pressure, and in patients with uremia. The major factor in Cheyne-Stokes respiration is a decreased blood flow to the medullary centers of the brain. Biot's respiration is seen most generally in patients with brain damage. Biot's respirations are similar to those of Cheyne-Stokes, except that there is no increasing depth of respiration. Respirations are simply interrupted by periods of apnea. Spinal meningitis is also a common cause for Biot's respiration. Kussmaul respiration is a slow, deep, regular pattern of breathing. It is commonly seen in patients with metabolic acidosis.

## POINT OF MAXIMUM IMPULSE

While inspecting, it is extremely helpful to look at the nonrespiratory movement of the thorax. The most important aspect of the nonrespiratory movement is the Point of Maximum Impulse (PMI) (see Fig. 5-6).

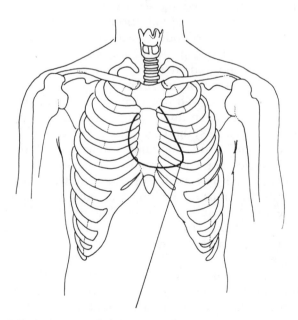

FIG. 5-6. Point of maximum impulse (PMI).

This is the area on the front of the chest wall where the left ventricle of the heart can be seen hitting the chest. The PMI occurs approximately 4-5 cm from the left sternum border and under the fifth intercostal space. It can be found by locating the midpoint of the left clavicle and moving down five intercostal spaces. This point should be approximately 5 cm from the sternum. Abnormal PMI pulsations can result from heart disease, lung disease, and major disorders of the skeletal structures in the thorax. Identification of the PMI is a unique clinical skill and a great deal of practice is necessary in order to become competent in the observation. The PMI can be found more easily during palpation.

## PALPATION

Palpation of the chest is helpful in identifying areas of tenderness, tone of chest muscles, respiratory excursion, and fremitus. When palpation is used during the physical exam of the chest, the therapist should be alert on four parameters: (1) tactile fremitus; (2) subcutaneous crepitus; (3) tracheal deviation, and (4) abnormalities of skeletal structures.

### TACTILE FREMITUS

Vibrations produced over the chest wall that can be picked up through palpation are called *tactile fremitus*. *Vocal fremitus*, a subdivision of tactile fremitus, is the vibrations that are felt over the chest wall and is created by vocal sounds. Vocal fremitus can be palpated by having the patient in a sitting position, placing the palm of the hand on the chest, and asking the patient to say "ninety-nine." The resulting vibrations are vocal fremitus. Abnormalities of the trachea, larynx, bronchi, lungs, pleura, and chest wall can change the intensity of the vibrations and thus be suggestive of an underlying disorder. Low-pitched voices will amplify the vocal fremitus; therefore, the patient should be instructed in repeating "ninety-nine" with the same intensity and the deepest voice possible. When testing for vocal fremitus, corresponding areas of each side of the thorax should be tested. For example, when testing for vocal fremitus of the apical regions of the lung, the hands should be able to note vibrations. While the patient is repeating "ninety-nine," the examiner should move his or her hands to the corresponding apical region on the other side of the chest and repeat this procedure so that he or she can make a comparison.

Any disease process that interferes with the transmission of sound vibrations will cause a decrease in vocal fremitus. Causes of a decrease in vocal fremitus include emphysema, tumors of the pleural cavity, bronchial obstruction, pneumothorax, and pleural effusion. Causes of an increase in the vocal fremitus are any underlying disorder that will increase the transmission of vibrations. Liquid and solid materials transmit vibrations more than air-filled spaces; therefore, increased vocal fremitus can be noted in the following conditions: pneumonia, atelectasis, lung masses, pulmonary fibrosis, and consolidation.

## SUBCUTANEOUS CREPITUS

Subcutaneous crepitus is the tactile sensation of cracking or bubbles under the skin. Subcutaneous crepitus is generally a result of subcutaneous emphysema and is often present in patients on mechanical ventilation, patients following thoracic surgery, and patients with gas gangrene. Subcutaneous emphysema is always considered an abnormal finding.

## TRACHEAL DEVIATION

Tracheal deviation can be tested for by having the patient sit in an upright position, if possible, and look straight ahead. The therapist places the index finger through the suprasternal notch (Fig. 5-1) and compares the space between the right clavicle and right border of the trachea and the corresponding left clavicle and left border of the trachea. Generally these two spaces should be equal. Tracheal deviation can occur in two categories: (1) those disorders that pull the trachea towards the abnormal side, which include atelectasis, unilateral pulmonary fibrosis, and pneumonectomy; and (2) those disorders that push the trachea towards the normal side, which include tension pneumothorax, pleural effusion, mediastinal masses, and disorders of the neck and thyroid.

In palpating the chest wall, the examiner should be aware of any abnormal masses. The temperature, moistness, and pliability of the skin should be noted. In addition, the therapist should be aware of any edema that might be present. Each rib should be palpated in order to determine any masses, sensitive areas, or structural abnormalities that might interfere with normal ventilation. During palpation the examiner should also observe the spinal column for deformities such as scoliosis, etc. (see Fig. 5-3).

# PERCUSSION

Percussion is useful in determining the nature of the underlying structures, the boundaries of organs, or areas of the lung which differ in density. Specifically, when percussing a patient one is interested in the amount of air or solid material present in a given area. In order for percussion to be a valuable tool for physical examination of the chest, it is necessary to have an understanding of the anatomy of the thorax. Figure 5-1 is a schematic representation of the thorax showing skeletal structures and other structures. It is also necessary to have a basic understanding of the physics of sound or at least the characteristics of each sound.

*Pitch* is the frequency of a sound wave. One can speak of a high-pitched vibration, a low-pitched vibration, or a normal-pitched vibration. The *amplitude* is simply the loudness of the sound, and it depends on the force used during percussion and the tissues that will conduct the sound. In performing a percussion, there are two techniques. The first is called *direct percussion,* where the examiner strikes the chest directly with one finger or slaps the chest with the hand. *Indirect percussion,* or mediated percussion, is the preferred method. In this technique, the middle finger of one hand is placed firmly against the chest wall in the intercostal spaces (see Fig. 5-7). A quick, sharp strike is made against this hand with the tip of the middle finger of the other hand, using a snapping motion of the wrist. This method, when performed correctly, produces a high quality percussion note and is more comfortable for the patient than the direct method.

Percussion is a clinical skill that requires a great deal of practice before significant validity may be placed upon interpretation of the percussion notes. Corresponding regions of the chest should be percussed, keeping in mind structural and anatomical differences that underlie those regions. Percussion over the normal air-containing tissues of the thorax produces a sound that is low pitched and long in duration. Percussion over areas of

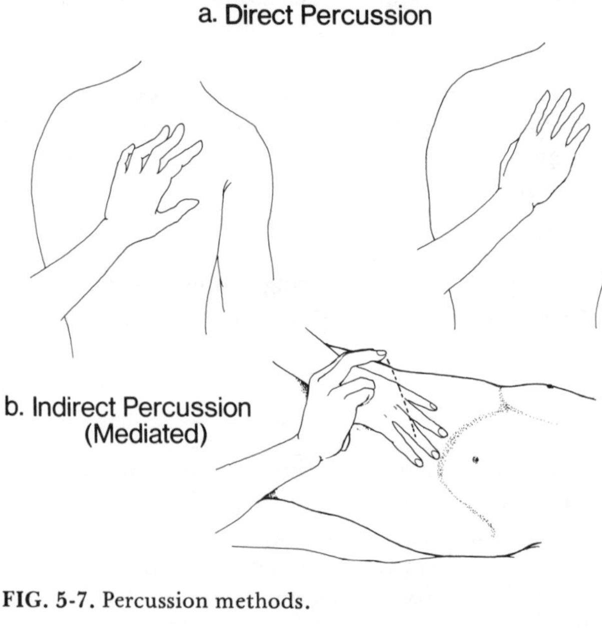

a. Direct Percussion

b. Indirect Percussion
(Mediated)

FIG. 5-7. Percussion methods.

the thorax where a large amount of air is present causes a sound that is lower in pitch and of a moderately long duration. Percussion over an area in which there is a large amount of solid tissue produces a high pitched or dull sound that is short in duration. Low-pitched long-duration sounds are normal; however, a great deal of variation in this normal sound may occur among patients. Dull percussion notes occur where the underlying tissue has a decreased air content. In the normal thorax, dullness is heard over the heart, spleen, scapula, spine, diaphragm, and liver. Abnormal causes of a dull percussion note include pneumonia, atelectasis, pulmonary edema, pulmonary fibrosis, pleural thickening, lung tumors, pleural effusion, and an enlargement of normal structures such as heart or liver. Low-pitched sounds that are moderately long in duration can be heard in emphysema and pneumothorax. A very high-pitched sound of long duration (often called tympanic) can be heard when there is a large pneumothorax, large emphysemic boli, or any large cavitation that is in the thorax.

The excursion of the diaphragm can be measured in many patients by percussion. The therapist performing the chest examination should ask the patient to inhale deeply and hold his breath. The change in percussion note between the resonant lung and the dull viscera of the abdomen will be obvious in a horizontal line across the patient's back (see Fig. 5-8). The patient should then be asked to exhale completely and hold his breath. A lower line of difference between pulmonary resonance and abdominal viscera can be noted, which establishes a second horizontal line. The difference between these two lines represents diaphragmatic excursion (Fig. 5-8). The technique has been one of moving from a resonant sound to a

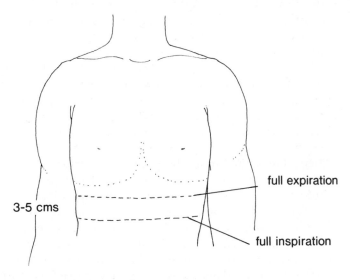

full expiration

3-5 cms

full inspiration

FIG. 5-8. Diaphragmatic movement.

dull sound for establishing the level of diaphragm. In the normal upright individual, the excursion of the diaphragm is from three to five centimeters. In patients with severe COPD, the level of the diaphragm will be depressed and the excursion will be reduced.

## AUSCULTATION

During auscultation of the lungs, three types of sounds can be heard: breath sounds, voice sounds, and extra or adventitious sounds. Auscultation of the chest can be done either directly or indirectly by using the stethoscope. The binaural stethoscope brings out detail at localized points in the chest. It is preferable to use a binaural stethoscope because it has both a bell and a diaphragm chest piece. The bell piece is extremely helpful in listening for low-pitched sounds and to the apices of the lungs and for placing the stethoscope in the intercostal spaces. The obvious advantage of the bell is that it allows the examiner to listen to areas that are less accessible. The diaphragm type of piece allows the examiner to listen to the higher pitched sounds which represent the majority of chest sounds. In most patients, the diaphragm piece is satisfactory for the entire auscultation process. On occasion, acceptable sounds may not be heard by using the stethoscope, and direct auscultation with the ear may be necessary.

During auscultation, it is best to have the patient in a quiet room so that extra noise will not interrupt the examiner. There are several sources of adventitious sounds of which the examiner must be aware. The examiner should not be breathing on the rubber tubing of the stethoscope because this will create noise and sound as though it were coming from the patient. In addition, when using a diaphragm, if the diaphragm is not held in place, chest hair against the diaphragm will produce sound and be a source of extraneous noise. Additional adventitious sounds can be created by contraction of muscles. Muscle sounds are typically rumbling distant types of sounds and often have a "drumming" quality. Whenever doing auscultation for breath sounds during the physical examination, the patient should be asked to breathe in and out in a forcible, deep manner. Normal respirations will not create a repeating quality sound. Whenever listening to the chest, the examiner should be aware of the anatomy of the patient. Obese and muscular patients will cause variation of loudness, and, therefore, affect the quality and intensity of the breath sounds. Patients who are thin and whose chest-wall musculature is poorly developed produce the most consistent quality of breath sounds.

When listening to the breath sounds, three qualities or parameters must be kept in mind: (1) the duration of the sound; (2) the intensity of the sound; and (3) the pitch of the sound. By using these three parameters, it is possible to diagram the breath sounds for comparison. Figure 5-9 depicts the representation of breath sounds.

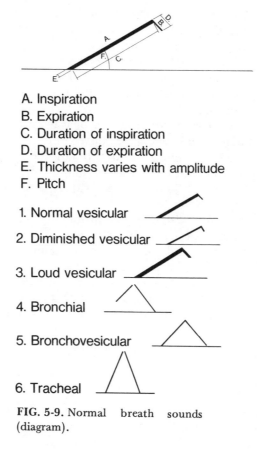

A. Inspiration
B. Expiration
C. Duration of inspiration
D. Duration of expiration
E. Thickness varies with amplitude
F. Pitch

1. Normal vesicular

2. Diminished vesicular

3. Loud vesicular

4. Bronchial

5. Bronchovesicular

6. Tracheal

**FIG. 5-9.** Normal breath sounds (diagram).

The breath sounds that are heard over the chest during auscultation show great variation. Those sounds heard over normal lung parenchyma are:

1. *Vesicular breath sounds.* Vesicular breath sounds are not heard in areas directly over the trachea, between the scapulae, or over areas directly on either side of the sternum. The inspiratory sound of vesicular breath sounds is more intense, longer, and higher pitched and thus more easily heard than the expiratory breath sounds. Vesicular breath sounds are described as breezy and resemble wind going through trees. The expiratory phase of a vesicular breath sound is about three times longer than the inspiratory phase, although sound is only heard during the early phase of expiration. This is due to the alveoli distending and separating during the inspiratory maneuver. In children, vesicular breath sounds are louder than in adults, while in obese patients, old patients, and muscular patients, the vesicular breath sounds are diminished.

2. *Bronchial sounds.* The bronchial sound is that sound which can be heard over the sternum in the normal patient. Bronchial sounds also have been called tubular sounds because of their resemblance to wind going through a long tube. In bronchial sounds, there is a pause between the inspiratory and expiratory phase during which no noise or no breath sounds are heard. Bronchial breath sounds are often associated with disease processes.

3. *Tracheal breath sounds.* Tracheal breath sounds are very loud, harsh, and tubular sounds which are heard only over the trachea. Trachea breath sounds have an increased duration of the expiratory phase, a higher intensity during both inspiratory and expiratory maneuvers, and a high pitch. Normally, there is a very short pause between the inspiratory and expiratory sounds.

4. *Bronchovesicular sounds.* Bronchovesicular sounds are a mixture of bronchial and vesicular breath sounds. Normally, expiration is longer, higher-pitched, and more intense than inspiration. Bronchovesicular sounds are heard where normal lung tissue overlies the large bronchi. There is no pause between inspiration and expiration. Vesicular, bronchial, bronchovesicular, and tracheal breath sounds are all normal breath sounds when heard in the appropriate area of the chest.

## THERAPEUTIC CONSIDERATIONS

### Abnormal Breath Sounds

Diseases or disorders of the respiratory system often cause alteration of breath sounds, the absence of breath sounds, or new sounds generally not heard with the normal patient. The absence of breath sounds can occur during obstruction of the larynx, trachea, and bronchi. This can result from the presence of a foreign body, mucus plugging, tumor, and excessive secretions. The accumulation of fluid, air, or solid tissue in the pleural cavity will result in a reduction or absence of normal breath sounds. Situations such as inflammation of the pleura, pneumothorax, malignant growth in the pleural cavity, and restriction will also result in diminished or absent breath sounds. In patients on mechanical ventilation, the absence of breath sounds on the left side most generally indicates endotracheal tube malpositioning (right bronchial intubation). Atelectasis, pulmonary fibrosis, and laryngeal spasm may also cause the reduction or absence of breath sounds.

Bronchial breath sounds are only heard over the manubrium of the sternum in the normal patient. Bronchial breath sounds are not heard over normal lung tissue except in pulmonary disease. This is generally an indication of solidification of underlying structures or infiltration. Bronchial breath sounds can be heard in atelectasis, lung tumors, pulmonary infarction, pneumonia, pleural effusion, and in patients with severe congestion and abscess. Bronchovesicular breath sounds are abnormal when they occur in the peripheral regions of the lung. Conditions which produce bronchovesicular sounds include pneumonia, tumors, pulmonary edema, and mild to moderate atelectasis.

Adventitious sounds are extra sounds. The examiner himself may cause these sounds by not correctly using the stethoscope or breathing on the tubing. Adventitious sounds may be sounds that are not normally heard in the chest and are extra sounds in addition to the breath sounds. *Rhonchi* are adventitious sounds that are produced by air moving through a narrowed tracheal-bronchial tree. Rhonchi may be heard throughout both the inspiratory and expiratory phase; however, they are more prominent during inspiration. Rhonchi have a very coarse quality to their sound. Typically, they are musical in nature and produced by air flowing through secretions in the tracheo-bronchial tree and even alveoli. A *rale* is a short, nonmusical, bubbling-type of sound that is heard generally during inspiration. Rales may be divided into two types—crepitant rales, fine moist cracking noises heard on inspiration, and subcrepitant rales, medium moist rales, noncracking in nature, heard during inspiration, and caused by air passing through the smaller bronchi, large bronchi, and trachea. The presence of rhonchi and rales denotes an abnormal condition of the lung. They are the result of either bronchoconstriction or increased secretions, or of a combination of both.

## BIBLIOGRAPHY

Cherniack, R.M., Cherniack, L. and V. Naimark, *Respiration in Health and Disease*, 2nd edition, Saunders, Philadelphia, 1972.

O'Connor, A.B., *et al.*, "Patient Assessment: Examination of the Chest and Lungs," American Journal of Nursing, Vol. 76, No. 9, September, 1976.

# CHAPTER
# 6

# Chest Physical
# Therapy

Chest physical therapy is provided by respiratory therapy personnel, nurses, and physical therapists. The service should be available on a 24-hour basis to the patient requiring it. The respiratory care practitioner provides some type of chest physical therapy with most primary respiratory care techniques. In the treatment of pulmonary disease, the purpose of chest physical therapy is both preventative and therapeutic. Chest physical therapy methods include postural drainage, percussion, coughing, breathing exercises, and ventilatory training.

## GOALS OF CHEST PHYSICAL THERAPY

1. To assist in the removal of bronchial secretions from the respiratory tract. Through the use of postural drainage techniques, patient training, and exercise procedures, chest physical therapy improves mobilization of bronchial secretions and prevents accumulation of secretions within the tracheobronchial tree.

128

**2.** To improve the distribution of ventilation within the lungs. Training and breathing exercises are used to improve movement of gas into the lungs. Secretion clearance with postural drainage techniques also will improve distribution of ventilation by eliminating potential airway obstructions.

**3.** To develop more efficient use of respiratory musculature and cardio-pulmonary reserve. Respiratory exercises and promotion of secretion removal from the lung are prescribed to allow physical conditioning of the patient to improve his or her physiological reserve. Exercises also may be used to improve or sustain a level of physical condition developed by the patient following the presence of acute or chronic respiratory disease.

## POSTURAL DRAINAGE

Postural drainage is the use of varying body positions to enhance the draining of secretions from the peripheral areas of the lungs. With the use of gravity, secretions are moved from peripheral areas of the lung into larger bronchi and bronchioles so that they may be coughed up or aspirated. The use of postural drainage requires the patient to be placed in a position so that the affected lung area is elevated, allowing drainage of the secretions in that area into the larger airways.

The affected areas of the lung to be drained are determined by chest physical examination and X-ray (see Chap. 5). Auscultation of the chest may be used to determine the presence of localized lung secretions and to evaluate lung sounds as the secretions are altered with postural drainage therapy. The figures included here illustrate the proper positioning of the patient to drain affected lung segments. (See Figs. 6-1 through 6-12.)

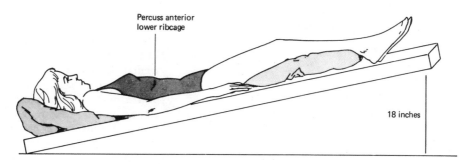

**FIG. 6-1.** Postural drainage position. Lower lobes (anterior basal segments). The patient is positioned supine with pillows under the head and knees. The foot of the bed is elevated to 18 inches.

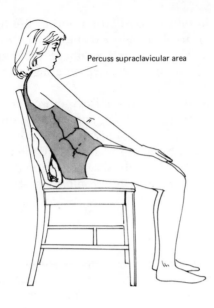

Percuss supraclavicular area

**FIG. 6-2.** Postural drainage position. Upper lobes (anterior apical segments).

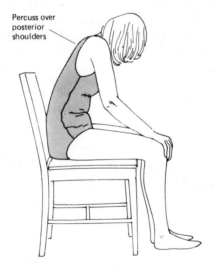

Percuss over posterior shoulders

**FIG. 6-3.** Postural drainage position. Upper lobes (posterior apical segments). Patient is seated in his bed or chair leaning forward at 20 degree angle. Patient may rest his elbows on pillows or the bed table. (Never percuss directly over the spinal cord.)

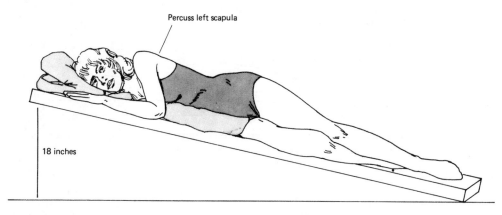

Percuss left scapula

18 inches

**FIG. 6-4.** Postural drainage position. Left upper lobe (posterior segments). The patient is positioned on his right side turned 45 degrees toward prone position with a pillow under head and along the spine. The head of the bed is elevated 18 inches.

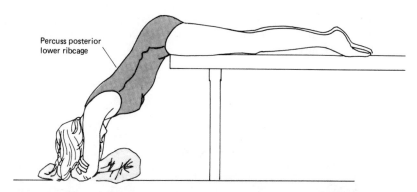

Percuss posterior
lower ribcage

**FIG. 6-5.** Postural drainage position. Lower lobes (posterior basal segments). Head down; hips at 60 degree angle off of bed or lying prone in bed with pillow under hips with thoracic cage at 45 degree angle. This can be done by elevating the foot of the bed by 18 inches.

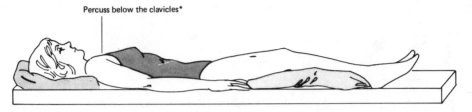

**FIG. 6-6.** Postural drainage position. Upper lobes (anterior segments). The patient is positioned supine with pillows placed under the head and knees.

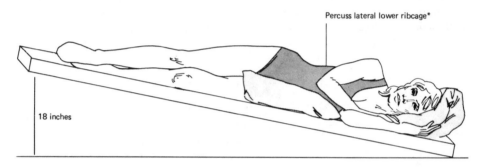

**FIG. 6-7.** Postural drainage position. Right lower lobes (lateral basal segments). The patient is positioned on the left side with pillows placed under waist and head. The foot of the bed is elevated 18 inches.

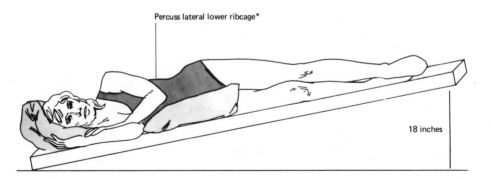

**FIG. 6-8.** Postural drainage position. Left lower lobe (lateral basal segments). The patient is positioned on right side with pillows placed under waist and head. The foot of the bed is elevated 18 inches.

132

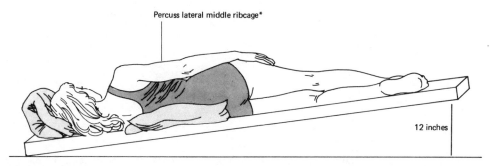

**FIG. 6-9.** Postural drainage position. Right middle lobe (medial and lateral segments). The patient is positioned on his left side turned 45 degrees toward the supine position with pillows* placed along spine and under head. (*Never percuss directly over the breast of women.)

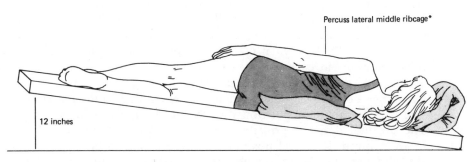

**FIG. 6-10.** Postural drainage position. Left upper lobe (superior and inferior segments—lingular area). The patient is positioned on his right side turned 45 degrees toward the supine position with pillows placed along the spine and under the head. The foot of the bed is elevated 12 inches.

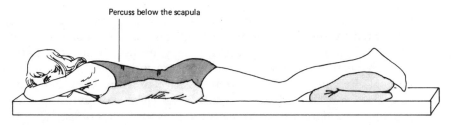

**FIG. 6-11.** Postural drainage position. Lower lobes (superior segments). The patient is positioned prone with pillows under the ankles and the waist.

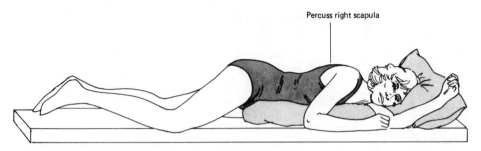

Percuss right scapula

**FIG. 6-12.** Postural drainage position. Right upper lobe (posterior segments). The patient is positioned on his left side turned 45 degrees toward the prone position with pillows placed under the head and along the spine.

## *THERAPEUTIC CONSIDERATIONS*

1. *Positioning.* Muscle relaxation must be obtained for the most effective delivery of postural drainage. The patient should be positioned to facilitate the maximum chest-wall expansion with his knees and arms gently flexed. Care must be taken to prevent pinching or twisting of the patient's arms or legs when placing him in a drainage position. Twenty to thirty minutes in each position should allow adequate time for passive drainage of pulmonary secretions. This drainage should be done at least two times a day and should be increased depending on the patient's needs. The patient should be positioned so that he is comfortable and supported. The postural drainage positions to be used are determined by the lung lobes involved. If several positions are necessary then the upper lobes that are affected should be drained first, working downward. Figure 6-13 illustrates the branching of the individual lung segments. Familiarity with this segmental anatomy is necessary for appropriate positioning of the patient to drain affected lung areas.

The patient may be placed in the appropriate postural drainage position by using an adjustable hospital bed, a tilt table, or a combination of blanket rolls and pillows to elevate the body into a position in which the lung is drained.

2. *Conditioning of the respiratory tract.* Postural drainage may be supplemented by the use of additional respiratory care modalities to improve secretion removal. Aerosol therapy may be used when the patient has thick, tenacious secretions to add moisture and reduce secretion viscosity. Aerosol therapy and intermittent positive pressure breathing treatments may also be used to deliver medication such as mucolytics, proteolytics, and bronchodilators to increase the removal of secretions. (see Chap. 4).

Secretions are removed from the lung more readily with appropriate hydration of the respiratory tract and the patient in general. To be most

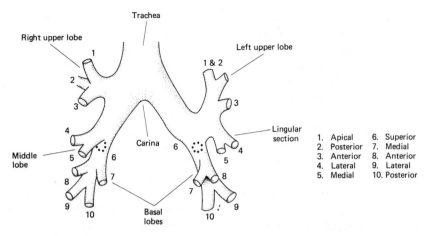

**FIG. 6-13.** Segmental branching of the lung. In the left lung the anterior-posterior segments (1,2) and the anterior-medial segments (8,7) are each combined with a common bronchus creating 8 segments in that lung.

effective, aerosol therapy or intermittent positive pressure breathing treatments should be done immediately prior to the postural drainage of the patient. Adequate fluid intake is mandatory to keep mucus thin. The patient's consumption of fluid should be the equivalent of at least 1½ l per day (approximately 1½ q).

3. *Breathing pattern.* While the patient is in a postural drainage position, he should be instructed to breathe appropriately. During inhalation the patient should breathe in through his nose, keeping his mouth closed and inhaling slow deep breaths. On exhalation, the patient should breathe out slowly through pursed lips. (Pursed-lip breathing will be described later in this chapter.) The patient should be encouraged to breathe at a slow, relaxed rate which should be monitored throughout the postural drainage procedure.

4. *Contraindications and modifications of postural drainage.* Postural drainage should never be done immediately following eating. The procedure should be administered at least one hour afterward. This is to prevent the patient from accidentally vomiting and to prevent nausea. Postural drainage also should not be administered just prior to a meal since the therapy may exhaust the patient, limiting his appetite and ability to eat immediately following therapy.

Stroke patients and post-operative craniotomy patients should not be positioned with their head down. Any position that requires the lowering of the patient's head below the horizontal axis of the body will produce an increase in intracranial pressure. This may be dangerous for the patient suffering from a head injury or intracranial injury since the maneuver will increase the cerebral pressure even more. Another consideration that may require modification of positions is that of the chronic obstructive lung-disease patient. The patient with chronic lung disease may become short of breath when placed in a position in which the head is lower than the horizontal axis of the body.

Modifications may also be necessary in postural drainage positions of patients on artificial mechanical ventilators or in traction. Others may include chest and abdominal surgery, pregnancy, gross obesity, and neuromuscular disease. If the patient requires postural drainage to promote the removal of secretions from the lung, adjustment should be made based upon his physical condition to place him in the most effective position possible that will not adversely affect his present condition. The length of time the patient stays in a particular position may also be changed so that the patient receives as much of the effect of that position as his physical condition can tolerate.

5. *Supplemental Oxygen.* If the patient is receiving oxygen, treatment should not be interrupted. The patient must be assured of the constant prescribed oxygen concentration at all times during the procedure. It also may be necessary to provide the patient with supplemental oxygen for use only during the therapy if dyspnea or shortness of breath occurs during the procedure. This is required more often with chronic lung disease patients and those with very low cardiopulmonary reserve.

6. *Coughing and/or mechanical aspiration of secretions.* Throughout the postural drainage procedure the patient should be encouraged to cough whenever he feels the need, or at least every five minutes during the therapy. This will improve the removal of secretions as they are drained from the lower respiratory tract. It will also limit the contamination of other areas of the lung with secretions from affected areas.

Preparation for postural drainage therapy should include instructing the patient in effective methods of coughing. If the patient is unable to cough, then the respiratory secretions should be mechanically aspirated. This may be necessary with very weak patients or those with an excessive amount of thick, tenacious secretions. Any time the patient begins uncontrolled coughing in a head-down position, he should be moved back into at least a horizontal position until he stops coughing. Coughing also causes an increase in intracranial pressure. Uncontrollable coughing can be very dangerous because of the excessive build-up of pressure.

7. *Monitoring postural drainage.* Throughout the procedure the patient's pulse should be monitored and the patient should be observed for increases in respiratory effort, anxiety, and diaphoresis. The secretions produced should be examined for color, texture, and amount. A change in pulse of more than 20 beats per minute or an excessive change in patient respiratory effort, anxiety, or diaphoresis may require that the postural drainage position be altered or discontinued.

# COUGHING

Coughing is the natural way to remove foreign substances from the lower respiratory tract. Development of a chronic respiratory disease may inhibit the patient's ability to cough. Respiratory infection can produce an excessive amount of mucus and the presence of mucus and infection may irritate the tracheobronchial tree, causing frequent involuntary coughing. This type of cough is normally very ineffective. For the most effective and efficient removal of secretions by coughing, it may be necessary to instruct the patient in proper coughing techniques.

The cough maneuver is a modification of the physiological Valsalva maneuver in which the diaphragm moves upward, compressing the inhaled gas volume against a closed glottis. In the normally healthy individual the amount of coughing necessary to clear the lower respiratory tract is limited; therefore, even when the normally healthy individual enters the hospital for a surgical procedure or nonrespiratory treatment, it may be necessary to instruct him in an appropriate method of coughing:

## THERAPEUTIC CONSIDERATIONS

1. *Position.* The patient should be placed in a position so that the arms and knees are slightly flexed and the abdominal muscles are also relaxed. The most effective position from which the patient can cough is the semi-Fowler's or sitting position. This is a comfortable position that facilitates maximal chest wall expansion.
2. *Coughing maneuver.* The act of coughing consists of three phases: inhalation, compression, and expulsion (See Fig. 6-14). The gas flows into

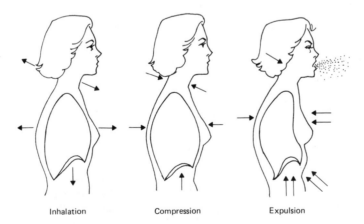

Inhalation      Compression      Expulsion

FIG. 6-14. Three stages of a cough.

the patient's lung as the diaphragm descends. After descent of the diaphragm, the glottis closes. Then the contraction of the accessory, abdominal, and thoracic muscles causes compression of air within the thoracic cavity against the closed glottis. Intra-pulmonary pressure rises, followed by a rapid opening of the glottis. The air is expelled with such force that foreign material from the tracheobronchial tree is ejected. Cough effectiveness is a combination of the inspired tidal volume and the velocity of the air flow.

The patient should be instructed to take slow, deep breaths, but not to breathe in as deeply as possible. The patient should be instructed to inhale until his lungs feel as if they are half-full of air. Then the patient should be instructed to hold his breath and compress his abdominal muscles. This may be easier for the patient if the therapist or the patient uses his hand as a reference point on the abdomen. As the abdomen is contracted, the glottis is rapidly opened and the gas expelled, creating the cough. The patient also should be instructed to cough only two or three short coughs, using a short, concise effort, and not coughing out as hard as possible.

3. *Splinting*. When coughing, the patient or the respiratory therapist should stabilize any abdominal or chest incision that may produce pain during the cough process. This allows the cough effort to be as effective and forceful as possible. Figures 6-15 and 6-16 illustrate how a pillow may be used or how the arms of a patient may be crossed across the chest wall to splint and stabilize the incised area. It may be necessary for the

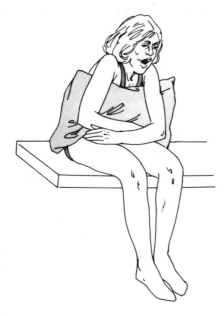

FIG. 6-15. Splinting with a pillow. Use of a pillow by a patient in a sitting position to stabilize (splint) a thoracic or abdominal wound and create a more forceful cough.

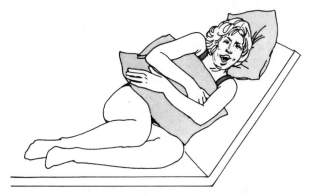

**FIG. 6-16.** Modified pillow splinting. If the patient cannot sit up in bed or in a chair the wound may still be splinted with the pillow with the patient in a modified elevated position to aid the production of a more forceful cough.

patient to receive pain medication to reduce splinting during coughing exercises.

4. *Humidification.* Humidification of the respiratory tract with humidity or aerosol therapy can be used to enhance the productivity of the cough.

**TABLE 6-1**

**Pulmonary Secretions**

| *Secretions* | *Characteristics* |
|---|---|
| Respiratory mucus | Thin, transparent; 95% water; normal respiratory secretion from goblet cells |
| Mucoid sputum | Sticky, translucent, very viscous, may be white or gray; difficult to expectorate; produced with bronchitis and pneumonia |
| Purulent sputum | Thick, opaque; reduced viscosity; more easily expectorated; yellow, offensive odor; green color, offensive odor is indication of infection; produced with bronchiectasis and lung abcess. |
| Mucopurulent sputum | Combination of the mucoid and purulent sputum commonly seen in disease process with the development of bacterial infection. |
| Pink, frothy sputum | Thin, water, foamy, pink; indicates pulmonary edema. |
| Hemoptysis | Frank bleeding, initially bright red, darkens and diminishes in few days; i.e., tuberculosis, bronchogenic carcinoma, bronchiectasis, pulmonary infarction |

5. *Suctioning.* If the patient cannot effectively cough, then oral or nasal tracheal suctioning must be performed to remove increased respiratory secretions from the lung.

6. *Evaluation.* The secretions should be evaluated and a notation made in the chart as to the color, consistency, and amount of secretions removed from the patient's respiratory tract. Changes in pulmonary secretions can be used to evaluate the progress of the patient's respiratory disease (see Table 6-1).

## PERCUSSION AND VIBRATION

*Percussion* is used after the patient has been placed in the desired postural drainage position. The hands are placed in a cupped position with the fingers and thumbs closed (see Fig. 6-17). Contact with the chest wall is only made with the heel and the corner of the fingers, simultaneously allowing the wrists and elbows to relax. Percussion is delivered at a consistent rate over three to five minutes on the affected area. Manual percussion is done by using the hands at a rate of at least 200 percussions per minute. These are delivered at a steady rhythmic rate. Percussion appears to create an increased vibration of the thoracic cage and lung, mechanically dislodging secretions from the bronchial walls. This increases mobility of secretions into the larger airways from which they may be expelled by coughing or mechanical aspiration.

*Vibration* is applied over the chest wall of the involved lung area during the exhalation phase. It is delivered to the patient by placing the hand on the chest wall with the elbows locked and rigidly vibrating the hands, causing a vibration to be felt through the thoracic boney structure and into the lungs. Vibration appears to increase the velocity of the expired tidal volume from the small airways of the lung and therefore loosens secretions.

### THERAPEUTIC CONSIDERATIONS

1. During the delivery of chest percussion and vibration, the chest wall area may be covered with a towel or hospital gown to prevent direct contact with the patient's skin, which can lead to irritation and redness.

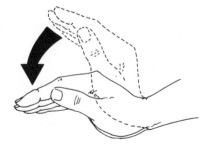

FIG. 6-17. Chest percussing. Illustrates the cupped position of the hands during percussion and the movement of the wrist with percussing of the chest wall as the hand contacts it.

2. Percussion and vibration should not be delivered over areas of incision, female mammary tissue, or any internal organs such as the kidneys, stomach, heart, liver, or spinal cord.

3. Percussion and vibration are contraindicated if the patient has acute chest pain, an acute cardiac condition, hemorrhage, or an acute inflammatory process that may spread to other areas of the pulmonary system.

4. Electrically driven mechanical devices have been developed to deliver vibration and percussion. Such equipment must be appropriately adjusted and adequately padded to prevent injury to the patient. The use of percussion and vibration equipment eliminates much of the physical strain of the procedure for the respiratory care personnel. Effective use of the equipment is at least equally as good as manual delivery of percussion and vibration. One drawback is an increased noise level. Use of such equipment depends on the user's knowledge and training and the psychological acceptance of the patient.

# DEEP BREATHING

Deep breathing promotes maximum alveolar inflation, helps to maintain normal functional lung capacity, and prevents atelectasis. Deep-breathing techniques sometimes use incentive devices to provide a stimulus for the patient and to provide a mandatory regime of breathing exercises. Incentive spirometry is included later in the chapter.

Post-operative patients often require deep-breathing exercises. Their pattern of breathing following surgery becomes shallow and monotonous tidal breathing. Post-operative pain and drug administration can also depress normal spontaneous deep breathing that usually occurs every four to five minutes in the normal healthy individual. If not restored within a few hours, atelectasis will form within the lung. Inhalation anesthesia given with general surgery reduces deep breathing post-operatively, as does restriction of movement with traction, bandages, or casts. Patients over 60 years of age or those that are weak and debilitated from body trauma or infection are especially affected by these limiting factors.

Specific respiratory therapy techniques and equipment are used to encourage deep breathing and promote ventilation of affected lung areas.

## DIAPHRAGMATIC BREATHING

Diaphragmatic breathing increases the downward excursion of the diaphragm and expansion of the lower costal areas of the thoracic cage. This increases ventilation of the lower lobes of the lungs by re-expanding alveoli and preventing the abnormal closure of alveoli, and assists in the removal of secretions by preventing pooling within collapsed alveoli.

The following is a procedure for diaphragmatic breathing:

1. *Instructions.* The patient should be instructed in the goals of the therapy and in the emphasis of effective ventilation using diaphragmatic breathing maneuvers. The patient's understanding of the specific exercise and the sequence of the maneuvers is important for the success of the exercise.

2. *Position.* The patient should be positioned so that his back and head are fully supported and his abdomen relaxed. If he is in bed, the patient should be sat up as high as possible in a semi-Fowler's position with his knees slightly bent, or if he is out of bed, the patient should be placed in an armless high-back chair (see Figs. 6-18 and 6-19).

3. *Movement.* The respiratory therapist or nurse should initially place his or her hands upon the anterior costal margin of the thoracic cage to stimulate and palpate the movement of the diaphragm (see Fig. 6-20). After the appropriate movement is checked, the patient may be instructed to feel the movement of the thoracic wall and diaphragm for himself.

4. *Inhalation.* The patient should be instructed to inhale slowly and to feel the lower costal area expanding as the air fills his lungs. The upper chest and shoulders should remain relaxed throughout the exercise. Emphasis for the patient should be placed on slow gradual filling of the lungs, using a minimum amount of effort.

5. *Common faults.* The patient should be observed and corrected if any of the following errors are made while breathing diaphragmatically:

   a) The patient should never exhale forcibly. During normal exhalation the airway shortens and becomes narrower. Therefore, a forced exhalation will cause the airway to narrow more rapidly and this may cause the airway collapse, leading to air being trapped in the lungs.

   b) Exhalation should also not be prolonged. The patient should be encouraged to breathe slowly with an even respiratory pattern. Care should be taken to observe the patient's use of his abdominal

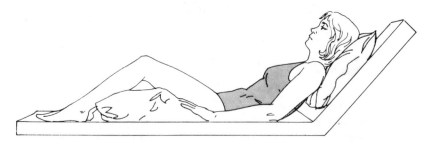

FIG. 6-18. Semi-Fowler's position for maximal diaphragmatic movement.

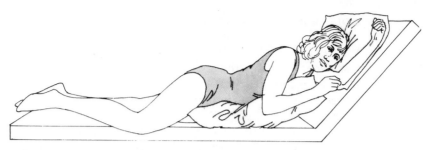

**FIG. 6-19.** Modified semi-Fowler's position. Illustrates a modification that allows effective diaphragmatic breathing.

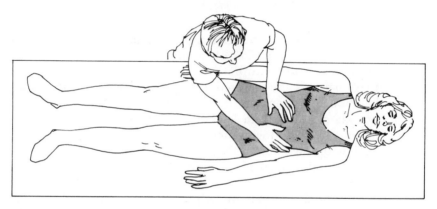

**FIG. 6-20.** Diaphragmatic breathing. Palpation of diaphragmatic movement by the therapist using the hands on the patient's thoracic cage.

musculature so that the patient is not allowed to move the abdominal muscles in and out without appropriately ventilating the lung. Observation also should be done to encourage the patient not to use accessory muscles in the upper chest wall and chest in an attempt to breathe deeply. Use of these accessory muscles inhibits downward movement of the diaphragm and limits the effectiveness of the diaphragmatic breathing exercises.

**6.** Diaphragmatic breathing should be used during all chest physical therapy exercises.

## SEGMENTAL BREATHING

By using the hands as a reference point for the patient to make him aware of the expansion of the chest wall, specific segments can be ventilated more readily. Placing the patient or therapist's hand over the affected area of the lung and asking the patient to breathe in slowly, while feeling the expansion and the pushing away of the hand from the affected area will increase the patient's awareness of lung expansion in that area and increase ventilation of the area. These localized breathing maneuvers assist in the expansion of specific affected areas of the lung. The hand of the therapist or the patient is placed on the affected area during each inspiratory phase. Following each inhalation, the patient should be encouraged to hold the breath for one to two seconds. This helps increase the distribution of gas within the lung and the affected area. The hands may be used individually over the basal, lateral, or apical sections to increase lung expansion.

### PURSED-LIP BREATHING

The purpose of this breathing technique is to prevent early airway collapse and the trapping of air during exhalation. Pursed-lip breathing is used most often with patients having chronic obstructive lung disease. In these patients the diseased airways tend to frequently collapse during exhalation and trap air in the alveoli. By creating a resistance with the pursing of the lips, air is allowed to be exhaled more slowly. Airway collapse is prevented with increased airway pressures created by retarding the airflow through pursed lips.

The following is a procedure for pursed-lip breathing:

1. *Position.* The patient is placed in a semi-Fowler's position with the abdominal muscles relaxed.
2. *Exhalation.* The patient is instructed to exhale through his mouth with his lips in a position similar to that of whistling or kissing. By shaping the lips into a whistling position, the patient can exhale through the mouth with his lips pursed. He can be instructed to whistle to make him aware of the appropriate position necessary, or to pretend your finger is a candle and to blow it out.

This will increase the length of exhalation so that exhalation is about twice as long as inhalation. Pursed-lip breathing should be encouraged with all patients that may be suspected of air trapping.

## INCENTIVE SPIROMETRY

Incentive spirometry is used as a goal-oriented inspiratory maneuver to encourage the patient to take slow, deep breaths. Incentive spirometry encourages deep breathing by using an incentive device such as a light or a ball rising in a tube to promote a maximum patient effort in achieving a slow, gradual, deep breath followed by a two to three second pause at end inhalation. Incentive spirometry devices are prescribed to encourage the patient to participate in intermittent deep breathing maneuvers. They also assure that the deep-breathing maneuver is of the appropriate depth and can be repeated by setting a prescribed volume of gas for the patient to inhale. The inspiratory maneuver is used to rehabilitate the patient until he can once again achieve his predicted inspiratory reserve volume or tested pre-operative volume. Incentive spirometry devices are prescribed by the physician with the following data:

> Type of equipment
> Number of maneuvers per hour
> Prescribed incentive reserve volume
> Number of days of therapy
> Physician prescribing therapy

The following is a procedure for using incentive spirometry devices:

1. *Respiratory evaluation and instruction.* In post-surgical patients the most effective procedure is to instruct the patient *prior* to surgery. This will allow the patient to become familiar with the device and allow evaluation of his inspiratory reserve volume when he is not in pain or is not restricted by binding dressings or other support equipment. The patient is instructed in the number of times per hour and/or per day that the incentive spirometry device is prescribed. The patient may also require instruction in appropriate diaphragmatic breathing and coughing techniques.

2. *Exhalation and Inhalation.* The patient is instructed to exhale slowly and completely. At the end of the quiet exhalation, the patient is instructed to inhale through the incentive device, taking a slow, deep inhalation.

3. *End inspiratory hold.* Following maximum inhalation, the patient is instructed to hold the deep breath for at least 3 seconds. This provides increased gas distribution in the lungs comparable to that of a deep yawn or sigh. This will also maintain the peak inspiratory position and create the maximum inspiratory pressures which will assist alveolar expansion and reopening collapsed alveoli.

4. *Incentive spirometry.* Following the end inspiratory hold, the patient should exhale normally. Between breaths the patient should relax and breathe normally. Incentive spirometry should be limited to four to five breaths per minute to prevent hyperventilation.

5. *Evaluation.* The patient's respiratory effort and inspiratory reserve volume should be evaluated at least once per shift. The patient's inspiratory reserve volume should be monitored with the incentive spirometry device and recorded. As the patient's effort and inspiratory reserve volume increases, the incentive spirometry equipment should be adjusted as neces-

sary. The patient should also be reinstructed in the use of the incentive device as necessary.

## THERAPEUTIC CONSIDERATIONS

1. Incentive spirometry devices are generally designed to provide an inspiratory reserve volume of between 500 and 2500 ml. The most effective method of determining the patient's inspiratory reserve volume is to measure it prior to any therapeutic or surgical procedure that the patient is to receive. The inspiratory reserve volume on the incentive spirometry device should be set at the maximum volume the patient can inhale and maintain for at least three seconds.

2. The inspiratory maneuver used with incentive spirometry devices is a normal inspiration that increases the movement of air into the lungs and increases the maximum inspiratory pressure within the patient's thoracic cavity. This can enhance alveolar expansion and venous blood return to the heart. Encouraging the patient to take slow, deep inhalations promotes a normal respiratory pattern. Using the incentive spirometry devices, this maneuver can be repeated and may be performed by the patient without direct assistance. In this manner the patient is encouraged to participate in his own therapy, and with the use of a goal-oriented device, the patient can observe his improvement.

3. Different incentive spirometry devices are designed with indicators for the approximate volume or flow the patient is attaining and an indicator to be observed for successful accomplishment of the set volume or flow. Some devices include a light, an illuminated panel, a float, or a ball moving up a tube to "reward" the patient. Figure 6-21 represents a drum-

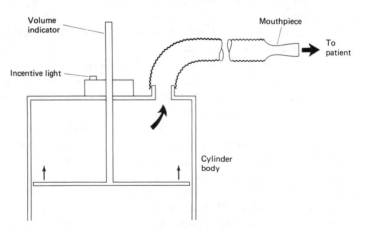

FIG. 6-21. Incentive spirometry device. This type design represents a drum type, volume measuring design.

type incentive spirometry device that measures volume. Some incentive spirometry devices have adjustable inspiratory reserve volumes that may be increased as the patient improves. Other devices are self-adjusting by using a combination of tubes containing balls that rise in tubes as a specific amount of gas in inhaled. These tube devices actually measure flow. It is recommended that volume-oriented devices be used to insure adequate lung expansion. Some devices can be combined with aerosol therapy to encourage hyperinflation of the lung and delivery of aerosol at the same time.

4. All incentive spirometry equipment that comes in direct contact with the exhaled tidal volume of the patient should be periodically sterilized or disposed of. This should be done at least every 48 hours. All other equipment that does not have contact with the patient should be kept dust-free and in accurate calibration.

## INTERMITTENT POSITIVE-PRESSURE BREATHING

Intermittent positive-pressure breathing (IPPB) therapy is a therapeutic modality that uses pressure higher than atmospheric to produce a flow of gas into the lungs during inhalation. This pressure is intermittently applied just as with positive pressure mechanical ventilation equipment. IPPB is prescribed in clinical situations requiring the patient to receive increased hydration, to receive aerosol medications and to hyperinflate the lung, and/or to decrease the work of breathing. A prescription for IPPB therapy or intermittent aerosol therapy without positive pressure should include the following:

> Type of Treatment
> Duration and Frequency of Therapy
> Type and Amount of Medication to be Delivered
> Oxygen concentration
> Physician's Signature

The IPPB prescription ideally would also include a preset pressure and tidal volume.

### GOALS OF IPPB THERAPY

1. To hyperinflate the tracheal/bronchial tree. Positive pressure breathing is used to encourage hyperinflation of the lung by using a preset positive pressure limit that must be met to cycle the pressure-cycled equipment to exhalation. Delivery of gas into the lungs at controlled levels of flow and volume is used to increase the patient's depth of ventilation and to im-

prove airway distribution of the inspired gas. The positive pressure level actually can work as an incentive to achieving the proper prescribed gas volume. By hyperinflating the tracheal/bronchial tree, the occurrence of post-operative atelectasis is reduced and re-expansion of areas of atelectasis is promoted.

Positive pressure breathing also may decrease the work of breathing of the patient similar to that of positive pressure mechanical ventilation, but the relief from the work of breathing would only be temporary and may only occur during the time that the IPPB treatments are being applied.
2. To improve delivery of medications into the lung. Nebulizers are incorporated in IPPB equipment to deliver aerosol medications to the patient's respiratory tract. The controlled flow and increased distribution of ventilation within the lung during effective IPPB therapy can enhance the delivery of aerosol medications into the lungs. In disease processes and post-operative conditions in which the patient is unable to breathe deeply or resists breathing deeply and so requires an incentive, intermittent positive pressure breathing may be indicated to allow more effective distribution of medications delivered as aerosols in the lungs.

In patients not needing assistance in decreasing the work of breathing or improving the depth and distribution of ventilation within the lung, intermittent aerosol therapy without pressure is adequate to deliver medication. IPPB should never be given just for the sake of delivering medication to the lung.

## IPPB TREATMENT PROCEDURE

1. *Instruction.* The procedure to be followed with intermittent positive-pressure breathing therapy should be fully explained to the patient. Emphasis should be placed on the fact that the patient's cooperation is necessary for the most effective therapy to be delivered. Proper explanation of the procedure will better assure such cooperation. During the explanation of the goals of therapy and how the patient may best receive an effective treatment, all equipment to be used should be left in the hallway or at the nurses's station. By first explaining the procedure to the patient before orienting him to the equipment, you can reduce the patient's anxiety about the procedure.
2. *Position.* The patient should be placed in a comfortable sitting or semi-Fowler's position. This position will allow the greatest diaphragmatic excursion, the maximum amount of chest expansion, and effective thoracic movement to allow coughing.
3. *Breathing pattern.* The patient should be encouraged to use diaphragmatic breathing during the treatment. The therapist's hands may be placed on the thoracic cage, as described earlier in diaphragmatic breathing, to encourage expansion of the thoracic cage and the full excursion of the diaphragm with each breath. Segmental breathing exercises may be used

to emphasize expansion of the affected areas. The patient should be instructed to breathe only through his mouth. By breathing through his mouth and not through his nose, less aerosol particles will be filtered out and therefore a greater number of aerosol particles will be delivered to the lower respiratory tract. It is also necessary to emphasize that the mouth must be completely sealed around the mouthpiece and no breathing must take place through the nose to allow the pressure cycled machine to reach the preset pressure and cycle to an off position. If there is a leak in the system, the preset pressure will not be met and the machine will not cycle off.

At the end of inspiration, the patient should be instructed to pause for two to three seconds to allow maximum gas distribution and aerosol deposition. This also will prevent the patient from cycling the equipment off by blowing back into the mouthpiece.

4. *Equipment adjustment.* When setting the equipment controls, the pressure limit should be set at a point at which the desired volume is delivered. With the cooperative, well instructed patient, this pressure limit will usually be between 10-15 cm of water pressure.

The *exhaled tidal volume* of the patient can be measured using a collecting bag or spirometry monitor to provide the prescribed tidal volume. The minimum volume to be prescribed can be estimated by using the following formula:

$$\text{prescribed volume} = 3\text{-}4 \text{ ml} \times \text{ideal body weight (lb)}$$

or

$$\text{prescribed volume} = 10 \text{ ml} \times \text{weight (kg)}$$

The *rate control* is not set during IPPB treatments. The patient triggers the machine to cycle "on" by creating a negative pressure within the mouthpiece. Therefore, the patient determines the respiratory rate. Since the patient is being encouraged to take full deep breaths at volumes of gas near his inspiratory capacity, his respiratory rate should be reduced to maintain a normal minute ventilation. The respiratory rate should be between eight to fifteen breaths per minute, depending on the physical condition of the patient. This must be encouraged to prevent hyperventilation.

The *flowrate control* on the IPPB equipment should be set at the minimum amount of flow necessary for the desired volume of gas. The flow setting should allow a slow, gradual inflation of the lung, providing the maximum amount of distribution of ventilation.

The *sensitivity* of the IPPB equipment should be adjusted if necessary so that the patient only has to create a negative pressure of 1-2 cm of water pressure to initiate the cycling "on" of the equipment.

5. *Medication.* Medication should be added to the nebulizer of the IPPB equipment in the prescribed dosage. The total amounts of medication received by the patient will depend on the stability of the aerosol and

the particle sizes and density delivered by the specific nebulizer. Ultrasonic nebulizers can be attached in line with IPPB equipment to provide a higher concentration of particulate water for humidification in the gas inhaled. This will better assure adequate hydration throughout the therapy and increase the level of moisture within the respiratory tract, aiding in the reduction of secretion viscosity and its removal. IPPB treatments should never be administered without a prescribed medication.

6. *Evaluation of the therapy.* During the IPPB treatment or aerosol therapy, the patient's exhaled volume should be measured to determine whether the prescribed gas volume is being delivered and to evaluate the effectiveness of this method of encouraging hyperinflation.

Pulse should be monitored with all IPPB treatment at least prior to and at the end of therapy. During the delivery of a bronchodilator, the pulse should be monitored at least three times; initially, during the therapy, and at the end. Also the blood pressure should be taken at least before and after the initial therapy to determine the patient's reaction to that particular dosage of bronchodilator, and whenever there is a pulse rate change of greater than 20 beats per minute. Bronchodilators may produce precordial distress, palpations, dizziness, nausea, and excessive perspiration, and therefore, may require close monitoring with therapy. The respiratory rate should also be counted. The respiratory rate should decrease while the patient is receiving the IPPB therapy because of the increased gas volumes with deep breathing.

Throughout the therapy the amount and characteristics of the secretions expectorated by the patient should be monitored to evaluate the effectiveness of the hydration being used with the IPPB therapy. Chest sounds also should be auscultated before and after therapy to evaluate improvements. (See Chest Physical Examination Chapter.) The patient's peak flowrate should be measured periodically with patient's receiving bronchodilator therapy to determine bronchodilator effect.

The preset pressure during the therapy and the negative pressure created by the patient during cycling of the machine also should be observed to assure the proper functioning of the equipment. The failure of the pressure-cycled equipment to cycle off can be caused by a leak in the equipment assembly or leakage from the patient's mouth or nose. There is also the possibility of an internal leak within a damaged part of the IPPB equipment, which would require replacement before therapy could be continued.

## CONSIDERATIONS OF IPPB THERAPY

1. *Delivery.* To deliver effective IPPB therapy requires a combination of a knowledgeable therapist who is skilled at proper evaluation of the therapy and the therapeutic goals, and the appropriately instructed,

cooperative patient who is aware of the breathing pattern that is necessary and who is instructed in the effective coughing techniques.

2. *Therapy.* IPPB therapy should never be used unless clinically indicated. Intermittent ultrasonic or hydronamic nebulization can be used for hydration and hand-held pneumatically-driven nebulizers for medications. Positive pressure is not necessary for those specific tasks. Positive-pressure breathing techniques may be used to encourage hyperinflation of the lungs in patients with inadequate muscle tone or integrity caused by poor physical condition or anesthetic, and who require assistance to inhale increased tidal volumes.

3. *Charting.* When charting IPPB or intermittent aerosol therapy, date, time, the type of therapy, equipment used, medication delivered, cycling pressure, duration of therapy, pulse, respiratory rate, exhaled volume or peak flow as indicated, characteristics of secretion and cough, and adverse or unusual reactions of the patient should be listed to provide a record of therapy.

4. *Contraindications of IPPB.* The major contraindication of IPPB is an uncorrected pneumothorax and/or massive hemoptysis. The delivery of positive-pressure breathing therapy to a patient with an uncorrected pneumothorax could force more air into the pleural cavity, compromising the patient's already limited pulmonary capacity and reducing the integrity of the cardiovascular system. Once chest tubes have been in place in the thoracic cavity to reduce the air in the pleura, then IPPB can be used in re-expanding any atelectic area caused by the pneumothorax compressing the lung tissue.

For patients with massive hemoptysis, positive pressure may force gas into arterial circulation creating air emboli, or further tear lacerated lung tissue. Treatment should be stopped immediately if fresh bleeding occurs.

Some physicians prefer that the patient who has received a lobectomy or pneumonectomy should not be given positive pressure-breathing therapy because of the potential of creating an air leak around the surgical stump prior to its healing. Also, patients undergoing needle biopsy should be closely observed and the use of positive pressure limited for at least 24 hours following the biopsy in case of a slight puncture of the lung tissue during the biopsy increasing the opportunity for pneumothorax.

In patients with active tuberculosis, the use of IPPB therapy should be limited because of the potential possibility of spreading the tuberculosis to other areas of the lung. Patients suffering from coronary angina should be closely monitored because of the possibility that the positive pressure could create a cardiac tamponade effect on the coronary circulation of the heart, leading to an increased incidence of angina.

5. *Hazards.* All of the hazards described in the chapter on mechanical ventilation are potential hazards of IPPB therapy. Although it is an intermittent therapy lasting 15–20 minutes and not a continuous therapy which reduces the overall long-term effects of positive pressure, it does

not reduce the potential of their occurring during intermittent therapy. These hazards include gastric inflation, pneumothorax, alkalosis, elimination of hypoxic drive in chronic lung patients, and an increased work of the heart caused by impeding venous return. Gastric inflations, pneumothorax, and the impeding of venous return are all described under the positive pressure effects in the intensive respiratory care chapter.

6. *Administering IPPB.* Therapy delivered by pressure-cycled equipment requires a closed system to provide the back pressure necessary to cycle the equipment off. The majority of patients receiving IPPB and intermittent aerosol therapy will be able to use a mouthpiece, following the proper instruction. It may be necessary to use noseclips even on cooperative, well instructed patients to prevent unconscious breathing through the nose. A phalange also may be attached to the mouthpiece of the patient's delivery circuit to create a seal around the edges of the mouth if the patient is unable to seal his mouth around the mouthpiece adequately (see Fig. 6-22).

Patients that are not alert or aware enough to use the mouthpiece may need to have therapy administered using a mask. The simple mask is designed to fit over the nose and mouth and must be held by the therapist to create a seal on the face. The mask should never be attached to the patient's face and left unattended. A clear mask is recommended to observe any secretions accumulating in the mask during the therapy and to prevent accidental aspiration of unwanted secretions into the respiratory tract during the positive-pressure inspiratory cycle.

When delivering intermittent positive-pressure therapy with a mask or by attaching the delivery system into an endotracheal or tracheostomy tube, it may be necessary to increase the flowrate of the gas delivered to the patient to compensate for minor leaks within the system around the mask or artificial airway. Delivery of IPPB therapy to patients with tracheostomy and endotracheal tubes requires that the cuff of the tube be inflated during the therapy.

7. *Delivered oxygen concentration.* IPPB equipment is usually pneumatically driven. Ideally, compressed air should be used to power IPPB equipment unless the delivery of oxygen is prescribed by the physician. The limited number of piped-in air systems within hospitals have led many facilities to the delivery of therapy with 100% oxygen. IPPB equipment is set on an air dilution, which means that the IPPB equipment is driven by 100 percent $O_2$ source gas and that this gas is diluted with room air prior to delivery to the patient. The setting of air dilution on IPPB equipment will deliver an oxygen concentration of greater than 40 percent $O_2$ to the patient during the therapy. This may be hazardous to chronic pulmonary disease patients and must be closely monitored.

Compressed air may be provided by a cylinder source or an electrically driven compressor. This will provide a delivery gas of 21 percent $O_2$. The

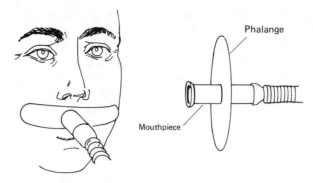

**FIG. 6-22.** Mouth seal phalange.

oxygen concentration must be analyzed using an oxygen analyzer to determine exactly how much oxygen the patient is receiving if more than air source gas is used. IPPB equipment delivering therapy to chronic obstructive lung disease patients with a hypoxic drive should never be powered with any greater than 21 percent $O_2$ unless specifically prescribed. The potential danger is that the increased oxygen concentration may eliminate the patient's hypoxic drive and produce apnea.

8. *Functioning.* The proper function of IPPB equipment requires that the equipment be calibrated at least quarterly to maintain an accurate flow control, pressure reading, sensitivity and pressure setting control. All permanent filters and removable valves should be cleaned at least quarterly or whenever the valve begins to stick. The gas going from the equipment to the patient should be filtered. Medical gas filters today can filter particle sizes down to 2-3 $\mu$. These in line filters should be changed as noted by the manufacturer.

The breathing assembly from the IPPB equipment to the patient should be sterilized at least every 24 hours. Disposable and nondisposable patient delivery circuits are available. The disposable patient delivery circuit eliminates the disassembly and assembly and resterilization of nondisposable circuits. Many departments have found them convenient and economical, depending on the number of therapies they deliver. The same patient delivery circuit should never be used by more than one patient. IPPB equipment is moved from patient to patient but the patient delivery system should be changed between each patient and a patient given a new system at least every 24 hours.

9. *Hyperinflation.* Hyperinflation of the lungs may be done in conjunction with postural drainage and percussion of the patient. By combining the aerosol therapy with the postural drainage and percussion, the patient receives the prescribed medication at the time that the secretions are being mobilized by the postural drainage. This may be effective in selective

patients to increase the amount of secretions removed with the combined therapy. Hyperinflation of the lungs may also be accomplished by manual ventilation with a resuscitating bag via mask or, endotracheal or tracheostomy tube. Any patient receiving continuous supplemental oxygen should have oxygen delivered to him while he is receiving IPPB or intermittent aerosol therapy. The oxygen concentration should be maintained at the prescribed concentration during the therapy.

## RESPIRATORY EXERCISES

Respiratory exericses are used to gradually develop body musculature, returning it to normal or improving it as much as possible to provide more effective pulmonary ventilation for the patient. Post-operative patients, patients receiving long-term continuous mechanical ventilation, and chronic obstructive lung disease patients often require retraining of respiratory musculature to provide effective ventilation and exercise tolerance necessary for daily living. Graded exercise will develop skeletal, heat, and cardiorespiratory muscles. Progressive exercise causes muscle fibers to become more efficient, requiring less oxygen for the same amount of work.

### ABDOMINAL MUSCLES

Strengthening of the abdominal muscles regains their capacity to relax and increases their elasticity, which will aid in effective coughing and diaphragmatic breathing. The abdominal muscles are improved by gradual active exercise. The following are three exercises to strengthen the abdominal muscles.

Abdominal Breathing

1.  The patient lays on his back with his knees flexed and his feet flat on the floor. A pillow is placed under his head (see Fig. 6-23).
2.  The exercise is begun by exhaling from the resting level through pursed lips. At the same time the patient is instructed to pull in his upper abdomen gradually with a conscious force, slowly exhaling, prolonging it as much as possible.
3.  The patient's hand is placed upon his abdomen, or some type of weight such as a book or a sandbag is placed there, to act as a reference to make him aware of the movement of the abdomen.
4.  At end exhalation he is told to inhale slowly through his nose, letting his upper abdomen balloon out. This is an active pushing out of the abdomen, pulling the diaphragm down and increasing its excursion.
5.  The patient should breathe in through the nose and out slowly through

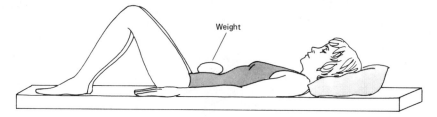

**FIG. 6-23.** Exercise position for abdominal breathing.

pursed lips. Near the end of each normal exhalation the patient should forcibly contract the abdominal musculature extending exhalation to the maximum. Then he should repeat Steps 2 through 5.

## Situps

1. The patient again lays on his back with his knees flexed and his feet flat on the floor, and a pillow is placed under his head.
2. His hands are placed behind his head, and on exhalation through pursed lips, he contracts his abdominal muscles, pulling himself to a semi-sitting position by raising his head and shoulders as far as he can.
3. This exercise is done with the patient breathing in through his nose and out through pursed lips. Each time he raises his head and shoulders, he should return to the initial starting position and repeat the exercise.

## Leg Lifts and Knee Bends

1. Assume position described under abdominal breathing.
2. While exhaling bring the left or right knee up to the left or right shoulders respectively, lifting the leg off the floor and flexing the knee toward the chin.
3. If this exercise is done on the floor, press the small of the back against the floor while raising the knee toward the chin. Raise the knee and the leg as high as possible, using a slow, gradual, lifting motion (see Fig. 6-24).
4. Lift each leg separately; alternating legs. Following the bending of the knee and lifting of the leg to this position, return to the initial starting position and relax. Repeat this for the right side and continue to alternate legs.

## COORDINATED WALKING

Walking is an essential part of a patient's exercise program. The development of walking techniques is also a gradual process. Walking itself stimulates deep breathing and increases ventilation, increasing venous blood return to the heart.

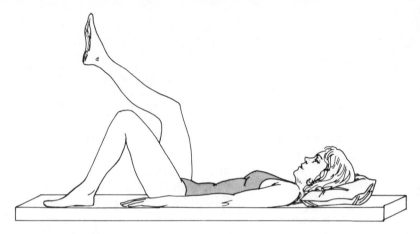

FIG. 6-24. Leg lift and knee bend exercise.

Walking requires a controlled breathing pattern and the use of proper techniques. The patient must be encouraged to use his arms to maintain his balance. Initially this may require special awareness for some patients and a permanent effort for many others.

1.  The patient should be first allowed to stand near the edge of his bed to gain his balance and the stability of standing.
2.  Once the patient is standing and balanced, then the procedure can continue. It may be necessary for the therapist or nurse to stabilize the patient by placing his hand on the shoulders of the patient to reinforce his presence.
3.  The patient is instructed to use abdominal breathing techniques while standing in place and walking. The use of abdominal breathing techniques should be practiced until the patient can complete the task while standing. The patient should also be instructed to breathe through his nose and exhale slowly through pursed lips while standing and walking.
4.  Initially the patient should walk on a flat surface and should be instructed to breathe in slowly and deeply while standing, then upon exhaling through pursed lips the patient should take two to three steps. This is followed by standing during inhalation and a repeat of two to three more steps. This exercise should be gradually increased until the patient can coordinate inhalation in the standing position, taking two to three steps during exhalation through pursed lips, and repeating this task by walking under supervision and then by himself.
5.  Walking up inclines or stairs should be practiced following appropriate coordinated walking techniques on horizontal surfaces. The patient is instructed to use the same abdominal breathing pattern when climbing stairs.

6. The patient standing at the foot of the stairs should take a slow deep breath in and on slow exhalation through pursed lips, walk up one or two steps, as tolerated. At end exhalation the patient should stop and inhale again through the nose.

7. Coordinated abdominal breathing should be continued with inhalation during standing and stepping during the exhalation.

8. As the patient develops a rhythmic pattern of abdominal breathing and movement during exhalation, the amount of time he must stop to breathe will be reduced.

## CONSIDERATIONS OF RESPIRATORY EXERCISES

1. All exercise maneuvers requiring patient effort should be performed during exhalation. This is a normal physiologic maneuver to stabilize the upper trunk of the body and is a basic step to accomplishing exercise and daily living tasks. The patient must be well-instructed and continually encouraged to complete the exercises and the exhalation maneuver when performing tasks. The patient is to take a deep breath and exhale through pursed lips while completing all tasks. Continual practice of this maneuver will create the desired habit.

2. During all exercise the patient should breathe in through his nose and exhale through pursed lips. Respiratory therapy should be used prior to the practice of all exercises, as needed to provide the maximum potential for effective ventilation and oxygenation.

3. Exercises that are performed while laying down may require modification if the patient is confined to the hospital bed. Exercises such as sit ups should be done on a hard surface. They may require that the positions be modified for the patient. The use of the exercises in modified positions is effective and should be used as necessary.

4. If the patient has pain caused by surgical wounds or broken or fractured bones and pain medication is prescribed, then the pain medication should be given at least 15–30 minutes before exercise practice is initiated, so that the patient can participate more actively in the exercises. If the patient is on a continuous oxygen concentration, then it should be used during all exercises. Oxygen also may be required for the patient during the exercises even though he may not be on continuous oxygen. The exercises will increase the consumption of oxygen initially and will require greater patient effort. This should be a consideration of the physician prescribing exercise techniques for the patient.

5. A record of changes showing progression or regression of the patient's exercise tolerance should be kept daily. Realistic goals should be prescribed to provide the patient with positive reinforcement for accomplishing the exercise task. Prescriptions should be based on the condition of

the patient and the rehabilitation limits of the particular patient. Notes should be used to record improvement and the patient should be encouraged and given support for his increasing improvement.

6. Exercises to strengthen the abdominal muscles should be done at least one hour after the patient has eaten to help prevent development of nausea or vomiting. The presence of food in the stomach would act as a restrictive factor during exercise and would be uncomfortable for the patient.

7. Successful completion of respiratory exercises is based primarily on the complete understanding and cooperation of the patient. The patient must be fully instructed in the appropriate maneuvers that are to be done, the number of repetitions to be performed, and the goals that are being accomplished by these exercises.

# BIBLIOGRAPHY

Bartlett, R.H., Gazzaniga, A.B., and R.T. Geraghty, "Respiratory Maneuver to Prevent Post-Operative Pulmonary Complications," *Journal of the American Medical Association*, 224:1017–1021, 1973.

Bendixen, H.H., *et al.*, *Respiratory Care*, C.V. Mosby, St. Louis, 1965.

Brunner, L.S. and D.S. Suddarth, *Lippincott Manual of Nursing Practice*, Lippincott, Philadelphia, 1974.

Bryan, C.D. and J.P. Taylor, *Manual of Respiratory Therapy*, C.V. Mosby, St. Louis, 1973.

Burton, G., *et al.*, *Respiratory Care: A Guide to Clinical Practice*, Lippincott, 1977.

Bushnell, S.S., *Respiratory Intensive Care Nursing*, Little, Brown, Boston, 1973.

Egan, F., *Fundamentals of Respiratory Therapy*, 3rd edition, C.V. Mosby, St. Louis, 1977.

Gaskell, D.V. and B.A. Webber, *The Bramptom Hospital Guide to Chest Physiotherapy*, Blackwell Scientific Publications, London, 1973.

Grenard, S., *et al.*, *Advanced Study in Respiratory Therapy*, Glenn Educational Medical Services, New York, 1971.

Johnson, R.F., *Pulmonary Care*, Grune and Stratton, New York, 1973.

Modrak, M., *et al.*, *Better Living and Breathing: A Manual for Patients*, C.V. Mosby, St. Louis, 1975.

Morrison, D.R., *et al.*, "A Proposal for More Rational Use of IPPB: Volume Orientation," *Respiratory Care*, 21:318, 1976.

Safar, P., *Respiratory Therapy*, F.A. Davis, Philadelphia, 1965.

Shapiro, B.A., *et al.*, *Clinical Application of Respiratory Care*, 2nd edition, Year Book Medical Publishers, Chicago, 1979.

Slonim, N.B. and L.H. Hamilton, *Respiratory Physiology,* 2nd edition, C.V. Mosby, 1971.

Taylor, J.P.: *Manual of Respiratory Therapy,* 2nd edition, C.V. Mosby, St. Louis, 1978.

Young, J.A. and D. Crocker, *Principles and Practices of Respiratory Therapy,* 2nd edition, Year Book Medical Publishers, Inc., Chicago, 1976.

# CHAPTER
# 7

# Airway
# Management

Airway management is an essential part of effective respiratory care. The airway connects the atmosphere with the alveoli of the lung, thus allowing for passage of gas in close proximity with the pulmonary blood flow. The primary goal of airway care is to prevent obstruction and restriction that will limit the movement of air into the lung, causing an increase in the work of breathing. The most common anatomical structure causing upper airway obstruction is the tongue. Other areas that can cause upper airway obstruction are inflammation of the epiglottis, vocal cords, and the laryngeal/tracheal area. Upper or lower airway obstruction may be caused by aspiration of foreign bodies, increased pulmonary secretions, or increased viscosity of secretions. An individual's normal clearing mechanisms include position changes, sneezing and coughing, and ciliary escalator functions.

## AIRWAY OBSTRUCTION

Table 7-1 lists probable sounds that occur when obstruction takes place in specific areas of the respiratory tract. The airway may be partially or totally obstructed. Partial obstruction is indicated by snoring, expiratory

160

**TABLE 7-1**

**Breath Sounds Associated with Airway Obstruction**

| *Breath Sound* | *Cause and Affected Area* |
|---|---|
| Sneeze | Stimulation of the Nasal Cavity |
| Gagging | Stimulation of the Pharynx |
| Snoring | Tongue against the Pharyngeal Wall |
| Hoarseness | Inflammation of the Larynx |
| Grunting | Narrowing of the Vocal Cords |
| Cough | Irritation of the Trachea and Bronchi |
| Wheezing | Narrowing of the Bronchioles |
| No Sound with Effort | Total Airway Obstruction |

stridor, gurgling, inspiratory squeaking, and audible breathing. Tachypnea and tachycardia also may be observed. With complete airway obstruction, there will be no sound; although the individual may make extreme efforts to move air into the lungs with deep substernal and intercostal retractions and contraction of accessory muscles. The patient will also appear anxious and be perspiring.

Accidental deaths caused by acute airway obstruction commonly occur when people are eating. This is referred to as *restaurant syndrome* or "cafe coronary." Complete occlusion of the respiratory tract occurs when food becomes lodged in the area of the epiglottis and the opening into the larynx. Inspiratory effort and anxiety of the individual can be observed, but the individual will be unable to make a sound or inhale air. This may be differentiated from a heart attack because the heart-attack victim will be able to talk or at least make sounds. If the obstruction is not removed, unconsciousness followed by death will occur within a few moments.

## GOALS OF AIRWAY MANAGEMENT

1. *To prevent or bypass upper airway obstruction.* Using specific artificial airways, obstruction of the upper airway is prevented or circumvented to allow for proper ventilation of the lung. An artificial airway is commonly required in patients who are under anesthesia or otherwise unconscious. Specific procedures and equipment to alleviate upper airway obstruction will be described in following sections.

2. *To protect the lower respiratory tract.* Artificial airway equipment is often used to seal off the upper airway from the lower airway to prevent the aspiration of foreign materials into the lower respiratory tract. Vomiting may occur during procedures such as anesthesia, CPR, mechanical ventilation, or with the elimination of muscle tone resulting from central nervous system dysfunction. These procedures involve depression of

normal pharyngeal reflexes of the upper respiratory tract, and therefore, increase the chances of aspiration of gastric content or foreign particles into the lower respiratory tract. Airway management techniques limit the possibility of this occurring.

3. *To assist with the removal of secretions.* Many primary and secondary pathological conditions such as bronchitis, dehydration, and pneumonia lead to an increase in the amount of secretions produced in the respiratory system and/or an increase in the viscosity of the secretions produced. Weak and debilitated patients also may require assistance with secretion removal, though his secretions are of a normal viscosity and amount. Airway management equipment and procedures are used to facilitate the removal of these secretions.

4. *To provide a closed system for the administration of prolonged ventilatory assistance.* Specific airway management equipment is used to attach patients to artificial mechanical ventilation systems. An artificial airway with a cuff is necessary to provide effective ventilation of the lung by mechanical ventilators. It also is necessary to provide a sealed system for the application of positive end expiratory pressure (PEEP) or continuous positive airway pressure (CPAP).

5. *To reduce the anatomical deadspace.* Insertion of an artificial airway such as an endotracheal tube or a tracheostomy tube reduces the anatomical deadspace of the respiratory system by 35–50 percent, thus improving alveolar ventilation and facilitating the more appropriate mixing of respiratory gases. This can be beneficial with patients having chronic lung changes that occur with emphysema and bronchitis or with acute respiratory disease to decrease the work of breathing.

## HAZARDS OF AIRWAY MANAGEMENT

1. *Infection and contamination of the respiratory system.* The placement of artificial airways extending into the trachea bypasses the upper respiratory system and the normal protective mechanism filtering inhaled gases. As a result of bypassing the upper airway defense mechanisms, unfiltered gas containing foreign bacterial microorganisms can enter the lower respiratory system. With insertion of artificial airways, normal microorganisms (flora) also are dislodged and carried into the normally sterile lower respiratory tract. Also, coughing, the normal clearing mechanism of the lower respiratory tract, is inhibited or eliminated by the placement of an artificial airway through the glottis. Without these normal defense mechanisms, infection and contamination of the lower respiratory tract are likely to occur. Ideally, all procedures dealing with artificial airways should be performed under sterile conditions.

2. *Dehydration.* Artificial airways that bypass the upper airway increase

the opportunity for dehydration of the respiratory mucosa. Whenever artificial airways bypass the humidification of the nasal cavity, some method of providing humidity to the inspired gas should be provided. 3. *Psychological depression.* Placement of artificial airway equipment in the oral cavity and/or through the vocal cords eliminates the ability of the patient to communicate normally. This can be a frightening situation for the patient. He can no longer ask questions about procedures being performed on his body or make requests. He may feel that he is less than a whole person. Some form of communication should be used to allow medical personnel, the patient, and his family to understand each other more clearly. A writing pad should be provided for the patient or if he is not able to write, an alphabet board or signs should be used.

## AIRWAY MAINTENANCE

The following are manual procedures for maintaining a patent airway:

1. *Positioning.* Proper positioning of a patient is the fundamental procedure used to maintain an open airway and to increase the effectiveness of ventilation. In the unconscious and/or anesthetized patient, upper airway obstruction can commonly be resolved in this manner. These patients should be lying on their side or in a prone position with their heads tilted back and facing to the side. This will prevent aspiration if vomiting should occur. It is often used as a temporary procedure in intensive care units and recovery rooms where the patient may be observed closely. Individuals suspected of vomiting should always be placed in these positions. The following are considerations of positioning:

   a) The tongue is moved forward by lifting at the ramus of the mandible and tilting the head back into a "sniffing" position (see Fig. 7-1). This will move the jaw forward and therefore pull the tongue off the pharyngeal wall. This maneuver extends the neck and can be done with the patient in a sidelying, prone, or supine position. A pillow or cloth roll can be placed under the shoulders to maintain the jaw in this upward position.

   b) An unconscious or comatose patient should be turned from side to side at least every two hours to prevent the pooling of secretions in the dependent areas of the lung and to provide effective ventilation to each lung. This maneuver also assists in the prevention of bedsores and pressure necrosis, which may occur with limited position changes. The better distribution of gas flow as well as pulmonary blood flow helps prevent atelectasis in dependent areas of the lung.

   c) Care must be taken so that the patient is never placed in a position that would obstruct the trachea. This is most apt to happen in

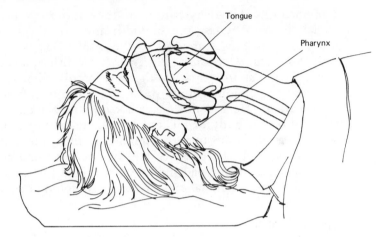

**FIG. 7-1.** Sniffing position. The tongue is moved away from the posterior wall of the pharynx by moving the jaw forward as illustrated.

weak, debilitated, or unconscious patients. It can occur when large, fluffy pillows are placed under the head to make the patient more comfortable. When a pillow is placed under the patient's head, it should be placed so that the patient's head *and* shoulders are on the pillow, keeping the trachea straight and the airway open (see Fig. 7-2).

2. *Obstruction removal.*  Remove all obstructions from the oral and nasal cavity. The upper airway should be cleared of all foreign or artificial articles such as false teeth, misplaced nasal packs, gum, food, or foreign objects. Examination of the oral and nasal cavity should be performed on all comatose and unconscious patients. Patients also should be suctioned

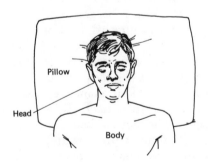

**FIG. 7-2.** Proper pillow position.

as necessary to prevent excess secretion buildup. Need for suctioning may be indicated by audible sounds (see Table 7-1).

3. *Heimlich Maneuver.* This procedure is used with acute airway obstruction to clear foreign objects from the airway. The maneuver is approved by the American Heart Association. Its common use is in situations described earlier as "cafe coronary" or *"restaurant syndrome."* The maneuver is performed by standing behind the individual who may be standing up or seated, and placing your arms around them similar to a bear hug. You do *not* squeeze the sides of chest at all. The hands are clasped together and placed between the substernal notch and the belly button. A quick forceful blow is delivered with the clenched hands to the substernal area (see Fig. 7-3). This will create a rapid movement of air out of the lungs, forcing the foreign object out of the airway. This maneuver can be easily performed by laymen without any specialized equipment.

4. *Coughing.* Patients can be trained in the effective way to cough to produce the most forceful expiratory flow of air, which assists in removal of secretions or other obstruction. Methods of training and reinforcing coughing techniques are described in Chap. 6.

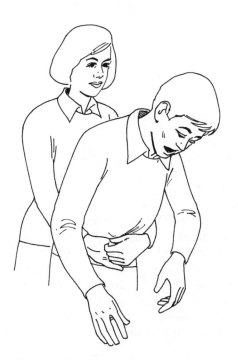
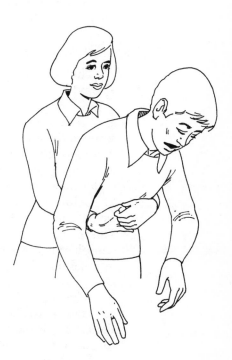

**FIG. 7-3.** Heimlich maneuver.

# ARTIFICIAL AIRWAYS

Fabricated airways have been designed for placement in the respiratory system to maintain patent communication between the atmosphere and the lower respiratory tract. These airways facilitate secretion removal and provide an open airway. They are rigid or semirigid tubes composed of rubber, metal, or plastic. They are designed specifically for temporary or long-term use. The following are types of artificial airways:

## PHARYNGEAL AIRWAYS

These airways are designed for nasal or oral insertion. They are used for temporary short-term maintenance of the airway and are usually made of plastic or rubber and range from neonate to adult sizes. They are inserted either through the nares into the nasal cavity extending down to the oral pharynx, (nasopharyngeal) or through the oral cavity extending down to and into the oropharynx (oropharyngeal). These pharyngeal airways hold the tongue away from the posterior wall of the pharynx. They are designed to allow air to move around or through them and into the lower respiratory tract. Proper placement of the pharyngeal airways requires that the head be tilted backwards and kept in this position while the airway is in place.

### Nasopharyngeal Airways

The following are therapeutic considerations of the nasopharyngeal airway:

1. These tubes are designed of soft rubber or latex material and placed through the nares into the oropharynx posterior to the base of the tongue. As described above, the head should be tilted backwards while the airway is in place (see Fig. 7-4). This is done by using a rolled towel or pillow under the shoulders of the patient.
2. Before insertion, the length of the airway required can be estimated by determining the distance between the nares and the tip of the ear lobe. This distance plus one inch should be the approximate length of the nasopharyngeal airway required for that particular patient. The largest internal diameter possible should be used. The external diameter of nasopharyngeal airway should be slightly smaller than the nare opening.
3. After the tube size is selected, lubricate the tube with a water soluble gel, and gently insert the tube through the selected nare. The airway should be visible through the mouth to insure that it extends behind the tongue in the oropharynx.

Many airways have a molded tip on the proximal end to prevent slipping. Once in place, gas exchange should be felt from the opening of

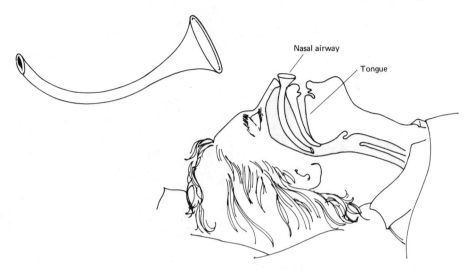

Nasal airway

Tongue

**FIG. 7-4.** Nasopharyngeal airway. The nasopharyngeal airway extends through the nasal cavity into the oropharynx to displace the tongue forward preventing airway obstruction.

the airway. Care must be taken to prevent mucosal injury during insertion of the tube. Lubrication with gel aids in preventing injury. The use of a water soluble gel is *not* irritating to the mucosa, will *not* act as a culture media, and eliminates potential mineral-oil aspiration from oil-based gels. Oil-based gels should never be used.

4. It is recommended that the airway be changed from one nare to the other every eight hours, and that adequate humidity be provided to insure normal secretion viscosity.

5. There are several disadvantages. This airway may easily kink, since it is made of a very soft material. The presence of the narrow airway also will increase airway resistance and, therefore, may increase the work of breathing. It should be used only in patients who may be closely observed, such as intensive care units or recovery rooms. Insertion also may cause trauma and bleeding.

6. The nasopharyngeal tube often is more easily tolerated by a conscious patient than the oropharyngeal airway. This is due to the presence of the normal gag reflex in an alert, conscious patient.

### Oropharyngeal Airways

The following are therapeutic considerations of an oropharyngeal airway:

1. This airway is designed to be inserted through the mouth and oral cavity into the oropharynx. A large phalange at the proximal end of the airway lies against the lips of the patient. The body of the tube lies against the roof of the mouth.

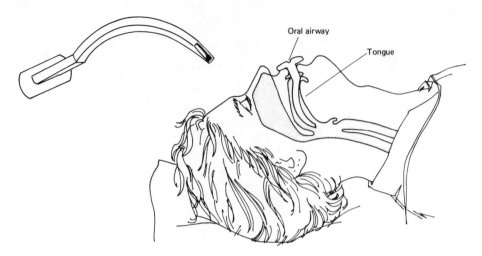

FIG. 7-5. Oropharyngeal airway.

2.  This tube is inserted by opening the mouth with the thumb and fore-finger and simultaneously pushing and rotating the tube into position. A firm, but gentle, force should be applied to the airway as it is inserted. It should be taped in place and it always requires close patient observation when in use, just as the nasopharyngeal airway does (see Fig. 7-5).

3.  With an unconscious or anesthetized patient, the airway can be used as a bite block with an endotracheal tube or to assure airway patency when ventilating a patient with a bag and mask.

4.  The oropharyngeal airways should be monitored continually for patency and should be suctioned as necessary. Humidification should also be used with this tube as necessary. If the oropharyngeal airway is not tolerated, it should be removed.

5.  There are several disadvantages. Insertion of an oropharyngeal airway in a semicomatose or anesthetized patient frequently may cause gagging and increase the potential of vomiting and aspiration. If gagging occurs, the airway should be removed. The conscious and alert patient usually cannot tolerate this airway.

6.  Pharyngeal airways are available as both disposable and nondisposable items and should be routinely changed when used for long-term airway maintenance (at least every 72 hours).

## ESOPHAGEAL OBTURATOR

The esophageal obturator is a temporary airway for short term use in emergency situations. It is composed of a hollow tube with a blind pouch at the distal end and open at the proximal end. Around the opening at the proximal end is a mask designed to fit over the face and nose of the pa-

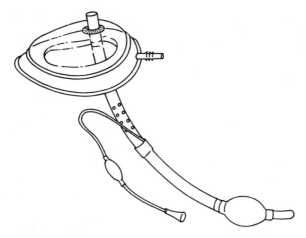

**FIG. 7-6.** Esophageal obturator.

tient. In the central portion of the tube, there are perforations to allow gas flow out of the tube. This airway is designed to be inserted *into the esophagus,* at which time a cuff at the distal end of the tube is inflated. Once the cuff is inflated, air forced into the top of the tube will move through the tube and out of the perforations into the oropharynx, permitting airflow into the trachea and the lungs. The airway may be inserted blindly into the esophagus. This airway can be used by emergency medical personnel where endotracheal intubation cannot be done (see Fig. 7-6). Its use is based on the assumption that it is easier to intubate the esophagus than the trachea of a patient.

## THERAPEUTIC CONSIDERATIONS

The following are therapeutic considerations of esophageal obturators:

1.  This tube is inserted into the esophagus. Immediately upon insertion and inflation of the cuff, the emergency personnel should evaluate the ventilation of the lung. Breath sounds should be checked by auscultation of the chest, and the chest should be examined for bilateral expansion.
2.  The mask of the esophageal obturator must be fitted tightly over the face and mouth of the patient, and the cuff must be inflated on the tube to provide ventilation to the patient.
3.  This type of airway is temporary. It is recommended only in emergency situations. It is designed to provide a rapid, blind method of airway establishment and to prevent gastric distention caused by manual artificial ventilation. Once the patient has been stabilized, endotracheal intubation can be done, if necessary. Orotracheal intubation is as rapid and is more effective if performed by a trained, practiced individual.

4. There are several disadvantages. The tube being placed in the esophagus may cause the patient to vomit. Although the cuff is inflated, the severe motion of vomiting may force vomitus past the cuff and into the patient's airway. When using the obturator tube, suction must be available immediately in case of vomiting. Also, this airway is not tolerated well by patients who are alert or semicomatose. Forceful bagging with a resuscitating bag may force air past the cuff into the stomach, eliminating one advantage of the tube. Since it requires a tight fitting mask, placement and drainage of nasal and oral gastric tubes also may be interrupted with the need for a tight mask to effectively ventilate the lungs.

## ENDOTRACHEAL TUBES

Endotracheal tubes (see Fig. 7-7) are hollow cylindrical airways bent to better adapt to the natural curvature of the upper respiratory tract. They are designed for nasal or oral insertion. They range in length from 12 cm (in neonates) to about 38 cm (adults), and they vary in internal diameter from 2.5 mm (in neonates) to about 11 mm (in adults) (see Table 7-2). Endotracheal tubes are made of rubber and several types of plastic materials including, polyvinyl chloride (PVC), silicone, nylon, teflon, and polyethylene. PVC is the most commonly used plastic for artificial airways. These materials, or their combination, are used to create a moldable, nontoxic, nonreactive tracheal device for use as artificial airways.

All tubes used in airway management must meet federal standards of implantation testing (I.T.) for toxicity and tissue reactivity set down by the Z-79 Committee for Anesthesia Equipment of the U.S. Standards Institute. Tubes meeting these requirements are permanently marked with Z-79 and/or IT. Tubes also should be labelled with the internal and ex-

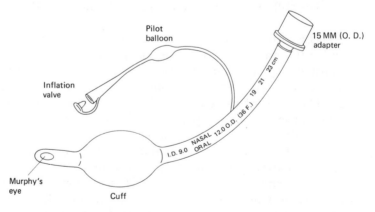

FIG. 7-7. Endotracheal tube.

**TABLE 7-2**

**Endotracheal tubes—Range of Tube Sizes and Types**

| French Gauge | English Size Magill Gauge | External Diameter (mm) | Internal Diameter (mm) |
|---|---|---|---|
| 12 | | 4.0 | 2.5 |
| 12–14 | 00 | ⌈4.5 | 3.0 |
| 14–16 | | ⌊5.0 | 3.5 |
| 16–18 | 0–1 | 5.5 | 4.0 |
| 18–20 | 1–2 | ⌈6.0 | 4.5 |
| 20–22 | | ⌊6.5 | 5.0 |
| 22 | 3–4 | ⌈7.0 | 5.5 |
| 24 | | ⌊8.0 | 6.0 |
| 26 | 4–5 | 8.5 | 6.5 |
| 28 | 5–6 | 9.0 | 7.0 |
| 30 | 5–7 | 9.5 | 7.5 |
| 32 | 5–8 | 10.0 | 8.0 |
| 34 | 8 | 11.5 | 8.5 |
| 36 | 9–10 | ⌈12.0 | 9.0 |
| 38 | | ⌊12.5 | 9.5 |
| 40 | 10–11 | ⌈13.0 | 10.0 |
| 42 | | ⌊13.5 | 10.5 |
| 42–44 | 11–12 | ⌈14.5 | 11.0 |
| 44–46 | | ⌊15.0 | 11.5 |

ternal diameter and the tubing length. Tracheal devices that have cuffs should have soft, high-volume, low-pressure cuffs.

Endotracheal intubation is the insertion of a flexible tube through the oral or nasal cavity into the trachea. The distal end of the tracheal tube rests in the midportion of the trachea. It is used for airway management that is considered to be necessary for up to 72 hours. Endotracheal tubes have been used for many years in anesthesia and in airway management for ventilatory insufficiency and failure.

## INTUBATION EQUIPMENT

The following is equipment used in endotracheal intubation:

1. *Laryngoscope.* This battery-powered instrument contains a curved or straight blade, with a built-in light to illuminate the laryngopharynx and vocal cords (see Fig. 7-8). The curved blade (MacIntosh) or straight blade (Miller) are used to move the epiglottis or other soft tissue from out of the line of sight to allow a direct view of the vocal cords. The Wis-Forregar blade is a combination of the straight and curved design. These blades are

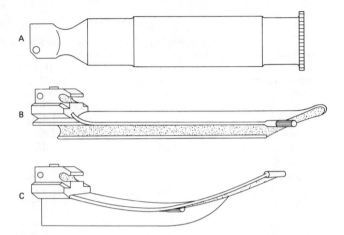

FIG. 7-8. Laryngoscope. (A) Handle, (B) Straight blade (Miller), (C) Curved blade (MacIntosh).

available in adult, pediatric, and neonatal sizes. They are designed to be held in the left hand so that insertion of the tube can be completed with the right hand (see Section on *Tracheal Intubation* in this chapter). It is recommended that no endotracheal tube be inserted without visualization of the vocal cords.

2. *Stylet.* This slender, flexible, soft metal rod is placed through the endotracheal tube. It is used to stiffen and shape the tube curvature to approximate the anatomical shape of the upper airway and facilitate inserting the endotracheal tube through the vocal cords. The stylet is inserted in the endotracheal tube so that the distal end of the rod is one half

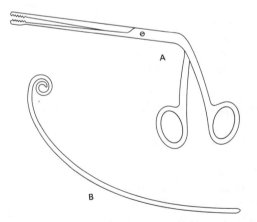

FIG. 7-9. Long-nosed (Magill Forceps (A) and stylet (B).

inch from the end of the endotracheal tube. This prevents damage to the tracheal wall by any protruding end of the rod. It is removed immediately after insertion of the tube (see Fig. 7-9B).

3. *Long-nosed-forceps (Magill) (see Fig. 7-9A).* This long, scissorlike device is used to grasp the endotracheal tube and guide it into the trachea when nasotracheal intubation is performed. It may be used with oral tracheal intubation if a stylet is not available and the tube is not rigid enough to be guided through the vocal cords by itself. The forceps should always be available when endotracheal intubation is performed. Its specific used is described in the section describing nasotracheal intubation.

## THERAPEUTIC CONSIDERATIONS

The following are therapeutic considerations of endotracheal tubes and endotracheal intubation equipment:

1. All standby intubation equipment should be checked at least once a week to see that it is in proper working order. This includes a check of the battery storage area in the handle of the laryngoscope. Also, a wide range of endotracheal tubes should always be available for intubation. Immediately prior to intubation, the cuff on the endotracheal tube should be checked to see that it is inflatable and that it does not leak.

2. Laryngoscopes and forceps should be sterilized periodically. Ideally this would be after each use. Endotracheal tubes are designed for either nondisposable or disposable use. Disposable tubes are packaged individually, then sterilized, and should be used once and then discarded. This eliminates the hazards caused by resterilization of endotracheal tubes.

If endotracheal tubes are to be sterilized, there are several special considerations. All tubes must be completely dried prior to ethylene oxide sterilization to prevent the formation of a toxic substance, ethylene glycol. Also, all endotracheal tubes must be completely aerated when gas sterilized to prevent any retention of ethylene oxide. Ethylene oxide is toxic to human tissue. Any polyvinyl chloride tubes that are sterilized by gamma radiation may form a toxic substance called ethylene chlorohydrin following resterilization with gas. It is recommended that tubes sterilized by gamma radiation should not be resterilized. Autoclaving may deform many types of plastic tubes and should be avoided.

3. Endotracheal tubes are chosen for insertion based on the size of the outer diameter of the tube in comparison with the size of the internal diameter of the tube and the length of the tube required. When inserting an endotracheal tube, the largest possible outer diameter should be used. In the adult, the narrowest part of the respiratory tract is at the vocal cords. The tube's outer diameter should be chosen to provide the maxi-

mum internal diameter to reduce airway resistance and to limit excess pressure on the vocal cords. Flexibility and rigidity of the tube should be considered when determining the outer diameter and internal diameter to be used to prevent crimping of the tube. Tube length must be adequate to allow insertion of the distal end of the tube through the vocal cords, extending down into the midportion of the trachea, to about one half inch above the carina. The length should also be adequate to allow connection via a 15 mm adaptor at the proximal end of the tube and to allow securing of the tube with bandages or twill tape.

4.   Cuffs on endotracheal tubes are very important. In selecting a cuffed endotracheal tube, the soft, pliability of a high-volume, low-pressure cuff is recommended. Cuff damage occurs when the lateral wall pressure created by the cuff against the tracheal wall exceeds tracheal capillary blood pressure, which is about 25 mm Hg. It has been found that pressures above this cause a decrease in local blood flow to the tissue, leading to pressure necrosis. Care must be taken to prevent accidental overinflation of the cuff. Some cuffs are designed to be self-inflating, such as the Bivona tubes, and these do not require the insertion of gas. The Bivona cuff inflation inlet should not be occluded while inflated (see Fig. 7-10).

5.   Some endotracheal tube designs also include an opening at the distal end of the tube between the cuff and the distal end of the tube, called a Murphy's eye (see Fig. 7-7). This opening is incorporated to prevent the accidental lodging of the tube opening against the tracheal wall. It provides collateral circulation of gas even if the opening at the distal end has become occluded (see Fig. 7-7).

6.   When endotracheal tubes are used, patients should be under close observation to limit the complications. Common problems with artificial air-

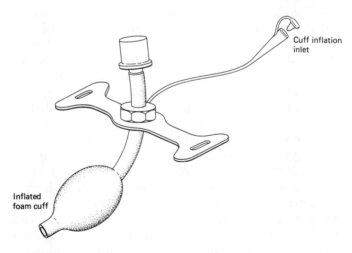

Cuff inflation inlet

Inflated foam cuff

**FIG. 7-10.** Bivona foam cuff.

ways occur at points at which the airway comes in contact with the larynx and trachea. The pressure caused by a rigid tube also may result in damage to the arytenoid cartilage. Long-term problems that may occur may include a deterioration of the vocal cords caused by increased pressure from an oversized tube. The cuff may cause tissue breakdown (necrosis) at the cuff site caused by surface irritation with tracheal movement and decreased tracheal capillary blood flow caused by excessive lateral wall pressure. Cuff-inflation pressures should be checked at least every eight hours *and* each time the cuff is inflated (see section on *endotracheal intubation*). Long-term damage to the trachea can lead to a tracheo-esophageal fistula and/or tracheal stenosis. Patient position changes should also be closely observed for obstruction of the artificial airway caused by kinking.

## TRACHEOSTOMY TUBES

Tracheostomy tubes are artificial airways designed to fit directly through a surgical opening in the trachea to provide a temporary or permanent connection between the lower respiratory tract and the atmosphere. These tubes may vary in length from approximately 2 to 6 inches and in internal diameter of about 2–12 mm (see Table 7-3). Their material design is similar to that of an endotracheal tube, with the exception of permanent tubes which are available in silver. Silver is nontoxic and does not react with tissue. Tracheostomy tubes are designed with both a single and double cannula. Double cannulas include an inner and outer cannula so that the inner cannula can be removed for cleaning and maintenance (see Fig. 7-11). Tracheostomy tubes are also designed with and without cuffs.

A tracheotomy is a surgical procedure in which an opening is cut into the trachea, usually for the purpose of inserting a tube to bypass upper-airway obstruction and to provide effective long-term airway management.

**TABLE 7-3**

**Tracheostomy Tubes—Range of Tube Sizes and Types**

| Jackson Trach Sizes | French Gauge | External Diameter (mm) |
|:---:|:---:|:---:|
| 4 | 24 | 8 |
| 5 | 27 | 9 |
| 6 | 30 | 10 |
| 7 | 33 | 11 |
| 8 | 36 | 12 |
| 9 | 39 | 13 |
| 10 | 42 | 14 |

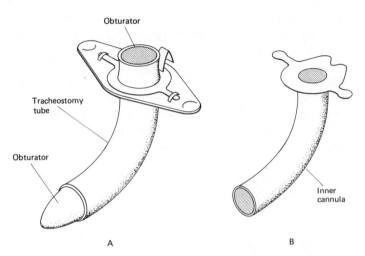

**FIG. 7-11.** Metal tracheostomy tube with obturator in place (A). Inner cannula to be inserted after removal of the obturator (B).

(In general, this is for a period longer than 72 hours.) The procedure for a tracheostomy will be described later in this chapter.

## TRACHEOSTOMY ACCESSORY EQUIPMENT

The following equipment is used with tracheostomy:

1. *Obturator (see Fig. 7-12).* This stylet-like post fits into the tracheostomy tube to increase its rigidity for insertion through the stoma into the trachea. A fitted obturator should be packaged with each tracheostomy tube and is designed for use with only one size of tracheostomy tube. Unlike the stylet, it protrudes beyond the tip of the tube. The obturator's rounded tip eliminates the blunt edge of the tracheostomy tube, which could scoop into the tracheal wall during tube insertion. This device should be kept wrapped at the bedside of the tracheostomy patient and be available if reinsertion is necessary.

2. *Tracheostomy button (see Fig. 7-13).* This is a teflon insert used to maintain the tracheal stoma by preventing it from closing. It is used in the process of weaning the patient with a tracheostomy, maintaining the stoma patency, and allowing gradual stoma closure. This insert includes a body that connects to the stoma by means of a flange. Spacers are included for proper fitting of the tracheostomy button into the tracheal epithelial layer. It also includes a 15-mm adaptor that decreases the stoma radius in half and may be used to connect respiratory therapy equipment to the tracheostomy button. It also includes a plug that may be inserted for total occlusion of the stoma.

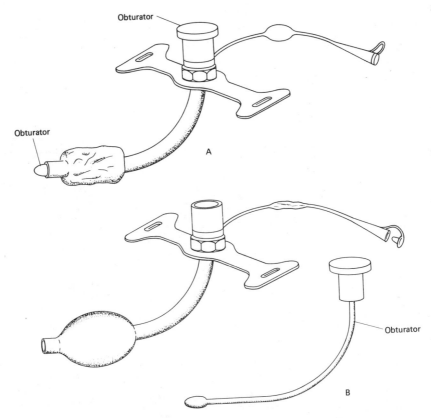

Obturator

Obturator

A

Obturator

B

**FIG. 7-12.** Standard tracheostomy tube. Obturator (A) illustrates the tracheostomy tube in place ready for insertion. (B) The obturator is shown separately.

These tracheostomy buttons range in length from 27 to 40 mm and in outer diameter from 9 to 14 mm. Their design is such that they do not extend into the trachea beyond the small flanged edge which rests on the stoma opening (see Fig. 7-13). Tracheostomy buttons are used to temporarily maintain the patency of the surgical stoma. Without the tracheostomy button in place, the stoma would close within 48 to 72 hours.

3. *Fenestrated tubes (see Fig. 7-14).* This tracheostomy tube is designed with an opening between the flange and the cuff of the tracheostomy tube. It is a double cannula tube used for weaning of a patient from a tracheostomy. When the inner cannula is removed, the patient may breathe through his upper airway allowing gas to pass through the fenestrated window. This is used to assist in weaning the patient from the tracheostomy tube and to allow use of the upper airway. The psychological advantage is that the patient still has a tracheostomy tube but can breathe and cough through his own upper airway.

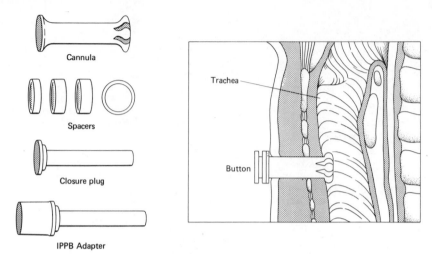

**FIG. 7-13.** Tracheostomy button.

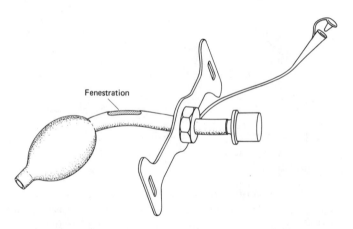

**FIG. 7-14.** Fenestrated tube with foam cuff.

## THERAPEUTIC CONSIDERATIONS

The following are therapeutic considerations of tracheostomy equipment:

1.  All surgical equipment required for a tracheostomy should be sterilized and available in the intensive care and operating-room areas. All tracheostomy tubes should be accompanied by matching obturator and a variety of tube sizes should be available. The standby equipment and tubes should be checked at least once a week.

2. Because insertion of the tracheostomy tube is not through the patient's vocal chords, it gains several advantages. It alleviates possible vocal cord damage that may occur with endotracheal intubation, and allows the patient to use his oral and nasal cavity normally. It reduces the stimulation of the patient's gag reflex, and also reduces the possibility of the patient's not tolerating the tube or vomiting.

3. Tracheostomy tubes are available in nondisposable and disposable units. The most practical type of unit is a disposable tube that can be used once and then thrown away. Silver tracheostomy tubes may be gas sterilized and reused, although care in handling should be observed to prevent denting or kinking of the tube. Tubes made of polyvinylchloride have the same resterilization hazards as endotracheal tubes.

The inner cannula of double cannula tracheostomy tubes should be cleaned as necessary at least every eight hours using 2 percent $H_2O_2$ (hydrogen peroxide) solution and a tracheostomy cleaning kit. The design of the inner cannula allows for easy removal for cleaning.

4. In selecting a tracheostomy tube size, the outer diameter must be fitted through the surgical stoma. The surgical stoma will depend on the size of the trachea and the incision made. The outer diameter of the tube should be such that no undue pressure is exerted against the site of the stoma. The internal diameter of the tube should be as large as possible to decrease airway resistance. Table 7-3 lists common tracheostomy tube sizes.

5. The tracheostomy tube cuffs are designed to be similar to that of endotracheal tubes. Tubes used for long-term and permanent tracheostomy do not have cuffs; therefore, they alleviate the damage possible with long-term use of the cuff. The uncuffed tube may be used with patients who have normal pharyngeal reflexes and normal use of their larynx and trachea which limits the hazard of aspiration.

6. Possible complications of tracheostomy tubes include tracheal stenosis caused by the build-up of scar tissue at the stoma. Complications of cuffed tracheostomy tubes are similar to that of cuffed endotracheal tubes. Patients with cuffed tracheostomy tubes should be observed continually for tracheal damage. Stenosis should be a consideration to be monitored during long-term tracheostomy tube placement and following tracheostomy extubation. Also, like endotracheal tubes, a tracheostomy tube increases the opportunity for respiratory infection.

## TRACHEAL INTUBATION

This section describes three methods of tracheal intubation: oral tracheal intubation, nasal tracheal intubation, and tracheostomy. These procedures should only be performed by trained, experienced individuals. The appropriate equipment should be available and all procedures should be done under sterile conditions.

## ORAL TRACHEAL INTUBATION

Oral tracheal intubation is the most rapid intubation technique and may be used in emergency situations in which an artificial airway is required. Oral tracheal intubation is normally limited to airway management for 72 hours or less. This procedure can be speedy and atraumatic. It is the technique of choice in airway management emergencies. The procedure is as follows:

1. *Explanations.* If the patient is conscious or semiconscious, the procedure should be explained to him, reassuring him of its efficiency of and need for intubation. The patient may also require mild sedation before undergoing the procedure.

2. *Position.* The patient should be placed in a supine position with the shoulders raised two to three inches above the level of the bed, allowing the head to be flexed backwards in a sniffing position. This position should allow for the upward movement of the tongue clearing the airway of soft tissue obstruction (see Fig. 7-1).

3. *Obstructions.* All visible forms of obstruction such as gum, food, and artificial airways should be removed from the patient's mouth. The patient also should be suctioned prior to intubation to remove any excess secretions that may inhibit insertion of the tube.

4. *Preoxygenation and hyperinflation.* Using a resuscitating bag and mask, the patient's lungs should be hyperinflated for at least one minute prior to intubation with an increased concentration of oxygen. It is recommended that 100 percent $O_2$ be delivered, if possible. This will provide an increased oxygen concentration and volume reserve that may supplement the patient's physiological needs during intubation.

5. *Preanesthesia.* If the patient is conscious it may be necessary to spray the upper airway with a topical anesthesia such as 2-4 percent Lidocaine in preparation for the insertion of the tube. If necessary, muscle relaxants such as succinylocholine also should be given to facilitate intubation. This will decrease the trauma to the patient during intubation and decrease the reflex contraction of muscles.

6. *Visualization of the vocal cords.* The mouth is opened by using the thumb and forefinger on the opposite rows of teeth to push the teeth and hold them apart. At this point the laryngoscope, held in the left hand, is inserted in the mouth. Great care must be taken not to strike the teeth with the laryngoscope blade. No pressure should ever be placed on the teeth of the patient. The blade of the laryngoscope is moved down the right-hand side of the mouth, pushing the soft tissue of the tongue to the left and identifying the anatomical landmarks (see Fig. 7-15).

These landmarks are the general anatomical structures that are visual-

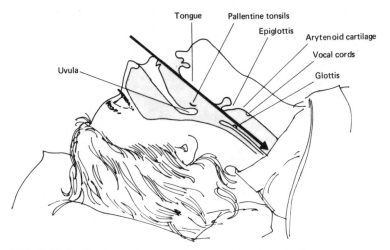

Tongue · Pallentine tonsils · Epiglottis · Arytenoid cartilage · Vocal cords · Glottis · Uvula

**FIG. 7-15.** Intubation of the trachea should only be performed under direct vision of the vocal chords.

ized on entry through the oral cavity. They may act as reference points for orotracheal intubation.

> Tongue
> Pallentine tonsils
> Uvula
> Epiglottis
> Esophagus
> Arytenoid cartilage
> Vocal cords
> Glottis

As the epiglottis is reached, the laryngoscope blade should be moved to the center of the pharynx, still keeping the soft tissue to the left of the blade. When using a curved blade, the tip of the blade should be inserted between the tongue and the base of the epiglottis (see Fig. 7-16). When using a straight blade, the tip of the laryngoscope blade should be placed below the base of the epiglottis (see Fig. 7-17). Once in position, movement of the epiglottis out of the line of site of the vocal cords is done by lifting the laryngoscope blade straight up. This is not a prying motion, but a lifting motion. Lifting of the epiglottis will give a direct view of the arytenoid cartilage and distal to them the vocal cords.

7. *Insertion of the endotracheal tube.* With oral tracheal intubation the endotracheal tube is inserted through the oral cavity and pharynx into the trachea through the glottic opening of the vocal cords. The endotracheal tube should only be inserted after the glottis is visible. This eliminates

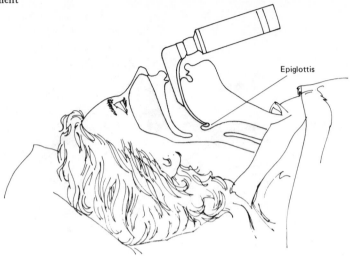

**FIG. 7-16.** Placement of laryngoscope blade when curved blade (MacIntosh) is used during intubation.

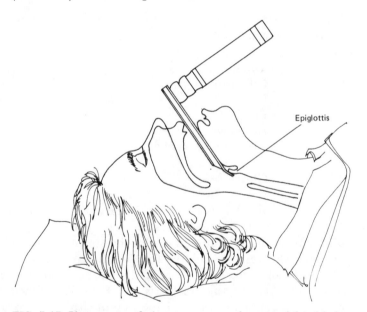

**FIG. 7-17.** Placement of laryngoscope when straight blade (Miller) is used during intubation.

accidental intubation of the esophagus. Prior to intubation, the cuff on the endotracheal tube should be completely collapsed. A stylet should be placed in the endotracheal tube to create a more rigid curved structure to assist with insertion of the tube. Prior to insertion into the endotracheal tube, the stylet and the tube both should be lubricated with a water soluble lubricant to facilitate the slipping through the upper airway and the vocal cords. Once the tube is inserted into the trachea, the stylet should be rapidly removed.

**8.** *Cuff inflation.* After insertion, while the tube is being held in place, the cuff of the tube should be inflated with just enough air to occlude the airway so that no leak may be heard during inspiration. That volume of gas is the *minimal occluding volume.* Once the cuff is inflated with the minimal occluding volume, a small amount of air may be withdrawn until only a slight leak is heard around the cuff. When a patient is being mechanically ventilated, it may be necessary to increase the tidal volume delivered to compensate for the minimal leak around the cuff. The minimal occluding volume and the minimal leak technique are used to limit the amount of local damage to the tracheal wall caused by possible excessive lateral wall pressure from the cuff.

**9.** *Tube placement.* The location of the tube should be immediately evaluated to assure that the tube is in the trachea and that the lungs are being ventilated. The endotracheal tube must not be inserted into the esophagus or too far into the trachea. The right mainstem bronchi is the most common bronchus cannulated by overinsertion of the tube resulting from its anatomical structure. Auscultation of the chest should be done immediately after intubation to check bilateral breath sounds. Also bilateral chest expansion should be observed with each inflation of the lungs. The chest should be uncovered to allow for an unobstructed view of expansion. If breath sounds are not heard and chest expansion is not observed, the tube should be immediately pulled back or removed. Proper placement of the tube is indicated in the spontaneously breathing patient by feeling warm exhaled air coming from the end of the tube.

Following stabilization of the tube, a chest X-ray should be taken to provide visual proof that the endotracheal tube is resting an adequate distance above the carina of the trachea. The tube should rest at least two to three centimeters above the carina. A patient should *never* be intubated without evaluation of where the tube is located and whether or not the patient is being ventilated through that airway. Inappropriate placement of the tube into the esophagus can lead to gastric distention and eructation if not immediately observed and altered. Tube placement should be reevaluated by auscultation and bilateral chest expansion at least once every hour.

**10.** *Securing the tube.* Once the cuff has been inflated and tube placement has been evaluated, the tube should be secured to prevent slipping or premature extubation. It may be secured by taping it to the maxillary area between the nares and lip or by using twill tape and securing it around the patient's head. Until it is secure, the tube should be held firmly and its position should be continually evaluated. The area that is to be taped on the face should be wiped with Benzoine to aid tape adhesiveness. Care should be taken *not* to get the Benzoine in the patient's eyes. The tape should be adhered securely to the tube and then to the face. The maxillary area is preferred because of the limited movement of that area of the skull. If necessary, the patient's hands should be restricted with ties to limit any attempt to dislodge the tube manually. Any equipment attached to the tube should be observed closely to prevent undue weight or pressure exerted on either side of the tube. Tubes in the mouth should be moved from one side to the other at least every 24 hours to prevent skin breakdown and to allow for skin care. Mouth and skin care should be performed at least every eight hours.

11. *Bite block.* Whenever an oral tracheal tube is used, an oral pharyngeal airway or bite block should be inserted and secured to prevent accidental severing of the tube caused by conscious or unconscious chewing by the patient. Intubated patients also should have a gastric tube inserted to remove air from the stomach and limit aspiration.

## NASAL TRACHEAL INTUBATION

1. *Explanations.* As with the oral tracheal intubation, explanations, preanesthesia, positioning, and hyperinflation and oxygenation should be completed prior to intubation of the patient. Equipment also should be checked to be sure it is in working order.

2. *Insertion of the tube.* The endotracheal tube is coated with a water-soluble anesthetic agent. During nasotracheal intubation, the endotracheal tube is inserted through the selected nare and nasal cavity into the pharynx.

3. *Visualization of vocal cords.* Following insertion of the nasotracheal tube into the pharynx, the mouth is opened by using the thumb and forefinger and the tip of the laryngoscope blade is inserted down the right side of the mouth, as in oral tracheal intubation. The epiglottis is lifted up, using a straight or curved blade to visualize the vocal cords. The nasotracheal tube is moved down using a gentle, firm force on the tube until it reaches the opening into the larynx. Using a pair of long-nosed forceps, the tube is grasped and further insertion is done by moving the tube forward with the forceps (see Fig. 7-9). Using the forceps, the nasotracheal tube is inserted through the vocal cords into the trachea. Care should be taken not to tear the cuff with the forceps.

4. *Cuff inflation.* The cuff is inflated and tube placement is immediately checked as described with the oral tracheal intubation procedure. The tube is then secured with tape to the bridge of the nose or the maxilla.

## THERAPEUTIC CONSIDERATIONS

The following are therapeutic considerations of nasal and oral tracheal intubations:

1. *Tube placement.* One of the most common errors of the endotracheal intubation is the accidental insertion of the endotracheal tube into the esophagus. It is recommended that the trachea should only be intubated when the vocal cords have been visualized and the therapist can observe the tube passing through the glottis. This is especially true in emergency situations.

2. *Blind intubation.* Blind nasotracheal intubation also can be performed. After preparation of the patient, the tube is passed into the pharynx, gently advanced until the reflex of coughing or the resistance of the epiglottis indicate its presence at the trachea. Pressure on each side of the thyroid cartilage with the thumb and forefingers allows the individual to feel the tip of the tube as it arrives in the larynx. At the trachea, a slight pressure may be placed on the larynx, depressing it and allowing the passage of the endotracheal tube into and through the vocal cords. Nasotracheal intubation under direct vision is preferred to limit unnecessary trauma to the larynx and to assure intubation of the trachea.

3. *Nasotracheal versus orotracheal tubes.* Nasotracheal intubation requires a smaller external diameter tube because of the difference in the sizes of the oral cavity and the nares, thus has greater airway resistance than oral tubes. Nasotracheal tubes have a more gradual sloping angle of insertion than the oral tracheal tube and are less likely to be kinked by the patient's changing positions. Oral tracheal tubes are at times more uncomfortable and less well tolerated by the conscious patient. Oral placement also may induce coughing and excessive salivation. Nasotracheal tubes are better tolerated by the patient and can be stabilized more easily.

4. *Mouth and nasal care.* Mouth and nasal care should be administered at least every eight hours. With the oral tubes, mouth care is more difficult to provide because of the presence of the tube and the bite blocks with nasotracheal tubes. Pressure necrosis in the nares is a potential hazard. Care should be taken so that minimal pressure is placed on the nose by the tube.

5. *Tube position.* The tube position must be checked and verified routinely. A mark can be placed on the tube at the point at which it enters the body. Any change in the position of this mark should be noted and the tube placement should be checked. If there is any doubt of tube position, an X-ray should be taken and the patient should be closely monitored to make sure that ventilation is occurring.

6. *Cuff leaks.* While checking the artificial airway, the cuff must be

checked to determine if it is inflated. If the cuff is ruptured or dislodged, it cannot seal off the lower respiratory tract. An excessive leak around the cuff will cause a reduction in the volume exhaled through the endotracheal tube. If the patient is on a volume-cycled ventilator, the prescribed volume may not be delivered to the patient's lungs. This may be indicated by a lower pressure reading on the ventilator manometer and gas being exhaled from the patient's mouth. If the patient is on a pressure-cycled ventilator, a large leak will cause the ventilator to not cycle off (to expiration) because the preset pressure cannot be reached. Overinflation of the cuff is also inappropriate and it is recommended that the minimum leak technique described earlier be used to prevent high-cuff pressures.

7. *Suctioning.* The endotracheal tubes should be examined and suctioned periodically to maintain their patency. Any increase in airway resistance causing an increase in the patient's ventilatory effort or in the ventilator pressure manometer reading should be checked. A whistling sound may indicate partial obstruction of the tube. Possible problems include secretion build-up or cuff dislocation over the end of the tube, blocking the airway. Evaluation of the patency of the tube should be constantly kept in mind since the patient is completely dependent on this artificial airway for all ventilation.

8. *Specimen culture.* When an artificial airway is placed into the trachea, a sterile tracheal specimen should be collected for culturing and testing. Cultures should be completed at least every 72 hours while an artificial airway is in place. Tracheal infection may result from contaminated respiratory care equipment, accumulation of secretions, and/or poor patient care techniques. Any equipment handling in contact with artificial airways should be done only after thorough handwashing. Sterile techniques should be followed when handling equipment to be inserted into the airway.

9. *Equipment monitoring.* Care should be taken to monitor proper equipment connection to the artificial airway. Equipment should not be allowed to pull or put any type of stress on the aritifical airway. Such stress can cause local pressure necrosis and epithelial damage. Equipment connections also should be checked to assure that equipment does not become disconnected. Disconnection from mechanical ventilation equipment can create a life or death situation.

10. *Hazards.* Problems that may occur with endotracheal intubation include injury to the teeth from the laryngoscope, lacerations of the mouth, pharynx, and larynx by "jabbing" with the tube, vomiting caused by pharyngeal reflexes when preanesthesia techniques are not used, failure to intubate in the appropriate amount of time, and bronchospasms and apnea. Figure 7-18 illustrates hazards of artificial airways including both endotracheal and tracheostomy tubes.

# TRACHEOSTOMY

A tracheostomy is a sterile surgical procedure. It is usually performed by the physician in the operating room on a patient that has been anesthetized and intubated. Tracheostomy is used for long-term airway management. This is generally considered when the airway will be needed for more than 72 hours. If at all possible, it should not be done as an emergency procedure. Oral tracheal intubation is the emergency procedure of choice for rapid, simple completion. A tracheostomy is considered to be the most effective and safe artificial airway for patients requiring long-term airway management.

The following is a procedure for tracheostomy:

1. *Preparation.* In an alert or semiconscious patient, the procedure and the advantages of a tracheostomy should be explained. The patient should be reassured continually prior to and throughout the procedure.

2. *Positioning.* The patient's head and neck should be extended with the patient lying in a supine position. The trachea and upper chest should be uncovered.

3. *Preanesthesia.* The trachea should be anesthetized by using a local anesthetic. Also, prior to the procedure, sedation or relaxants should be given to the patient to quiet and calm him.

4. *Surgical incision.* Ideally, the surgical incision should be made over an endotracheal tube that has been inserted into the trachea. This will guarantee a patent airway throughout the procedure. The incision may be made transtracheal (horizontal) or midline between the second and fifth tracheal rings. The transtracheal incision is commonly used because it both eliminates large areas of scarring and exposes less of the trachea. Care must be taken to prevent severing nearby arteries or lacerating the thyroid gland.

5. *Insertion of the tube.* If the tube has a cuff it should be inspected and tested. The cuff must be completely deflated during insertion to avoid damage to the cuff and for ease of insertion. An obturator should always be in the tube during insertion. The tube should be inserted by using a gentle, but firm, rotating motion.

There is always the possibility of cannulating the subdermal layer above the trachea if care is not taken. Auscultation and examination for the chest bilateral expansion should be done immediately to guarantee proper tube placement. In the apneic patient, a resuscitating bag may be attached to the 15-mm connector on the tube and the patient is given a volume of air through the bag to test the patency of the airway and to assure its location within the trachea.

6. *Cuff inflation.* The cuff on the tracheostomy tube should be inflated

using minimal leak technique (see the sections on *cuff inflation* and *oral tracheal intubation*).

7. *Securing the tube*. The tube should be tied using surgical tape around the patient's neck with a square knot. A bow-tie knot should *never* be used. The tape also should be attached so that only one knot is necessary. The tracheostomy tube must be secured to prevent accidental extubation by the patient.

8. *Reassurance*. The patient should be reassured continually of the patency and productivity of the tracheostomy tube placement.

## THERAPEUTIC CONSIDERATIONS

The following are therapeutic considerations of a tracheostomy:

1. *Observation*. Following the procedure the patient should be closely observed. The tracheostomy procedure creates the danger of post-surgical hemorrhaging and pneumothorax and tracheal damage caused by insertion of the tube. Bleeding should be closely monitored and treated as necessary. The use of the tracheostomy airway does limit the possibility of vocal-cord damage, since the tube is inserted into the trachea below the vocal cords. The major long-term complications are infection resulting from the direct connection of the trachea with the atmosphere and tracheal stenosis due to scarring. All equipment and procedures used should be sterile.

2. *Obturator*. The obturator used with a tracheostomy tube should be kept at the head of the bed in case of accidental extubation. Also, a tube of the same size should be kept near the patient's bedside.

3. *Tube changes*. Routine tube changes are not recommended. Tube changes within the first 24 hours also should be avoided because of the possible instability of the new surgical opening. If the cuff leaks or the tube becomes obstructed, the tracheostomy tube may have to be changed; especially if a sealed cuff is needed to prevent aspiration and to deliver mechanical ventilation and other types of positive-pressure therapy.

4. *Tracheostomy stoma care*. The stoma should be cleaned with hydrogen peroxide at least every eight hours. Hydrogen peroxide should be applied, followed by a rinsing with a normal saline and the placement of a fresh sterile dressing over the wound. Care should be taken not to use sterile dressings with cut, ragged edges because the fibers may get into the tracheostomy causing inflammation. Tracheal secretions should be collected and cultured immediately after a tracheostomy and as needed while the tracheostomy is in place.

5. *Tube connections*. All attachments of respiratory equipment to the tracheostomy tube connection should not pull on the tracheostomy tube. Any excessive pressure placed on the tube will cause erosion of the stoma and trachea wall.

6. *Securing the tube*. The tube should be secured with surgical twill tape

using *only* square knots. This tape should also be changed whenever it is soiled. Changing of these tracheostomy ties should be done by two people to assure against accidental extubation.

## EXTUBATION

Tracheal extubation is indicated when the reason for placement of the artificial airway has been relieved. This includes the ability of the patient to effectively remove secretions from his lungs and the return of normal pharyngeal reflexes. Normal pharyngeal reflexes are indicated by the return of the patient's ability to swallow. If a patient has required mechanical ventilation, then the necessity for artificial ventilation must no longer exist. Upper airway obstruction, such as with central nervous system disorders, and infections, such as epiglottitis or laryngotracheobronchitis (croup) must be decreased in severity. There must be overall improvement of the patient, reducing his need for an artificial airway.

### NASAL AND ORAL TRACHEAL EXTUBATION

The following is a procedure for nasal and oral tracheal extubation:

1. *Preparation for extubation.* The patient should be placed in a sitting or semi-Fowler's position in the bed. This will allow him full use of respiratory muscles and assure a more open airway once the artificial airway is removed. The procedure should be explained to the patient.
2. *Tracheal aspiration.* The artificial airway should be suctioned for removal of any excess secretions from the airway and the respiratory tract. Following tracheal suctioning, the pharyngeal and the laryngeal areas above the cuff also should be suctioned. The airway also may be suctioned again as the tube is removed.
3. *Preoxygenation and hyperinflation.* The patient should be given large breaths using a resuscitating bag or an artificial mechanical ventilator with an increased concentration of oxygen. It is recommended that 100 percent $O_2$ be delivered to the patient as he is "sighed" for at least one minute prior to extubation.
4. *Deflating the cuff.* Once hyperinflation and oxygenation has been completed and the patient's ability to ventilate and clear his lungs for himself has been assessed, the cuff of the artificial airway should be deflated and the ties securing the artificial airway should be detached. Care must be taken to assure that the cuff is completely deflated to reduce the possibility of vocal-cord irritation with the withdrawal of an endotracheal tube or trauma to the stoma from withdrawing a tracheostomy tube.
5. *Removal of the tube.* The patient should be encouraged to take slow, deep breaths. Upon inhalation, at the point of peak inspiration, the airway

should be removed. This will allow for removal of the tube at the point of maximal airway dilatation.

6. *Observation.* Following extubation, the patient should be observed for any difficulties in ventilating his lungs. Inspiratory stridor or any difficulty in breathing should be noted. The major hazard of extubation is irritation to the vocal cords leading to laryngospasms. Following extubation, the patient's ability to cough also should be evaluated and the patient should be encouraged to take at least 10–15 deep breaths followed by firm, forceful short coughs. (See technique for coughing in Chap. 6.)

7. *Oxygen.* The patient should receive supplemental oxygen and aerosol with his inhaled gas following extubation via a face mask. The oxygen concentration should be at least as great as that which he was receiving prior to extubation.

8. *Blood gas analysis.* It is recommended that arterial blood gases be drawn one-half hour after extubation to evaluate the ability of the patient to ventilate himself and to maintain an adequate oxygen level within the blood.

## TRACHEOSTOMY EXTUBATION

The following is a procedure for tracheostomy extubation:

1. The procedure for removal of a tracheostomy tube is similar to that of an endotracheal tube with one exception. Following removal of a tracheostomy tube, stoma care is required.

2. Once the tracheostomy tube has been removed, there is to be no trial period, then a sterile dressing is placed over the stoma allowing it to heal. The stoma will heal and closure will be complete within 48–72 hours following tube removal. If infection is present, this process may be slower.

3. If a trial period is desired for the patient without closure of the tracheostomy, then a fenestrated tracheostomy tube or trach button may be used to maintain stoma patency and allow the patient to use his upper respiratory tract. This allows evaluation of his ability to clear secretions and to breathe through his upper respiratory tract. Fenestrated tubes and stoma buttons are temporary and used to prepare the patient for permanent closure of the tracheostomy.

## THERAPEUTIC CONSIDERATIONS OF EXTUBATION

1. *Reintubation.* Anytime extubation is performed, both the equipment and the trained personnel necessary for reintubation must be present. Only individuals trained and practiced with the ability to reintubate should extubate the patient.

2. *Laryngospasm.* The persons extubating the patient should always be aware of the possibility of laryngospasm. This is the most common hazard of extubation. It may be indicated by inspiratory stridor, crowing, extreme difficulty in breathing, and anxiety. It should be treated immediately with an aerosol of 0.5 ml racemic epinephrine diluted in a 1:8 solution and delivered at the lowest flowrate tolerated by the patient. To help reduce the patient's effort in breathing, assist the patient with ventilation using a resuscitating bag and mask delivering 100 percent $O_2$. If laryngospasms persist, the patient will have to be reintubated. Muscle-relaxing drugs also may be used to treat the spasms. The patient then also may require ventilatory support. Topical and systemic steroids are sometimes prescribed prior to extubation to limit the possibility of laryngospasm.

3. *Follow-up.* The patient should be closely observed for at least two hours after extubation, at which time his ability to clear secretions should be re-evaluated. The patient should also be encouraged to breathe deeply and should be instructed, as necessary, in breathing exercises. (See Chap. 6.)

4. *Long term observation.* Long-term observation following extubation should be a consideration when a patient returns to the hospital or clinic. A patient with a history of intubation who has a persistent breathing problem due to obstruction should be suspected of having damage in the area of the previous cuff site or the vocal cords. Susceptibility to tracheal damage caused by intubation is an individual consideration and in some patients the time required for damage to take place may be as short as 6–12 hours following intubation and it may not occur at all in others.

## ARTIFICIAL AIRWAY COMPLICATIONS

Endotracheal intubation and tracheostomy tubes both involve possible serious side effects resulting from their presence in the airway. Only close observations and respiratory care can help prevent and minimize complications (See Fig. 7-18).

1. *Pressure necrosis.* Pressure necrosis occurs most commonly at the cuff site with tracheostomy and endotracheal tubes. Cuff-site damage may be due to over inflation and/or prolonged use. This damage is lessened by using the minimum-leak technique for cuff filling and aggressively treating the problems necessitating an artificial airway. Endotracheal intubation can also include vocal-cord damage resulting from the pressure of oversized tubes or when inflammation and swelling reduces the airway size, causing the tube to irritate the cords. The planned use of an artificial airway for more than 72 hours should be an indication for the use of a tracheostomy

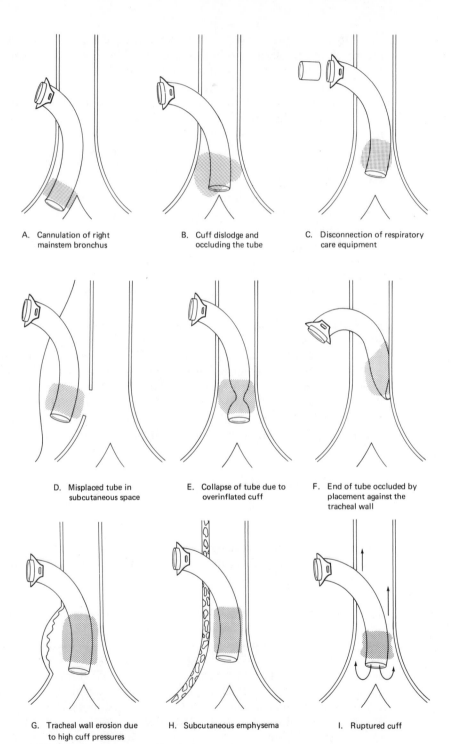

A. Cannulation of right
mainstem bronchus

B. Cuff dislodge and
occluding the tube

C. Disconnection of respiratory
care equipment

D. Misplaced tube in
subcutaneous space

E. Collapse of tube due to
overinflated cuff

F. End of tube occluded by
placement against the
tracheal wall

G. Tracheal wall erosion due
to high cuff pressures

H. Subcutaneous emphysema

I. Ruptured cuff

**FIG. 7-18.** Airway complications.

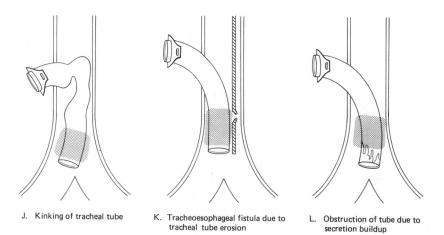

J. Kinking of tracheal tube    K. Tracheoesophageal fistula due to    L. Obstruction of tube due to
                                  tracheal tube erosion                    secretion buildup

**FIG. 7-18.** (Continued.)

tube as a means to eliminate vocal-cord damage. Other areas affected by endotracheal tube intubation include the arytenoid cartilage, the oro-pharynx, and, with a nasotracheal tube, the external nares. The tips of endotracheal tubes and tracheostomy tubes also can cause gouging of the tracheal wall especially when the patient changes position. All movement of the patient should be performed deliberately and gently.

2. *Dehydration.* Humidification must be supplied to the patient while an artificial airway is in place. If humidification is not provided, respiratory mucosa can be permanently damaged from excessive drying, and secretion viscosity will increase, causing problems with secretion removal and potential artificial-airway obstruction.

3. *Premature extubation.* Premature extubation can create a life or death situation for a patient with a limited cardiopulmonary reserve, therefore all artificial airways must be secured. Patients must be restrained if they try to pull out the airway. If a patient makes a conscious effort to extubate himself, tube placement should be re-evaluated and an effort should be made to develop the patient's psychological acceptance for the airway.

4. *Accidental disconnection.* (see Fig. 7-18C). This situation also may be life-threatening, especially if the patient is connected to a mechanical ventilator. Disconnection can lead to dehydration of the patient, hypoxia, increased work of breathing, anxiety, and death. Alarms should be used with life support systems to signal disconnection.

5. *Airway obstruction.* (see Fig. 7-18L). Once the patient has an artificial airway in place, airway patency depends on the open artificial passage. If the endotracheal tube or tracheostomy-tube tip is pushed against the tracheal wall, ventilation will be reduced. Reduced ventilation also occurs with kinking of the tube or obstruction of the tube with secretions. Pos-

sible signs of obstruction include an increased work of breathing, anxiety, or the failure in passing a suction catheter through the tube. Obstruction requires immediate action. If the patient cannot be ventilated with a mechanical ventilator or resuscitating bag, the tube should be removed and replaced.

**6.** *False security.* One of the major complications of artificial airways is the over-assurance of personnel that the airway is continually patent, based only on the presence of the artificial airway. Just because the artificial airway is in place does not mean that the patient is being ventilated or is ventilating adequately or that his airway is patent. It is necessary to periodically evaluate the openness of the airway and the ability of the patient to ventilate himself. It is recommended that an artificial airway be evaluated at least once every hour.

## SECRETION CLEARANCE

A major goal in airway management described earlier was the need to assist in the removal of respiratory secretions in an effort to prevent and correct airway obstructions. Under normal physiological conditions, the lungs maintain secretion clearance. Cilia line the upper and lower respiratory tract except for the area of the oral pharynx and the alveoli. These cilia work in a brushlike manner to propel respiratory secretions toward the larger airways and oral pharynx, where the secretions are coughed up and expelled through the mouth or swallowed. Three conditions may exist in which secretion removal becomes difficult. These are an increase in secretion production, an increase in secretion viscosity and/or a decrease in the ability of the patient to remove secretions. Such incidents are especially common in the weak and debilitated patient.

Secretion removal as a part of airway management is done not only as a therapeutic modality, but also as a diagnostic modality in an effort to study respiratory secretions to determine the presence of abnormal cellular changes, to culture and determine the presence of infection, and to identify drug sensitivity.

## COUGHING

Coughing is a normal physiological function for the clearing of the lower respiratory tract. Often the patient's ability to cough is compromised by the presence of respiratory disease or physical conditions that result from trauma or a surgical procedure. A cough can be described in three phases: inhalation, compression, and expulsion. (The instructural procedure of coughing is described in Chap. 6).

## THERAPEUTIC CONSIDERATIONS

The following are therapeutic considerations of coughing:

1. The patient must have the ability and the awareness to be fully instructed and encouraged in appropriate methods of coughing. The explanation and instructions should be realistic in relation to the patient's disease or physical state. If patient comprehension is not possible, tracheal aspiration may be necessary.

2. The patient should be positioned in a semi-Fowler's position (a 45° angle, sitting position). The patient's knees should be slightly flexed to relax the tension that having the legs straight would cause on the abdominal muscles. This will help to increase the force of the abdominal muscle in an effort to cough.

3. The patient should be encouraged to take a normal breath followed by a pause, during which time the abdominal muscle should be contracted, followed by the patient's coughing two or three short, forceful coughs (see Chap. 6). The patient should *not* be encouraged to take a large deep breath prior to coughing, or to cough as hard and loud as possible. This type of coughing is actually ineffective and may lead to a coughing spasm.

4. If there is pain (for example, as a result of surgery of the abdomen or a chronic lung condition), the patient should be encouraged to cough using some type of support. Suppression of coughing occurs if the patient is not encouraged. The therapist can assist with bracing or splinting the patient by the use of a pillow held over the area of pain.

5. Periodic coughing should be encouraged during every aerosol therapy and IPPB treatment. It should be especially encouraged in patients who are bedridden because of traction, post-operative surgery, or chest injuries. All surgical wounds should be dressed with the least possible amount of bandage adhered to the chest wall. This is so chest expansion is not restricted.

6. Aerosol therapy with mucolytics and effective humidification should be delivered to patients as necessary to decrease the secretion viscosity and increase the productivity. Chest percussion and postural drainage also may be used to move respiratory secretions to the larger airways where they may be more easily coughed from the lower respiratory tract.

## TRACHEAL ASPIRATION

Tracheal aspiration is the use of suction to facilitate the removal of secretions from the respiratory tract. It has become a common modality in respiratory care for use in airway management.

Under normal circumstances, patients with normal coughing do not have difficulty in removal of secretions. Tracheal aspiration is indicated in conditions in which the patient's normal ability to cough has been removed. Situations decreasing the effectiveness of the cough include: central nervous system depression, such as with anesthesia or with diseases such as myasthenia gravis; and the placement of an endotracheal tube or tracheostomy tube into the airway, thus decreasing the compressibility of the gases within the thoracic cavity and eliminating the effectiveness of the patient's cough. Disease conditions in which a patient becomes very weak and debilitated, thus eliminating his strength to cough, also may be indications for tracheal aspirations.

## VACUUM EQUIPMENT

(See Fig. 7-19). To perform tracheal aspiration, a vacuum source is needed. A suction-pump system produces a vacuum and, when applied to the airway, can be used to assist in the removal of secretions. Hospitals today may have either piped-in high-pressure vacuum systems that create up to 600 mm Hg negative pressure or mobile suction-pump units that may be rolled from bedside to bedside into any area that has a standard electrical outlet. These units operate off regular grounded hospital electrical outlets. Both the piped-in systems and the mobile suction pumps must produce an adequate supply of negative pressure to be used with mechanical aspiration equipment.

Each unit should include an adjustable pressure regulator and secretion reservoir container. Containers are constructed of either plastic or glass, and are available in disposable or nondisposable units. This equipment produces a continual flow of negative pressure. The units have a connecting tube that attaches to the vacuum equipment and is long enough to reach the patient's bedside from the wall outlet or mobile stand. The connecting tubing attaches to a suction catheter at the bedside of the patient. This connecting tubing must be made of noncollapsible durable plastic to allow flexibility in movement and use and to prevent the negative pressure from collapsing the tube.

### THERAPEUTIC CONSIDERATIONS

The following are therapeutic considerations of vacuum equipment:

1. Vacuum equipment, including pressure gauge and adjustable regulators, must be in good repair to provide a safe, adequate level of negative pressure suction and to control suction levels within a safe therapeutic range. The safe therapeutic ranges for tracheal aspiration are: adults—between 120 and 150 mm Hg; pediatric—between 80 and 120 mm Hg, and neo-

natal—between 60 and 80 mm Hg. Proper operation of the equipment should be checked prior to suctioning by checking the tubing connections and adjusting the regulator pressure.

2. Connection tubing and reservoir jars from the vacuum equipment to the suction catheter should be changed at least every forty-eight hours or whenever they become extremely soiled. This will inhibit the growth of micro-organisms.

3. A series of reservoir jars may be used to act as a collection area and an overflow to protect the suction source from contamination. A common combination is a two-jar system, in which the first jar acts as the collection jar and the second jar acts as the overflow. Disposable reservoir collection containers are manufactured today with a one-way ball or flapper-type valve in the system to prevent aspirants from reaching the negative pressure regulator and the vacuum source, thus eliminating the need for two-jar systems. In older systems, two-jar systems may still be used.

4. How rapidly the maximum negative pressure is achieved depends on the size of the reservoir jar or jars used. The larger the volume of the reservoir jar, the longer the time required to allow pressure build-up. It is recommended that the volume of reservoir collection containers be less than two liters to facilitate more rapid build-up of maximum negative pressure.

## SUCTION CATHETERS

Suction catheters (see Fig. 7-19) are hollow, cylindrical tubes incorporating an opening or series of openings at the distal end for secretion removal from the lower respiratory tract and an attachment fitting at the proximal end to attach to the connecting tubing from the vacuum equipment. Most catheters also incorporate a vent at the proximal end to regu-

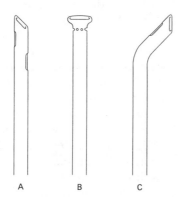

**FIG. 7-19.** Suction catheter tip designs. (A) Standard straight catheter tip with beveled edge and collateral parts, (B) Ring tip with multiple collateral parts, (C) Coudé (angled) tip.

late the intermittent application of negative pressure. This is a thumb port that may be easily operated with one hand during actual suctioning of a patient. These tubes are made of soft, pliable, plastic, nontoxic materials. They also are disposable, single-use products. Their design includes sizes ranging from neonates to adults.

## THERAPEUTIC CONSIDERATIONS

The following are considerations for use of suction catheters:

1.  The aspiration of the trachea using negative pressure (vacuum) should be a sterile procedure. Suction catheters are designed for one-time, single use. Nondisposable catheters are available but not recommended because of risk of contamination of the lower respiratory tract resulting from improper re-sterilization. Normal upper airway bacteria may contaminate and infect the lower respiratory tract of the weak and debilitated individual, therefore catheters used for suctioning the pharynx, oral cavities, or nasal cavities should never then be used for suctioning the lower respiratory tract. Used suction catheters also should never be kept and reused for aspiration of the trachea.

2.  It is recommended that all suction catheters be equipped with a thumbport vent for intermittently controlling the application of negative pressure (vacuum). This control allows the application of negative pressure only while withdrawing the catheter. As the vent is occluded with the thumb, the negative pressure increases. Complete removal of the thumb from the vent should stop the negative pressure flow occurring at the distal end of the suction catheter.

3.  The distal end of the suction catheters are designed to reduce the trauma that occurs both from the physical presence of the tip of the catheter in the respiratory tract and the negative pressure "suction" on the respiratory tract (see Fig. 7-19). The conventional catheter tip is a straight tube with a blunt or rounded bevel edge having a hole (fenestration) 1–2 cm from the distal end of the tube. Another design uses a bent tip at an angle called a Coudé tip. This slanted tip allows for more direction of the catheter into the desired bronchi. Because of this tip's design, insertion through artificial airways may be more difficult and require a greater amount of force. Second, this type of tip must be moved gently through the respiratory tract because of its potential for gouging the respiratory mucosa, causing vocal damage. Another special tip (roll doughnut) design has been incorporated in catheters to limit the accidental grabbing of epithelial mucosa. It is a roll-tip design that has been shown to reduce significantly local damage caused by catheter insertion.

The presence of one or more holes in the lateral wall of catheters acts in a similar way to that of a Murphy's eye in an endotracheal tube, allow-

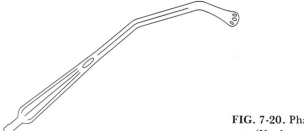

**FIG. 7-20.** Pharyngeal suction catheter (Yankauer).

ing collateral circulation to occur. If the catheter becomes lodged against the tracheal wall, the holes decrease the chance of excessive negative pressure being felt on the respiratory epithelium.

4. A common catheter design limited to pharyngeal suction is a hard plastic tube called a Yankauer suction catheter (see Fig. 7-20). This catheter may be used for emergency upper airway clearance, dental suction, or routine mouth care. This has nondisposable or disposable design and normally does not have a thumb-control vent. It is particularly effective for suctioning food and vomitus.

## SPUTUM COLLECTION CONTAINERS

Sputum collection containers (see Figs. 7-21 and 7-22) are sterile plastic containers that are included in-line for suction sputum induction or voluntary coughing to produce tracheal secretion samples. The in-line single-use design may be inserted between the connecting tubing and the catheter to allow collection of individual secretion samples for laboratory testing.

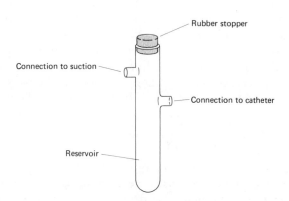

Rubber stopper

Connection to suction

Connection to catheter

Reservoir

**FIG. 7-21.** Specimen container (Lukin's tube).

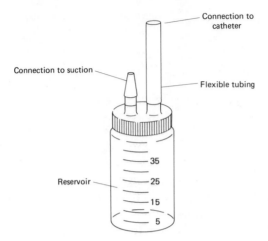

FIG. 7-22. Sputum specimen container.

## THERAPEUTIC CONSIDERATIONS

The following are therapeutic considerations for sputum collection containers:

1. These containers are sterile and should be handled in a manner that prevents contamination of the interior of the container. Any contamination may cause false test results. Handling of the containers should include careful handwashing procedures prior to sputum collection.
2. The sputum collection container should be clearly marked with the patient's name, room number, date, and time of collection, and should be taken to the medical laboratory as soon as the specimen has been collected. It is not recommended that the specimen be kept in the patient's room or that the patient be allowed to independently collect the sputum, since this would not assure proper sterile techniques.
3. Specimen traps or Luken's tubes are used as described above with a suction catheter or bronchoscope in the collection of an in-line sample of respiratory secretions. Care must be taken to keep specimen containers upright or the specimen will be lost through the vacuum system.

## SUCTIONING OF THE AIRWAY

Airway management uses mechanical aspiration of the airway as a modality in the maintenance and prevention of airway obstruction. Procedures using mechanical aspiration include suctioning of the oral and nasal pharynx, oral and nasal tracheal suctioning, and suctioning of artificial airways.

## AIRWAY SUCTIONING PROCEDURE

The following is a procedure for airway suctioning:

1. *Explanation.* The procedure should be clearly explained to the patient so that he will fully understand what you are about to do. Respiratory care personnel should assure the patient of the necessity to effectively accomplish the procedure and should briefly describe the importance of maintaining a clear airway. The patient's cooperation throughout the procedure will depend on this reassurance and a full understanding of this procedure.
2. *Positioning.* This is important for successful completion of the suctioning procedure. The patient should be placed so that the trachea is straight and the upper airway is completely open. A sitting position at a 45° angle (semi-Fowler's) will facilitate the alignment of the airway and the straightening of the trachea assuring greater patency.
3. *Preoxygenation and hyperinflation.* If the patient to be suctioned is not receiving continuous oxygen therapy, then supplemental oxygen should be set up to be used with suctioning. If the patient is receiving oxygen, then to prepare the patient for suctioning, the oxygen concentration should be increased to 100 percent for at least one minute prior to suctioning. This will help to avoid the occurrence of hypoxia and atelectasis (see section on *complications of suctioning*). The patient also should be encouraged to take five to ten slow deep breaths spontaneously or with a resuscitating bag prior to suctioning.
4. *Insertion of the catheter.* After the patient has been positioned, preoxygenated and hyperinflated, the suction catheter should be inserted using a slow, gentle motion. No vacuum (suction) should be applied on insertion. The catheter should be inserted into the airway as far as it will advance, then withdrawn slightly before the suction is applied. The size of the suction catheter to be inserted should be no greater than 1/2 the internal diameter of the artificial airway or the nare in which it is to be inserted. (see section on *suctioning with and without an artificial airway*).
5. *Applying suction.* Negative-pressure suctioning should only be applied during the withdrawal of the catheter from the airway. Application of suction should be intermittent, never continous, to prevent the catheter from "grabbing" the tracheal mucosa. The catheter also should be rotated 360° between the fingers as it is withdrawn from the airway. The negative pressure suction should be applied for no longer than 10–15 seconds as the catheter is withdrawn. The total procedure from insertion to complete withdrawal should take no more than 20 seconds. The suction procedure

should be stopped immediately if arrhythmias or severe tachycardia should occur. If either occurs, the patient should be ventilated as needed using 100 percent $O_2$ until the vital signs have returned to normal.

6. *Reoxygenation and hyperinflation after suctioning.* The patient should receive oxygen and hyperinflation for at least one minute following suction. The patient's heart rate, blood pressure, and rhythm also should be observed until he has returned to his pre-suction limits.

7. *Repetition.* The above steps of the suction procedure should be repeated each time the suction process is done.

## SUCTIONING THROUGH AN ARTIFICIAL AIRWAY

The following are therapeutic considerations for tracheal suctioning through an artificial airway:

1. The size of the suction catheter should be no more than 1/2 the internal diameter of the artificial airway to be suctioned. Coudé catheters may require lubrication for insertion through artificial airways because of their angle tip design. The largest internal diameter catheter possible meeting the above requirements should be used to aid removal of secretions (see Table 7-4).

2. Suctioning should be done above the cuff of artificial airways prior to deflation of the cuff. This will prevent secretions from being deposited all at once in the lower respiratory tract and will limit the possibility of the upper airway contaminating the lower respiratory tract.

3. Never store or reuse a suction catheter following a suctioning procedure. Disposable suction catheters and all contaminated equipment should be thrown away following each procedure. Non-disposable catheters should be sterilized after each use. All procedures must be sterile to maintain the sterility of the lower respiratory tract. Never suction the trachea with the same catheter that was used to suction the upper respiratory tract.

4. Color, amount, and viscosity of secretions removed from the airway and any problems encountered during the procedure should be noted with each suctioning procedure and recorded.

## SUCTIONING WITHOUT AN AIRWAY

The following are therapeutic considerations of oral or nasal tracheal suctioning without an artificial airway:

1. Insertion of the tube may be done most effectively through the nasal cavity. Through the nasal cavity there is a better natural slope of the

**TABLE 7-4**

**Guide for Appropriate Suction Catheter Sizes
for Various Tube Sizes**

| Suction Catheters (French Gauge)* | Tracheal Tubes (French Gauge)* |
|---|---|
| | 12 |
| | 12–14 |
| 5 | 14–16 |
| 5 | 16–18 |
| 6 | 18–20 |
| 6 | 20–22 |
| 8 | 22 |
| 8–10 | 24 |
| 10 | 26 |
| 12 | 28 |
| 12 | 30 |
| 12–14 | 32 |
| 14 | 34 |
| 14 | 36 |
| 14 | 38 |
| 16 | 40 |
| 18 | 42 |

*French guage may vary slightly from one style of tracheal tube to another because of differences in construction of tube wall thickness.

pharynx leading into the opening of the trachea. Prior to insertion, the catheter should be lubricated using a water-soluble gel, and it should be gently passed into the nasal cavity using a slight downward angle through either nare. Forcing the catheter may cause vascular mucosal damage and should never be done. Always be aware of the possibility that the patient has a deviated septum and/or nasal passages may be obstructed. Suctioning through the upper airway can cause contamination of the lower respiratory tract with upper respiratory tract normal bacteria. This may be limited by having the patient rinse his mouth with an antiseptic mouthwash and brushing the teeth prior to the suctioning procedure if this time allocation is feasible.

2. The catheter should be passed down into the pharynx, which may cause a slight retching by the patient from the normal pharyngeal gag reflex. Ask the patient to open his mouth and extend his tongue. The tongue may be held forward using a gloved hand or sterile 4 × 4 gauge to prevent the natural retraction of the tongue with gagging.

3. Instruct the patient to take slow, deep breaths or to cough gently. This will cause the epiglottis to retract, allowing insertion of the catheter through the vocal cord into the trachea. Pass the catheter as far into the

lower respiratory tract as possible until obstruction is met, then withdraw the catheter 2 or 3 cm and apply suction. Continue to apply intermittent suction on withdrawal.

For insertion into the left mainstem bronchi, a Coudé tipped tube is recommended. This also may be assisted by turning the patient's head to the right, giving more alignment of the natural bend of the suction catheter to move into the left mainstem bronchi, and by turning the patient's head to the left, to give a better alignment of the trachea for insertion of the catheter into the right mainstem bronchi. Under normal circumstances a catheter will enter the right mainstem bronchi more than 80 percent of the time unless a Coudé tip is used.

## ORAL AND NASAL PHARYNGEAL SUCTIONING

The following are therapeutic considerations of oral and nasal pharyngeal suctioning:

1. The patient should be placed in a sitting position if possible. The patient is asked to open his mouth, or if unconscious, the mouth should be opened for him, using the thumb and forefinger. If conscious, the patient then should be asked to stick out his tongue. The suction catheter is inserted and an intermittent suction upon withdrawal is used to suction out the oropharynx and mouth. Care should be taken not to probe within the mouth or to suction for a prolonged period of time in any one area.

2. Following suctioning of the mouth, the catheter should be rinsed with sterile water and cleaned and lubricated with a water-soluble gel. Then the catheter should be inserted into each of the nares and the nasal cavity should be suctioned.

3. When suctioning the nasal cavity, do not force the catheter. This will cause unnecessary vascular mucosal damage. Only apply intermittent negative suction during withdrawal of the catheter while it is being rotated.

4. Never suction the trachea with a catheter used for suctioning the upper respiratory tract.

5. Again, note and record the color, amount, and viscosity of the secretions during the suctioning procedure.

## COMPLICATIONS OF SUCTIONING

1. *Hypoxia.* Tissue hypoxia may result from the evacuation of oxygen-enriched air from the lung during the suctioning procedure. This is very hazardous with patients on mechanical ventilation and/or supplemental oxygen-enriched atmospheres. Significant changes in heart rate, rhythm, or blood pressure during suctioning should be considered an indication for hypoxemia. A 20 percent change from the patient's normal limits should

be considered significant. Arrhythmias result from myocardial tissue hypoxia and it has been noted that many cardiac arrests occur shortly after patients have been suctioned. Cardiac reactions may be avoided by suctioning the patient for no longer than 10 seconds. Preoxygenation of the patient and hyperinflation of the lung prior to the suctioning procedure will also help avoid hypoxia. Interruption of mechanical ventilation should be done for only as long as is critically necessary for the suctioning procedure to be completed, and the cardiac status always should be monitored.

2.  *Vagal stimulation.* Suctioning in the area of the pharynx, larynx, and trachea, may also cause stimulation of branches of the vagus nerve. This parasympathetic stimulation may lead to bradycardia and hypotension during suctioning. This can be limited by the gentle catheter insertion and limited application of suction. These recommendations will not guarantee that side effects will not occur, but they will assist in preventing or limiting their reactions.

3.  *Atelectasis.* The negative pressure applied to the respiratroy system during suctioning causes the inadvertent removal of residual gas volume. Excessive removal of residual volume can lead to alveolar collapse and atelectasis. This volume removal may be limited by using a tube with an external diameter that is less than 1/2 the internal diameter of the artificial airway or the nare. Atelectasis is caused by the inadequate entrainment of air around the tube as the patient is being suctioned. Thus residual volume is removed and is not replaced by incoming air. The hazard of atelectasis will also be limited by preoxygenation and hyperinflation prior to suctioning and by suctioning the patient for less than 10 seconds using an intermittent suction technique.

4.  *Trauma to the airway.* Because of probing and forcing the catheter and repeated suctioning procedures, the airway can be damaged, causing hemorrhage, epithelial destruction, and local inflammation. Damage can be limited by the use of intermittent suction and continual rotation of the catheter during withdrawal. The catheter also should never be forced. It should only be inserted gently.

5.  *Infection is a major complication of suctioning.* Only the stringent use of sterile equipment and strict handwashing techniques reduce this hazard. Although repeated suctioning enhances the probability of complication, it is necessary for the patient to have an open airway to maintain ventilation of the lungs and therefore suctioning should be completed as often as is necessary. Periodic laboratory testing of secretion will aid in monitoring the presence of infection.

## BIBLIOGRAPHY

Bendixen, H.H., *et al.*, *Respiratory Care*, C.V. Mosby, St. Louis, 1965.

Brunner, L.S. and D.S. Suddarth, *Lippincott Manual of Nursing Practice.* J.B. Lippincott, Philadelphia, 1974.

Burton, G., *et al.*, *Respiratory Care: A Guide to Clinical Practice*, J.B. Lippincott, Philadelphia, 1977.

Bushnell, S.S., *Respiratory Intensive Care Nursing*, Little, Brown, Boston, 1975.

Egan, S.F., *Fundamentals of Respiratory Therapy*, 3rd edition, C.V. Mosby, St. Louis, 1977.

Garrett, D.F. and W.P. Donaldson, *Physical Principles of Respiratory Therapy Equipment*, Ohio Medical Products, Madison, Wisconsin, 1975.

Grenard, S. *et al.*, *Advanced Study in Respiratory Therapy*, Glenn Educational Medical Services, New York, 1971.

Hedley-White, J., *et al.* *Applied Physiology of Respiratory Care*, Little, Brown, Boston, 1976.

Heimlich, H.J., "A Life Saving Maneuver to Prevent Food Choking," *Journal of the American Medical Association*, 234:398, 1975.

Heimlich, H.J., *et al.*, "Food Choking and Drowning Death Prevented by External Subdiaphragmatic Compression: Physiologic Basis," *Annals of Thoracic Surgery*, 20:188, 1975.

Hunsinger, D.L., *et al.*, *Respiratory Technology: A Procedure Manual*, 2nd edition, Reston Publishing Company, Inc., Reston, Virginia, 1976.

Slonim, N.B. and L.H. Hamilton, *Respiratory Physiology*, 2nd edition, C.V. Mosby, St. Louis, 1971.

Taylor, J.P., *Manual of Respiratory Therapy*, 2nd edition, C.V. Mosby, St. Louis, 1978.

Wade, J.F., *Respiratory Nursing Care*, 2nd edition, C.V. Mosby, St. Louis, 1977.

Young, J.A. and D. Crocker, *Principles and Practices of Respiratory Therapy*, 2nd edition, Year Book Medical Publishers, Chicago, 1976.

# CHAPTER

# 8

# INTENSIVE RESPIRATORY CARE

Intensive respiratory care requires the total commitment of the critical care team. Experienced respiratory care professionals can be valuable resource persons to the physician and are an integral part of the critical care team. This chapter presents information on therapeutic modalities for patients who require artificial mechanical ventilation and emergency cardiopulmonary support. Initially, the reversibility of the disease must be determined to assess the benefit of artificial cardiopulmonary support. Such support is not meant to prolong life uselessly, but to provide temporary support during which time the body can recover to a point that spontaneous physiologic function returns. This does not exclude extended ventilatory care needed because of partial or total paralysis.

## MECHANICAL VENTILATION

*Ventilation* is described as the movement of gas into and out of the lungs. Effective ventilation of the lungs maintains a $P_aCO_2$ in a normal healthy patient between 35 and 45 torr.* As a result of disease, post-surgical con-

*torr = mm Hg

ditions, and trauma, some patients need mechanical ventilatory support to assist them temporarily with their ventilatory requirements. Artificial mechanical ventilation is most effective with early intervention. It requires periodic close analysis of laboratory and clinical information to evaluate its effectiveness.

Artificial mechanical ventilation is the movement of gas into the lungs by artificial means. Today positive pressure is the primary method of delivering mechanical ventilation. The two predominant types of positive-pressure ventilators are volume-cycled and pressure-cycled ventilators. This chapter pertains to positive pressure ventilation equipment only. In the following sections volume-cycled and pressure-cycled ventilators will be distinguished when necessary in any explanation of equipment.

## GOALS OF MECHANICAL VENTILATION

The following goals of artificial mechanical ventilation are based on the kinds of commitment, not specifically on disease entities. The accomplishment of the goals requires an accurate clinical assessment and intervention.

1. *To decrease the work of breathing for the patient.* Disease processes such as status asthmaticus, crushed chest injury, or respiratory distress syndrome increase the energy and oxygen consumption required for breathing. The patient uses more and more effort to ventilate his lungs. Increased use of the accessory muscles, intercostal retractions, nasal flaring, pursed-lip breathing, diaphoresis (sweating), tachypnea, and/or tachycardia may be observed.

Mechanical ventilation is used to prevent acute respiratory failure by intervening before the patient is completely exhausted. Early intervention with mechanical ventilation can reduce energy requirements and act as a temporary support so that the primary disease may be treated. Arterial blood gas values identifying respiratory insufficiency will indicate a decreased $P_aCO_2$ with an increased or normal pH and a decreased $P_aO_2$ (respiratory alkalosis with mild to severe hypoxia). For example, $P_aCO_2$ 28; pH 7.52; $P_aO_2$ 55.

2. *To ventilate the patient's lungs.* Effective ventilation is *always* a goal of mechanical ventilation. If the patient is suffering from respiratory failure, he is no longer able to produce the necessary inspiratory effort for adequate ventilation. Respiratory failure may result from severe acute or chronic respiratory diseases and may accompany or be accompanied by cardiac failure. Other contributing factors may include over-sedation, shock, anesthesia, and drug overdoses. Arterial blood gas measurements with respiratory failure indicate an increased $P_aCO_2$ with a decreased pH

and a decreased $P_aO_2$ (respiratory acidosis with severe hypoxia). For example, $P_aCO_2$ 58; pH 7.23; $P_aO_2$ 42.

3. *Improved oxygenation.* By effective mechanical ventilation of the lung, oxygenation of the blood can be improved with more appropriate matching of alveolar ventilation and pulmonary blood flow ($V/Q$ ratio). Increasing inspired oxygen concentrations delivered by mechanical ventilation also can improve diffusion and oxygenation. It should be noted that adequate oxygenation is most accurately evaluated by measuring arterial oxygen saturation and tension ($P_aO_2$), and effective ventilation is most accurately evaluated by measuring the $P_aCO_2$. These two values are evaluated individually to determine the adequacy of oxygenation and ventilation.

## THERAPEUTIC CONSIDERATIONS OF MECHANICAL VENTILATION

1. *Personnel and equipment.* Use of mechanical ventilation equipment demands respiratory care personnel with a thorough knowledge of and experience with critical care equipment and patient evaluation and observation techniques. Hospitals providing this type of patient care must have 24 hour respiratory care services and adequate equipment to provide effective mechanical ventilation. Laboratory and other support facilities also must be adequate to provide close clinical and laboratory testing.

2. *Accidental disconnection.* A mechanical ventilation system is a closed high-flow gas system; therefore, the patient will receive all of his ventilatory gas needs from the system. If for any reason the ventilation system fails to deliver gas to the patient or the patient becomes accidentally disconnected from the system, the results may be physically harmful and ultimately fatal to the critically ill patient. Disconnection should be limited to tracheostomy or endotracheal-tube care and airway suctioning. At least every two hours the entire physical ventilator system should be checked, including the equipment connection to the patient. It is recommended that alarm systems be used to continually monitor the ventilatory circuit and the patient connection.

3. *Cardiovascular effects.* Because of the possible cardiovascular effects of positive-pressure ventilation, the patient's cardiovascular status should be evaluated. Continuous electrocardiograms and periodic arterial blood pressures should be monitored to indicate any changes occurring while the patient is on mechanical ventilation.

4. *Infection control.* Infection control must be observed closely. Several sources of potential infection are associated with mechanical ventilation. There is the possibility of the transmission of microorganisms by the humidification system caused by the growth of microorganisms within the

water-filled reservoir. Also, since the artificial airway into the trachea bypasses the upper respiratory tract defenses, it increases the chance of infection. To limit possible cross-contamination and infection during mechanical ventilation, strict handwashing procedures should be followed. Only sterile techniques should be used with tracheostomy or endotracheal tube care. All equipment should be sterilized every 24 hours, and only sterile water and sterile equipment should be used in connecting the patient to the mechanical ventilation system.

5. *Spontaneous breathing.* Any patient effort to breathe must be coordinated with the mechanical ventilation system to reduce the detrimental effects of the patient "fighting" the ventilator. The synchronization of the patient's respiratory pattern and the ventilator must be evaluated with each ventilator check. It may be necessary to use drug therapy or supplemental methods such as assist-control or intermittent mandatory ventilation to provide an appropriate patient-ventilator interface.

6. *Closed system.* Artificial mechanical ventilation can be delivered most effectively through cuffed endotracheal or tracheostomy tubes. It is necessary to have such a closed system to assure the delivery of a specific tidal volume into the patient's lungs. The cuffed tube should be filled, using the minimum volume necessary to prevent a large leak from around the cuff. All therapeutic considerations and hazards of these artificial airways also must be considered during mechanical ventilation (see Chap. 7).

## HAZARDS OF POSITIVE-PRESSURE VENTILATION

1. *Pulmonary circulation.* Depending on the compliance of the lungs and the airway resistance, it is possible that the positive pressure during mechanical ventilation may have a detrimental effect on the pulmonary circulation. Excessive positive pressure can cause increased resistance in pulmonary vessels by over-distended alveoli expanded by the positive pressure. This can lead to increased pulmonary artery pressures producing shunting and increased cardiac work. The pulmonary circulation is affected most by the mean positive airway pressure and not by the peak positive airway pressure. This effect may be monitored by measuring the pulmonary arterial pressure. Normal pulmonary blood pressure is 25 mm Hg systolic and 8 mm Hg diastolic with a mean arterial pulmonary pressure of 15 mm Hg.

2. *Decreased cardiac output.* Transmission of positive pressure through the thoracic cage also can reduce the normal venous blood return to the right side of the heart, causing decreased cardiac output and possible systemic hypotension. Increased thoracic pressures also may cause cardiac tamponade. Depending on the health and age of the patient, such physical

insults of this type will be compensated by an increased pulse and blood pressure. The ability of the aged and critically ill to compensate is limited and a decrease in pulse and/or blood pressure may be observed.

Under normal circumstances, venous return to the heart is increased during inspiration because of the thoracic pump effect of the decreased pressure in the thoracic cavity. During positive-pressure ventilation, the inspiratory phase becomes a positive-pressure phase, and there is no longer a normal decrease in the pressure within the thoracic cavity. The normal thoracic pump effect is reduced or completely inhibited. Cardiac output and venous return may be effected and should be monitored by measuring arterial pressure and central venous pressure (CVP), pulse, and EKG. CVP measurement should be done with the patient off the ventilator, so that positive pressure ventilator cycling does not cause error in measuring.

3. *Systemic circulation.* The systemic circulation also may be affected by the positive pressure. The effects of positive pressure on the circulatory system may lead to a decreased renal output caused by inappropriate baroreceptor stimulation in the aortic arch. These baroreceptors note a decrease in blood volume with decreased cardiac output that may occur with positive-pressure ventilation. The message sent to the brain is evaluated and the decreased cardiac output is equated with a decreased blood volume that results in the release of ADH (antidiuretic hormone). This leads to a retention of body fluid by the kidney to increase blood volume. This condition should be monitored by measuring and comparing daily fluid intake and output and daily weight change.

4. *Cerebral circulation.* Cerebral circulation can also be influenced by mechanical ventilation. Changes in $P_aCO_2$ blood levels cause changes in cerebral blood flow. Decreases in $P_aCO_2$ cause cerebral vasoconstriction, and increases in $P_aCO_2$ cause cerebral vasodilation. These may be therapeutically beneficial in head injuries and stroke patients, but are unhealthy for all patients if the $P_aCO_2$ is extremely high or low. $P_aCO_2$ levels below 20 mm Hg increase the possibility of seizures or tetany and possible death.

5. *Pneumothorax.* The use of positive-pressure mechanical ventilation can cause a pneumothorax. The effects of excessive pressure and volume combined within the alveoli can lead to rupture of the membrane. This risk is reduced by using the lowest mean positive airway pressure possible to deliver the desired volume to the patient.

6. *Decreases in lung compliance.* The monotonous ventilatory pattern of artificial mechanical ventilation equipment can lead to a reduction in pulmonary tissue compliance. Periodic sighing (deep-breathing) of the patient using a resuscitating bag or a sigh hyperinflation mechanism within the ventilation system can help to reduce this by delivering an increased volume of gas periodically to re-expand dormant alveoli and stimulate the production of surfactant. Intermittent mandatory ventilation can also be used to provide periodic hyperinflation.

7. *Gastrointestinal distention and bleeding.* Many mechanical ventilation patients develop gastrointestinal bleeding. This is checked by monitoring the presence of blood in stools and gastric drainage. The presence of occult bleeding may indicate such a condition. Also, abdominal distention inhibits the downward movement of the diaphragm and appropriate lung expansion, increasing the pressure necessary to deliver the set volume to the patient. This should be monitored by daily measurement of the abdominal girth. Also, a nasogastric tube should be in place to allow air and gas to escape from the stomach.

## MECHANICAL VENTILATOR ADJUSTMENTS

The following are guidelines for initial ventilator control adjustments. Specific controls vary between different models of ventilators. (See Chap. 9 for specific lists of ventilator controls.)

### VENTILATOR SYSTEM COMPLIANCE CALCULATION

$$\text{System Compliance} = \frac{\text{Exhaled Tidal Volume (ml)}}{\text{Pressure Reading (cm } H_2O)}$$

*System compliance* is the factor that reflects the amount of gas compressed in the ventilator circuit for each centimeter of water pressure generated by the ventilator to deliver at set volume. This compliance factor will fluctuate and must be calculated with each ventilator circuit.

EXAMPLE: The ventilator tidal volume is set at 200 ml. With the patient connection occluded, a volume of 200 ml is measured at the exhalation port. The pressure manometer reading is 50 cm $H_2O$.

$$\text{System Compliance} = \frac{200 \text{ ml}}{50 \text{ cm } H_2O} = 4 \text{ ml/cm } H_2O = \text{System Compliance}$$

4 ml of gas volume is compressed in the tubing system for each centimeter of water pressure generated.

### COMPRESSED GAS VOLUME AND PATIENT TIDAL VOLUME CALCULATION*

Compressed Gas Volume = Pressure Manometer Reading × System Compliance

Patient Tidal Volume = Exhaled Tidal Volume – Compressed Gas Volume

*Patient Tidal Volume* is that gas volume delivered by the ventilator that actually is delivered to the patient's respiratory system.

---

*Exhaled tidal volume is more accurately measured directly at the patient connection by placing a respirometer in line momentarily. When measured directly the monitoring device can only be used with one patient until resterilized to avoid cross infection. Direct measurement also allows accurate measurements with IMV gas flow in the main patient circuit, and does not require calculation of the compressed gas volume to determine the actual patient tidal volume.

*For example;* if a ventilator is attached to a patient and a volume of 612 ml is measured at the exhalation port of the patient circuit and the pressure manometer reading is 30 cm $H_2O$, then:

Compressed Gas Volume = 30 cm $H_2O$ $\times$ 4 ml/cm $H_2O$

Compressed Gas Volume = 120 ml

Patient Tidal Volume = 612 ml − 120 ml

Patient Tidal Volume = 492 ml

During a delivery of 612 ml into this ventilator patient circuit that has a system compliance of 4 ml/cm $H_2O$ the volume compressed in the delivery circuit is 120 ml, therefore 492 ml is the actual patient tidal volume.

**1.** *Minute volume.* Minute volume equals tidal volume times respiratory rate: $(MV = V_T \times f)$ Tidal volume should be measured at the exhalation port or at the patient connection. Tidal volume should be measured as close to the patient as possible and should be measured on the exhalation side of the patient to judge the patient's exhaled gas volume. Minute ventilation is the most accurate calculation to monitor consistent lung ventilation, since it incorporates all changes in tidal volume and rate (see Table 8-1). A patient's approximate minute volume may be calculated from body surface area.

**TABLE 8-1**

**Minute Ventilation = Rate $\times$ Tidal Volume**

| | Tidal Volume | Rate | | Minute Ventilation | |
|---|---|---|---|---|---|
| A | ▨ 600 ml. | $\times$ 10 | = | ▨ 6000 ml | |
| B | ▨ 500 ml. | $\times$ 12 | = | ▨ 6000 ml | |
| C | ▨ 600 ml. | $\times$ 12 | = | ▨ 7200 ml | |

*A* and *B* show a constant minute ventilation through rate and tidal volume change. *C* reflects a change in minute ventilation (an increase) caused by a change of rate with no adjustment in tidal volume.

MINUTE VENTILATION CALCULATION

Minute Ventilation $(MV)$ = Body surface area $(m^2)$ $\times$ Conversion Factor

Conversion factor – female  3.5
male    4.0

Body surface area (BSA) calculated from DuBois nomogram (Table 8-2)

Ideal body weight = male 106 + (6 $\times$ no. inches over 5 ft.)
female 105 + (5 $\times$ no. inches over 5 ft.)

EXAMPLE: Height = 5 ft. 1 in.
Weight = 100 lbs.
Body surface area = 1.4 $m^2$
Patient sex = male
Ideal body weight = 106 + (6 $\times$ 1 in.) = 106 + 6 = 112

Minute Ventilation 1.4 $m^2$ $\times$ 4.0 = 5.6 LPM (5600 ml)

Tidal Volume = 112 lb $\times$ 4 ml/lb = 448 ml

Respiratory Rate 5600 ml $\div$ 448 ml = 12.5 (12) breaths per minute

*Respiratory rate.* The respiratory rate determines the number of respiratory cycles per minute of the ventilator. It is set by adjustment of the inspiratory time or inspiratory flowrate and expiratory time controls depending on the ventilator used. In the control ventilation mode, this would be the total number of respiratory cycles delivered by the ventilator per minute. If the ventilator is set so that the patient may assist, this may become the back-up rate for the patient. This rate is the total number of cycles per minute that the ventilator initiates without the assistance of the patient. For example, if the control rate of the ventilator is set at 10 but the patient is "triggering" the ventilator at 18 respiratory cycles per minute, then 10 becomes a back-up rate to reinforce the patient if he fails to create an inspiratory effort to cycle the ventilator on.

Setting the respiratory rate also determines the length of the respiratory cycle. For example, at a rate of 10, the respiratory cycle length is established at 6 sec or the rate of 10 divided into the 60 sec in 1 min. Normal adult respiratory rate is between 12 and 18 breaths per min, depending on age and physical health. As the person becomes older, his respiratory rate increases gradually. Respiratory rate is calculated by dividing predicted minute ventilation by tidal volume.

*Tidal volume.* Tidal volume determines the volume to be delivered from the mechanical ventilator to the patient. The normal adult tidal volume ranges from 3 to 4 ml per pound of ideal body weight. For example, if a patient weighs 100 lb, then he would have a tidal volume of between 300 and 400 ml. Tidal volume also may be calculated using the Radford nomogram (Table 8-3).

It must be considered that part of the gas volume delivered from the mechanical ventilator will be compressed within the tubing and the machine deadspace of the mechanical ventilator and will not go to the patient. This is described as *compressed* volume. This is relatively constant within the system and only fluctuates to a limited degree with the water level within the humidifier and temperatures in the ventilator system. The system compliance of the tubing is calculated by occluding the tubing at

# TABLE 8-2

## Dubois Body Surface Chart (As Prepared by Boothby and Sandlford of the Mayo Clinic)

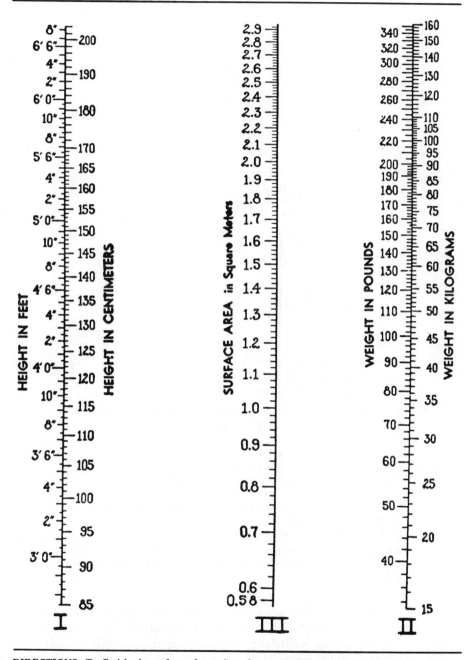

**DIRECTIONS:** To find body surface of a patient, locate the height in inches (or centimeters) on scale I and the weight in pounds (or kilograms) on Scale II and place a straight edge (ruler) between these two points which will intersect Scale III at the patient's surface area.

# TABLE 8-3

## Predicted Tidal Volumes (Radford Nomogram)*

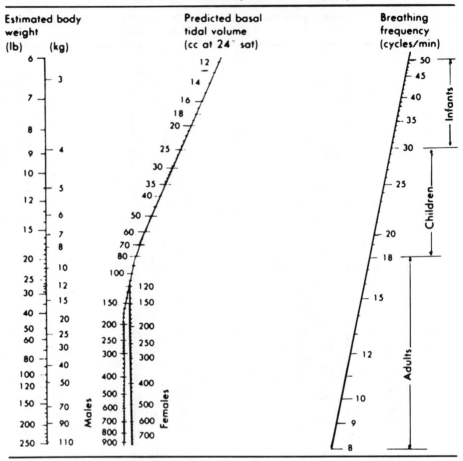

| Estimated body weight (lb) (kg) | Predicted basal tidal volume (cc at 24° sat) | Breathing frequency (cycles/min) |
|---|---|---|

Corrections of predicted basal tidal volumes.

For patients not in coma: add 10%

Fever: add 5% for each °F above 99 (rectal)
  add 9% for each °C above 37 (rectal)

Altitude: add 5% for each 2000 feet above sea level
  add 8% for each 1000 meters above sea level

Intubation: subtract volume equal to one half body weight in pounds
  subtract 1 cc/kg of body weight

Dead space: add equipment dead space

*(Adapted from Radford, E.P., et al. "Clinical use of a nomogram to estimate proper ventilation during artificial respiration." *New England Journal of Medicine,* vol. 21, no. 22, 1954, with permission.)

the patient connection and measuring the volume exhaled, while observing the pressure on the manometer on the ventilator. The amount of gas compressed in the ventilator depends on the specific ventilator design and patient circuit used. The specific tidal volume going to the patient should be measured with each ventilator check, and the compression factor for the tubing should be measured at least each time a new patient circuit is placed on the mechanical ventilator.

2. *Inspiratory/expiratory ratio (I:E ratio).* The inspiratory/expiratory ratio describes the relationship between the inspiratory time and the expiratory time. The normal I:E ratio for adults is 1:2 to 1:3. Physiologically, twice as much time is given for exhalation as for inhalation. A patient breathing 10 breaths per minute would have a total respiratory cycle of 6 seconds (60 sec divided by 10 breaths per minute). If the I:E ratio is 1:2, then the inspiratory time would be approximately 2 sec and the expiratory time 4 sec (6 ÷ 3 = 2 and 6 − 2 = 4). When a patient is on mechanical ventilation, the I:E ratio should be maintained near a normal 1:2 to 1:3 ratio. The I:E ratio must not be less than 1:1 when a patient is being supported solely by the mechanical ventilator. I:E ratio adjustment may be done by the combined adjustments of tidal volume, inspiratory time, and inspiratory flowrate.

Some mechanical ventilators have specific I:E ratio controls.

3. *Inspiratory flowrate.* Some mechanical ventilators are designed so that the flowrate varies automatically, while other ventilators incorporate a flowrate control that sets the peak inspiratory flowrate. Flowrate is equal to volume delivered per unit time (l/min. or ml/sec). The internal design of the ventilator system will vary the flow pattern delivered. (For flow-curve variations, see Chap. 9.) Adequate inspiratory flowrate must be provided to deliver the prescribed tidal volume in an inspiratory time that will maintain an I : E ratio for the patient at greater than 1 : 1 and preferably 1 : 2 or 1 : 3.

### CALCULATION OF THE MINIMUM GAS FLOWRATE REQUIRED IN A HIGH FLOW GAS SYSTEM

The minimum flowrate is calculated from the estimated peak inspiratory flowrate of the patient. For example:

A patient with the following clinical measurements:

| | |
|---|---|
| Respiratory rate | 15 |
| Tidal Volume | 600 ml |
| I:E (normal adult) | 1:2 |

Length of respiratory cycle = 60 sec/min ÷ 15 breaths/min = 4 sec

Inspiratory time = 4 sec ÷ 3 (based on the I:E ratio of 1:2) = 1.33 sec

Inspiratory flowrate = 600 ml/1.33 sec (amount of tidal inhaled during the inspiratory time)

Required inspiratory flowrate = 450 ml/sec

450 ml/sec × 60 = 27.0 l/min

Minimum flowrate into a high-flow system to meet the above tidal volume inspiratory flowrate at a 1:2 I:E ratio = 27.3 l/min

If the patient is assisting, then the minimum inspiratory flowrate must be high enough to meet the peak inspiratory demands of the patient, while still maintaining his I : E ratio above 1 : 1. The inspiratory flowrate needed will depend on the prescribed tidal volume and the respiratory rate of the patient-ventilator system.

4. *System pressure.* The pressure is the total system impedence to the movement of gas from the ventilator into the patient's lungs. It includes both airway resistance and lung compliance. When using a volume-cycled ventilator, the pressure must not be limited to a level below that necessary to deliver the preset volume. For example, if the ventilator requires a delivery pressure of 40 cm of water pressure to deliver a prescribed volume of 500 ml, then the pressure-limit control should not be set below 40 cm of water pressure. If the ventilator is a pressure-cycled ventilator, the upper pressure limits must be set so that the prescribed tidal volume is delivered at that pressure setting. Volume is only delivered until the preset pressure is reached. With a volume-cycled system, the pressure will vary, but the prescribed volume will always be delivered from the ventilator. With the pressure-cycled ventilator, the pressure is limited and preset and will not vary, and changes in airway resistance and compliance can reduce or increase the volume, varying the volume delivered to the patient. The most accurate measurement of proximal airway pressure is performed by recording the airway pressure at the patient connection.

The pressure limit on a volume-cycled ventilator should be set 10–15 cm above the cycling pressure required to deliver the prescribed volume (see the section on *Ventilator Monitoring* in this chapter). With the pressure-cycled ventilator and volume-cycled ventilator, the exhaled tidal volume of the patient should be measured with each ventilator check to determine the tidal volume being delivered.

5. *Inspiratory plateau.* This is created by temporarily holding the delivered tidal volume in the lung following the inspiratory cycle to allow more time for even distribution of gas throughout the lungs and equilibration of inspiratory pressures within the alveoli. This mechanism is used to enhance the recovery from and prevention of atelectasis. This control, when available on a ventilator, is used to momentarily prevent exhalation of tidal volume gases following end inspiration. This is sometimes described as prolonged inspiration or inspiratory hold. Inspiratory plateau settings range from 0.2 to 2 seconds. Adjustment of the inspiratory plateau control may affect either the inspiratory or the expiratory time, depending on the ventilator design.

6. *Sigh volume and frequency.* "Sighing" is the periodic delivery of increased gas volumes (greater than normal tidal volume) to hyperinflate the lung and reduce the monotony of set tidal breathing. During spontaneous breathing, such increased volumes are provided by individuals yawning, sighing, or deep breathing. When a patient is placed on a mechanical

ventilator, this periodic sighing or deep breathing is lost. It appears that this sighing increases the production of surfactant in the alveoli because of the elastic movement of Type II alveolar membrane cells. Some mechanical ventilators are equipped with sigh volume mechanisms. The periodic mechanical "sighing" also prevents peripheral milliary atelectasis that otherwise could develop with monotonous ventilation patterns. The sigh volume should be approximately 1.5 to 3 times the prescribed tidal volume. If the sigh mechanism is not incorporated into the ventilator design, then the patient should be hyperinflated periodically, or sighed, with a resuscitation bag. This should be done at least every hour if a sigh mechanism is not available. When hyperinflating a patient using a resuscitation bag, all prescribed levels of $FiO_2$ and PEEP should be maintained the same as on the mechanical ventilator. It is recommended that the patient be "sighed" at least every 4-6 minutes when using an automatic sigh mechanism.

7. *Humidification and temperature control.* All mechanical ventilators must have some type of heated humidification system. A humidifier rather than a nebulizer is preferred to limit the potential transport of microorganisms into the patient's lower respiratory tract. Adequate humidity will prevent dehydration and thickening of tracheal bronchial secretions. It is also necessary to provide heat to the inspired gas to limit both the humidity and temperature deficit of the dry medical gas. The gas should be delivered to the patient 100 percent saturated at a minimum temperature of 30°C (87°F) measured at the patient ventilator connection. Care also must be taken to prevent inhaled gas temperatures from exceeding 38°C. Above this temperature the gas may cause tracheal burns.

8. *Oxygen concentration.* Most modern ventilator systems have adjustable oxygen controls that provide consistent specific oxygen delivery to the patient. The amount of oxygen necessary in the inspired gas depends on the physiological need of the patient. Arterial blood gas values should be monitored to maintain the $PaO_2$ and the $SaO_2$ within normal or predetermined ranges.

9. *Positive-end expiratory pressure.* Positive-end expiratory pressure (PEEP) may be incorporated into mechanical ventilation systems to provide positive pressure in the lung throughout the expiratory phase of the mechanical ventilator. The presence of positive pressure during exhalation acts to stabilize the alveoli and prevent their collapse. Alveolar collapse at end exhalation is caused by diseases that affect the surfactant production of the alveoli, such as respiratory distress syndrome. PEEP creates a higher than atmospheric pressure and establishes a new pressure baseline above 0 cm $H_2O$ in the alveoli. The normal range of PEEP used is between 0 and 20 cm of water pressure. Physiologically, PEEP increases the functional residual capacity, increases alveolar ventilation and decreases pulmonary vascular resistance. It also improves the matching of ventilation with

pulmonary blood flow and by doing so, improves oxygenation of the arterial blood. Increases in $P_aO_2$ can allow lower oxygen concentrations to be used. When PEEP is used, consideration must be given to maintain cardiovascular integrity, with appropriate fluid levels and pharmacologic support as necessary.

10. *Alarm systems.* Mechanical ventilation systems should incorporate audible and visual alarms to act as immediate warning signals of abnormal and unwanted ventilator changes. Alarms are incorporated into mechanical ventilation systems to increase ventilator efficiency and patient safety. Low and high-pressure alarms and low-volume alarms act to assure appropriate delivery of the prescribed tidal volume. I:E ratio alarms guarantee at least a ratio of 1:1. An alarm system also should include oxygen alarms that warn of inappropriate oxygen concentrations. A final basic alarm is a fail-safe alarm, which must be battery-operated, to warn of a disconnected and unplugged ventilator.

## MAINTAINING MECHANICAL VENTILATION

Maintenance of mechanical ventilation requires 24-hour monitoring. Mechanical ventilation equipment must be checked physically and the patient-ventilator interface must be evaluated at least every two hours or whenever any changes occur. Monitoring of mechanical ventilation and the patient ventilator interface is based on change. Checks should be done to determine whether any desirable or undesirable changes have taken place. There should be a consistent monitoring pattern that is followed by all the respiratory-care personnel. Table 8-4 lists therapeutic parameters to be monitored with mechanical ventilation.

1. *Patient assessment.* With each check the patient's stability in relationship to mechanical ventilation should be evaluated. Personnel should be alert to changes in patient consciousness and awareness. This should include the patient's alertness to the respiratory therapist's or nurse's presence, the presence of the mechanical ventilator, and the patient's present hospital surroundings. If the patient is "fighting" the mechanical ventilator, the condition of the patient should be assessed so that corrections and adjustments can be made to the ventilator or reassurance be given to the patient to limit this struggling. A patient should never be allowed to struggle against the mechanical ventilator because of the dangers of pneumothorax, cardiovascular collapse, and airway trauma. If necessary pharmacological agents should be used to prevent "fighting." (Methods of coordinating patient and ventilator interface will be discussed later in this chapter.)

**TABLE 8-4**

**Frequency of Routine Monitoring of Patient Receiving Mechanical Ventilation**

| *Continuous* | *At Least Daily* | *At Least q2h* |
|---|---|---|
| EKG | – Hemoglobin and | – Blood pressure and pulse |
| | – Hematocrit | – Chest sounds |
| | | – Respiratory rate |
| Arterial pressure | – Weight | – Tidal volume |
| Ventilator alarms | – White blood count | – Minute ventilation |
| | – Electrolytes, BUN | – Effective dynamic compliance |
| | – Arterial blood gases (at | – Inspired oxygen concentration |
| | least once per day and | – Central venous pressure (left |
| | whenever ventilator is | atrial pressure) |
| | changed or clinical con- | – Ventilator settings and |
| | dition changes) | assembly |
| | – Chest x-ray | – System pressures |

2. *Equipment assembly and ventilator settings.* All connections of the ventilator system and all control settings should be inspected and recorded to note whether any accidental or prescribed changes have taken place. Movement of the patient, the heat from the system gas, and the accumulation of humidity and condensate may cause slipping or accidental twisting of patient-delivery tubing. These inconsistencies can be corrected with each ventilator check. Equipment assembly and control settings require close checking at least every two hours.

3. *Minute ventilation.* Minute ventilation may be measured at the exhalation port or the patient connection. The minute volume measured at the exhalation port of the mechanical ventilator will include both the patient's exhaled tidal volumes as well as the gas compressed within the mechanical ventilation system during the cycling of the ventilator. The compressed gas volume should be subtracted from the total exhaled volume at the exhalation port to determine the approximate exhaled minute volume of the patient. The minute ventilation and tidal volume measured directly from the artificial airway is most accurate. Minute ventilation or tidal volume may be calculated by counting the respiratory rate and using the following formula:

$$MV = V_T \times R$$

When using a volume-cycled ventilator, a drop in exhaled tidal volume may indicate a leak in the patient-delivery system such as at the humidifier or the tubing connection to the patient. Drops in exhaled tidal volume also will be seen when there is a leak around the artificial airway cuff or if there is a volume loss through chest tubes. Losses of volume should be carefully examined and corrected whenever possible. When using a pressure-cycled ventilator, a drop in exhaled tidal volume can be caused by a decrease in lung compliance or an increase in airway resistance. An increase in lung compliance and a decrease in airway resistance will be reflected in an increased exhaled tidal volume when the patient is on a pressure-cycled ventilator. One of the limitations of the pressure-cycled ventilator is that it cannot deliver a constant tidal volume to the patient as compliance and resistance change.

4. *Airway placement and patency.* With each ventilator check the artificial airway placement and patency should be assessed. Airway placement is checked by evaluating bilateral chest sounds, and routine examination of bilateral chest expansion. The evaluation of chest sounds should determine whether they have changed, are normal or abnormal, and absent or present. A chest x-ray should also be taken if there is any doubt as to adequate airway placement or patency.

Patient-ventilator connection also should be checked. The connection of the patient to the mechanical ventilator system should allow for movement of the patient's head and thoracic area and limit the amount of pressure that the equipment puts on the patient connection by pulling or unnecessary weight caused by position. Equipment should be checked to guarantee that the artificial airway is not in a position that may kink or occlude the airway or damage the tracheal wall. Need for suction also should be assessed and appropriate airway suctioning techniques should be followed.

5. *Airway pressure.* Peak inspiratory pressure should include both the dynamic and static measurements of pressure on the ventilator pressure manometer. The volume-cycled ventilator will have varying pressure readings depending on the amount of pressure it takes to deliver the prescribed tidal volume. Once the tidal volume has been set on the mechanical ventilator, the proximal airway pressure will be relatively constant. Increases in airway resistance and/or decreases in lung compliance will cause an increase in the pressure reading on the manometer, reflecting an increase in the amount of pressure needed to deliver the gas into the patient's lungs. This must be carefully evaluated and changes in pressure must be monitored with each ventilator check (see Table 8-5). High and low pressure alarms can be used to signal that there has been a change in airway pressure and that the system needs to be re-examined.

With a pressure-cycled mechanical ventilator, the pressure is preset and will remain constant. Any change in airway resistance or lung compliance will be reflected by a variation in the delivered tidal volume. If the patient becomes disconnected from the pressure-cycled ventilator, the ventilator will fail to cycle because the preset pressure will not be reached. This will vary depending on the model of the ventilator. (See Chap. 9.)

6. *Oxygen concentration.* The ventilator check should include oxygen analysis. The actual oxygen concentration delivered by the system should

## TABLE 8-5

### Causes of Pressure Manometer Changes

| *Increases in Pressure Reading* | *Decreases in Pressure Reading* |
|---|---|
| Build-up of secretions | Improvement in airway patency |
| Increase in secretion viscosity | Leak in patient delivery system |
| Obstruction of the artificial airway | Leak around the cuff of the artificial |
| Kinking of airway due to patient position | airway |
| Bronchospasms | Improvement of pulmonary |
| Atelectasis | condition |
| Consolidation | Disconnection of patient |
| Pulmonary edema | |
| Pleural effusion | |
| Patient "fighting" ventilation (usually causes rapid increase) | |
| Tension pneumothorax (usually causes rapid increase) | |

be analyzed to assure proper oxygen concentration delivered by the ventilator. An analyzer can be used in-line on the inspiratory side of the patient delivery tubing. Most ventilator systems do not have oxygen built-in analyzers, but actually have a mechanical apparatus to create an oxygen concentration calibrated to the dial on the control panel of the ventilator. Therefore, delivered gas concentration must be analyzed.

The example below describes the calculation of a ratio between the inspired oxygen concentration $(F_IO_2)$ and the arterial oxygen tension $(P_aO_2)$. The ratio of a healthy individual who is breathing room air would be 400–500. Unlike arterial-alveolar gradients, this ratio remains constant and can be used to compare $F_IO_2$ and $P_aO_2$.

CALCULATION OF $P_aO_2/F_IO_2$ RATIO

$$P_aO_2/F_IO_2 \text{ ratio} = \frac{P_aO_2}{F_IO_2}$$

i.e., $\quad P_aO_2 = 80 \text{ torr } F_IO_2 = 0.5 \quad \dfrac{80}{0.5} = 160$

$$P_aO_2/F_IO_2 \text{ ratio} = 160$$

*Positive End Expiratory Pressure.* Positive end expiratory pressure levels also should be carefully noted. The addition of positive end expiratory pressure will cause an increase in the pressure baseline of the ventilator when it cycles off. For example, if the patient is on a positive end expiratory pressure of +6, then the pressure necessary to deliver the volume during that cycle will be reflected by a change in pressure from the new baseline of +6 to whatever the peak inspiratory pressure reading is on the manometer.

If the positive end expiratory pressure appears to be decreasing, or "bleeding off" during the exhalation phase of the patient once it has been set, then there is a leak in the patient-ventilator system. This must be corrected for the prescribed positive end expiratory pressure to be delivered. A common cause of leaks in patients receiving positive end expiratory pressure is at the cuff site of the artificial airway.

7. *Arterial blood gas measurements.* Ideally, an arterial blood gas measurement should be obtained as normal baseline values prior to placing the patient on mechanical ventilation. This measurement would act as a guide to follow the progress of the therapy instituted. The pH and $P_aCO_2$ are correlated with minute ventilation. $P_aO_2$ and $S_aO_2$ and arterial oxygen content $(C_aO_2)$ are correlated with the $F_IO_2$ and PEEP that the patient is receiving. An arterial blood gas measurement should be measured within 1/2 hour of the initiation of mechanical ventilation and 1/2 hour after each mechanical ventilation setting change to determine the physiological effect. Small gradual changes may only require immediate observation of pulse, blood pressure, patient anxiety levels, and the patient's physical reaction but more accurate assessment requires blood gas analysis.

Placement of an arterial line into the radial or femoral artery is most efficient for measuring serial arterial blood gases in the critically ill patient because of the projected need for numerous samples to evaluate the patient's ventilation and oxygenation during the first 3–4 days of required therapy.

8. *Alveolar-arterial gradient.* The *A-a* gradient is a comparison of the oxygen tension within the alveoli and the oxygen tension within arterial blood and may be used in the clinical setting to evaluate the amount of shunting present in the cardiopulmonary system. The example below illustrates the calculations of *A-a* gradients using 100 percent $O_2$ and using the prescribed oxygen setting the patient is on. If possible, the *A-a* gradient should be determined using 100 percent $O_2$ with the patient inhaling this oxygen concentration for at least seven minutes prior to drawing of the arterial blood sample. The normal range of *A-a* gradient in a healthy individual is 30–50 mm Hg (on 100 percent $O_2$).

CALCULATION* OF *A-a* GRADIENT $(A\text{-}a\ DO_2)$
WITH 100% $O_2$

$$A\text{-}a\ DO_2 = P_AO_2 - P_aO_2$$

$$P_AO_2 = P_B - P_{H_2O} - P_aCO_2$$

$P_B$ equal atmospheric pressure in torr (760 torr at sea level)

$P_{H_2O} = 47$ torr BTPS

*Assume respiratory quotient (R) equals to 1.0.

EXAMPLE: If $P_aO_2 = 210$ torr, $P_B = 760$ torr, $P_aCO_2 = 40$ torr, $F_IO_2 = 1.0$ then,

$P_AO_2 = 760 - 47 - 40 = 673$ torr   $P_aO_2 = 210$      $673 - 210 = 463$

$A$-$a$ gradient = 463 torr

CLINICAL CALCULATION AT ANY OXYGEN CONCENTRATION:

$P_AO_2 = F_IO_2 (P_B - P_{H_2O}) - P_aCO_2$   $F_IO_2$ equal functional concentration of inspired oxygen

EXAMPLE: If $P_aO_2 = 210$ torr, $P_B = 760$ torr, $P_aCO_2 = 40$ $F_IO_2 = 0.6$ then,

$$P_AO_2 = 0.6 (760 - 47) - 40 = 428 - 40 = 388 = P_AO_2$$
$$= 388 - 210 = 178$$

$A$-$a$ gradient = 178 torr

9. *Arterial pressure.* An arterial line through the radial artery can be used to continuously monitor arterial pressure. Mean arterial pressure may drop with mechanical ventilation and especially with the application of positive end expiratory pressure. Mean arterial pressure ranges from 70–100 torr. Arterial pressure measurements are affected by blood volume, peripheral resistance, blood viscosities, and cardiac output. Changes in these parameters will be reflected in arterial pressure fluctuation. Table 8-6 indicates arterial pressure changes and the probable causes of those changes. A fall in arterial pressure also may be an early sign of a tension pneumothorax.

If an arterial line is not in place, systemic arterial pressure should be measured at least every two hours over the brachial artery using a sphyg-

TABLE 8-6

**Arterial Pressure Changes**

| Change in Pressure | Probable Cause |
| --- | --- |
| ↓ | Decreased blood volume |
| ↓ | Decreased cardiac output |
| ↓ | Decreased blood viscosity |
| ↓ | Decreased peripheral resistance |
| ↑ | Increased blood volume |
| ↑ | Increased cardiac output |
| ↑ | Increased blood viscosity |
| ↑ | Increased peripheral resistance |

momanometer. Systemic arterial pressures during systole and diastole measured with the sphygmomanometer range from 140/100 to 100/60 in the normal healthy patient.

**10.** *Pulmonary wedge pressure.* Pulmonary artery catheterization with a Swanz Ganz catheter will allow continuous monitoring of mixed venous oxygen and pulmonary artery wedge pressure. Mixed venous oxygen content is monitored to observe blood oxygen-level changes. The normal mixed venous oxygen content is 15 volumes percent. Pulmonary artery wedge pressure is monitored to observe pressure fluctuations. Wedge pressure approximates left atrial pressure and can be used as a guide to the appropriateness of blood volume, adequacy of the filling of the left ventricle, and/or the presence of left heart failure (see Table 8-7). Left-ventricle failure is reflected in a high left atrial pressure (greater than 13–15 torr). Wedge pressure measurements also can be used to estimate hydrostatic causes of pulmonary edema. Pulmonary edema occurs when pulmonary capillary pressures are greater than the colloid osmotic pressure (greater than 20–25 torr).

When a patient is on a mechanical ventilator, measurement should be done in the exhalation phase of the ventilator cycle. Each measurement should follow the same procedure to maintain consistency of results. It also should be noted that when a patient is on a positive end expiratory pressure greater than 10 torr, the pulmonary artery wedge pressure may not correlate well with the left atrial pressure.

**11.** *Central venous pressure.* Central venous pressure measurements estimate the proper functioning of the right heart and reflects the right-atrial filling pressure. Central venous pressure is measured through a catheter-manometer system that must be placed level to the patient's heart. The catheter is inserted into the superior vena cava. All manometer readings should be taken with the patient in the same position (usually flat in bed). Normally the central venous pressure ranges from 3–10 cm of water pressure. The central venous pressure reflects a combination of the adequacy of cardiac pumping action, blood volume, and vascular tone (see Table 8-8). The course of serial central venous pressure values is fol-

**TABLE 8-7**

**Changes in Pulmonary Wedge Pressure (PWP)**

| *Increased PWP* | *Decreased PWP* |
|---|---|
| Increased blood volume | Decreased blood volume |
| Increased pulmonary vascular resistance | Decreased pulmonary vascular resistance |
| Inadequate filling of left ventricle | Decreased cardiac output |
| Right and/or left heart failure | Decreased venous return |

**TABLE 8-8**

**Changes in Central Venous Pressure**

| *Increased CVP* | *Decreased CVP* |
|---|---|
| Increased blood volume | Decreased blood volume |
| Increased pulmonary vascular resistance | Decreased pulmonary vascular resistance |
| Increased vascular tone | Decreased vascular tone |
| Right and/or left heart failure | |

lowed to observe changes with disease development and/or mechanical ventilator adjustment.

**12.** *Humidification and gas temperature.* The ventilator check should include a check of the water level in the humidification equipment. The reservoir of the system must be kept full of water for the most efficient operation of the humidification system. The water and gas temperature in the humidifier should be adequate to provide a gas temperature at the patient connection of at least 30°C. Temperature of the inspired gas should be continually monitored with a temperature probe as close to the patient connection as possible.

Water condensing into the delivery tubing may create an obstruction of the gas flow and cause a sudden flooding of the trachea. This should be prevented by periodic draining of the tubing. Water should be drained during exhalation into an empty waste container or bucket.

**13.** *Positioning of the patient.* The patient's position should be changed on an hourly basis to provide better distribution of ventilation and perfusion within the lung and to limit the pooling of secretions. The patient should be sat up, turned from side to side, and turned to his back at least every four hours as tolerated. These position changes assure more effective ventilation of the lower lobes. Pooling of secretions and reduced ventilation lead to an increased possibility of pneumonia.

**14.** *Renal output.* The renal output and weight of the patient should be checked daily. These should be compared with daily intake and the previous days weight. The adult patient receiving parenteral nutrition can be expected to lose about 1/2 pound per day. Based on this information, a constant daily body weight would indicate fluid retention. An increase in body weight and interstitial pulmonary edema due to fluid retention are frequent problems with mechanical ventilation. Prevention and treatment is most successful with early recognition of renal output decreases and fluid build up. Renal output ranges from 1000–1500 ml per day in the normal patient and fluctuates with the patient on mechanical ventilation depending on the fluid input.

**15.** *Fluid and electrolyte balance.* (*See* Table 8-9.) Intracellular and extracellular ions must be within normal ranges for effective acid-base

**TABLE 8-9**

**Diagram of Normal Electrolytes Values**

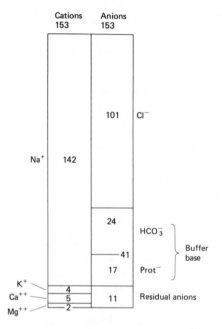

buffering, enzyme functioning, and muscle contraction. Measurement of electrolyte levels within the blood reflects the levels within the intracellular and extracellular body cavity. Sodium, potassium, chloride, calcium, and bicarbonate are especially important for acid-base and muscle function. Abnormal levels may lead to cardiac arrhythmia or standstill and acidosis or alkalosis. Increased electrolyte concentrations also may indicate reduced fluid level (hypovolemia) while decreases in their levels may indicate hypervolemia.

**16.** *Effective Compliance.* The tidal volume is the patient's exhaled tidal volume. This is minus the compressed gas volume in the patient circuit. The pressure is read from the ventilator pressure manometer. By momentarily occluding the exhalation valve and creating a pressure plateau at end inspiration, the pressure reading will represent the approximate pressure necessary to expand the lung with the delivered tidal volume. This is a static pressure reading when an inflation hold is used. A reading taken at peak inflation pressure also would include the pressure necessary to overcome airway resistance. By occluding the exhalation valve, the plateau inflation pressure is not influenced by airway resistance.

A dynamic airway pressure measurement may also be used to calculate the effective compliance, but it will include changes in airway resistance.

Effective Compliance = Tidal Volume (ml) ÷ pressure (cm $H_2O$)

Static compliance is normally larger than dynamic compliance and more meaningful. Static compliance ranges from 50–100 ml/cm of water pressure or 0.05 to 0.1 l/cm of water pressure. The routine measurement of either static or dynamic compliance allows the therapist to follow changes in the lung and is a valuable information source for monitoring therapy. Compliance should be calculated at least every two hours.

Static compliance also is useful in identifying optimal levels of PEEP. Optimal levels of PEEP can be established at levels which result in the highest values of lung compliance.

**17.** *Deadspace measurement.* The physiological deadspace represents wasted ventilation occurring within the lung. This deadspace or $V_D/V_T$ is measured by collecting a 3–5 minute sample of exhaled gas in a reservoir and by measuring the $P_E CO_2$ of this sample. Arterial $P_a CO_2$ should also be measured simultaneously. The deadspace ratio is then calculated with the following formula:

$$V_D/V_T = \frac{P_a CO_2 - P_E CO_2}{P_a CO_2}$$

Physiological deadspace increases with respiratory disease. These increases are normally caused by development of alveolar deadspace due to airway obstruction or shunting within the cardiopulmonary system. The normal range of physiological deadspace is between 0.25 and 0.4 of the patient's tidal volume. In the clinical situation, if carbon dioxide production and delivered tidal volume remain unchanged, then increases in respiratory rate and minute ventilation required to maintain a constant $PaCO_2$ indicate increases in physiological deadspace.

## CHANGES IN MECHANICAL VENTILATION

The adjustment of mechanical ventilation controls are prescribed to provide effective ventilation and adequate oxygen to the patient. Ideally, only one parameter of mechanical ventilation should be changed at a time to evaluate the effect of each change. All major changes in mechanical ventilation should be done in conjunction with the measurement of arterial-blood gases 20 to 30 minutes after the change. Table 8-10 lists changes in mechanical ventilation with the predicted results of change in $P_a CO_2$ and $P_a O_2$. These mechanical ventilator changes are described in the following section.

### Changes to Increase $P_a CO_2$

An increase in $P_a CO_2$ in the arterial blood will cause an increase in the hydrogen ion concentration, which is reflected by a decrease in pH. The

TABLE 8-10

Predicted Arterial Blood Gas Changes with
Mechanical Ventilator Adjustments

| *Decrease* $PCO_2$ | *Increase* $PCO_2$ |
|---|---|
| Increase respiratory rate | Decrease respiratory rate |
| Increase tidal volume | Decrease tidal volume |
| Remove mechanical deadspace | Add mechanical deadspace |
| | |
| *Decrease* $PO_2$ | *Increase* $PO_2$ |
| Decrease $F_IO_2$ | Increase $F_IO_2$ |
| Decrease PEEP | Increase PEEP |

following mechanical ventilator adjustments should cause an increase in $P_aCO_2$.

1. *Decrease minute ventilation.* Changes in ventilation that decrease the minute ventilation may be completed by reducing the patient's tidal volume or decreasing the patient's total respiratory rate. A decrease in the minute alveolar ventilation of the patient causes an increase in arterial $PCO_2$.

Regulating the respiratory rate of the mechanical ventilation system of the patient is the most effective means of altering $P_aCO_2$. A decrease in the patient tidal volume also may reduce the matching of alveolar ventilation with pulmonary perfusion, and, therefore, cause a change in arterial oxygen levels that may not be desirable.

Ideally, changes in tidal volume should be made in increments of 50–75 ml and changes in respiratory rate should be limited to increments of 2–3 cycles per minute. This allows gradual physiological adjustment with each change. All these changes should be monitored by evaluation of pulse, blood pressure, and patient observation and by arterial blood gas measurements.

2. *Add mechanical deadspace (see Fig. 8-1).* A tubing extension may be placed between the patient's delivery connection and the artificial airway to increase the amount of total deadspace of the patient's cardiopulmonary system. This increases the mixing of exhaled carbon dioxide with the inhaled gas from the mechanical ventilator, and, therefore, increases the alveolar $PCO_2$ concentration with the arterial $P_aCO_2$. This only occurs if the patient's minute ventilation remains constant. If the patient is assisting on the mechanical ventilator and increases his respiratory rate, the placement of deadspace on the mechanical ventilator is compensated and the $P_aCO_2$ remains the same. The advantage is that it allows the patient to continue to create his own inspiratory effort and maintain central nervous system stimulation of respiration. Mechanical deadspace should be

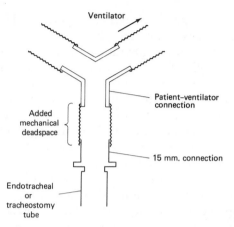

**FIG. 8-1.** Mechanical deadspace.

added in increments of 25–50 ml and monitored by arterial blood gas measurements.

### Changes to Decrease $P_aCO_2$

Decreases in arterial carbon dioxide tension cause a decrease in the hydrogen ion concentration of the blood which is reflected by an increase in pH. The following mechanical ventilator changes may be made to cause a decrease in arterial carbon dioxide tension:

1. *Increased minute ventilation.* The minute ventilation of the patient is raised by increasing the patient's tidal volume or increasing the patient's total respiratory rate. An increase in alveolar ventilation causes a reduction of alveolar $PCO_2$ and therefore a decrease in arterial $PCO_2$.

Patients on controlled mechanical ventilation may have their tidal volume or total respiratory rate increased by a definite ventilator control. When the patient is assisting on mechanical ventilation, the patient will establish his own respiratory rate and the tidal volume control may be used to decrease the $P_aCO_2$ by increasing the delivered tidal volume. $P_aCO_2$ will decrease only if the patient does not decrease his total minute ventilation by reducing his own respiratory rate.

2. *Reduced mechanical deadspace.* If it is present this should be the first change that should be done to reduce the $P_aCO_2$. If any mechanical deadspace has been placed within the patient ventilator delivery system, it should be removed to limit the patient deadspace and decrease the mixing of exhaled carbon-dioxide tension with the inhaled gas.

### Changes to Increase $P_aO_2$

These changes are made to maintain the patient within a "normal" range of $P_aO_2$ (in healthy individuals 80–100 torr, in the chronic respiratory disease patient, 40–60 torr).

1. *Increase the inspired oxygen concentration ($F_IO_2$)*. The need for an increase in oxygen tension is indicated when the $P_aO_2$ falls below the patient's normal range. In healthy individuals the normal range is greater than 80 torr. Changes in $F_IO_2$ should be done in increments of 0.1 to 0.2 (10-20 percent) $O_2$ concentration levels. All changes should be monitored by arterial blood gas analysis 20-30 minutes following the change. Increases in inspired oxygen concentration will not greatly increase the arterial oxygen tension when significant shunting is present within the respiratory system. If arterial oxygen does not increase with increases in inspired oxygen, PEEP should be used.

2. *Increased positive end expiratory pressure (PEEP)*. Positive airway pressure exerted throughout the respiratory system during the expiratory phase of the patient prevents the alveolar collapse. PEEP improves the matching of alveolar ventilation with pulmonary perfusion by reducing the shunting within the cardiopulmonary system. It also increases the functional residual capacity, returning it to normal. It is used with mechanical ventilation to supplement and reduce the oxygen concentration necessary to maintain a normal $P_aO_2$. PEEP is indicated when the $F_IO_2$ required to maintain a normal $P_aO_2$ is greater than 0.5 (50 percent). PEEP can be changed in increments of 3-5 cm of water pressure with the continual monitoring of pulse, arterial pressure, and cardiac rhythm. Changes in PEEP also should be followed within 20-30 minutes by arterial blood gas measurements. High levels of PEEP may require the administration of cardiovascular drugs to support the circulatory system.

## Changes to Decrease $P_aO_2$

1. *Decrease the inspired oxygen concentration ($F_IO_2$)*. Decrease in arterial oxygen tension is required as the patient's respiratory disease is reduced and normal lung function returns. The inspired oxygen concentration should be decreased in increments of 0.1 to 0.2 (10-20 percent). Again, arterial blood gases, pulse, arterial pressure, and cardiac rhythm is monitored with all changes in inspired oxygen concentration.

2. *Decrease positive end expiratory pressure (PEEP)*. As surfactant production and alveolar stability returns to normal, the need to maintain a specific level of PEEP is reduced. This allows a decrease in PEEP as the $P_aO_2$ is maintained within a normal range by an $F_IO_2$ less than 0.5. If the reduction of positive end expiratory pressure causes a drop in the $P_aO_2$, then the alveoli may still be unstable, collapsing upon exhalation. The PEEP should be returned to its original level. Also, if the pulse or arterial pressure changes by more than 20 beats per minute or 20 mm Hg with a change in PEEP, it should be returned to its original level. This also requires close monitoring of arterial pressure and cardiac pulse and rhythm.

## METHODS OF SYNCHRONIZING THE
## PATIENT WITH MECHANICAL VENTILATION

When a patient is placed on a mechanical ventilator, his inspiratory effort should be evaluated. If he is able to produce an inspiratory effort, then the mechanical ventilator should be coordinated with the patient's effort to provide smooth delivery and acceptance of ventilation. The following are methods to synchronize patient effort and ventilator cycling.

### Intermittent Mandatory Ventilation

Intermittent mandatory ventilation (IMV) flow systems are incorporated in ventilator delivery circuits' to allow the patient to continue spontaneous breathing with only periodic volumes of gas being delivered by the mechanical ventilator (Fig. 8-2). These high gas-flow systems are used with a set gas volume being delivered at a set time from the mechanical ventilator into the patient's circuit. The ventilator's cycling sensitivity is reduced so that the patient cannot "trigger" the ventilator. The patient must accept the ventilator "breath" when it is delivered. Some IMV systems allow the patient to "trigger" the mechanical ventilator to cycle to inspiration. These are described as intermittent demand ventilation.

The mechanical ventilator rate is set to support the patient's ventilatory needs. This is the rate the patient requires in addition to his own

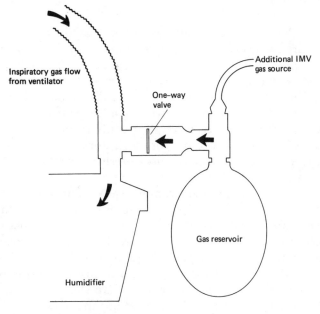

Inspiratory gas flow from ventilator

Additional IMV gas source

One-way valve

Gas reservoir

Humidifier

**FIG. 8-2.** IMV connection.

respiratory rate to maintain his normal $P_aCO_2$. The patient may breathe spontaneously through the high-flow gas system and at his own respiratory rate and depth of ventilation. At set intervals the mechanical ventilator will cycle on, delivering a prescribed tidal volume into the ventilator system and to the patient. For example, if the ventilator rate is set at 12 cycles per minute, the ventilator will deliver a set tidal volume every 5 sec. Between the ventilator cycles, the patient may breathe spontaneously through a high-flow system. The oxygen concentration in the high-flow gas system must be maintained at the same gas concentration as the mechanical ventilator. An IMV system allows the patient to continue to actively use his respiratory muscles, and it can reduce the total work of breathing for the patient.

IMV should be monitored the same as a mechanical ventilator. Arterial blood gases should be measured with all changes in IMV settings or changes in clinical conditions of the patient. The IMV rate should have to be changed to maintain the $P_aCO_2$ within a normal range. As the patient's respiratory disease improves, the rate may be reduced gradually to a rate near zero when the patient no longer requires mechanical ventilator or IMV assistance. Removal also may be done between rates of 2–4 cycles per minute, but this will depend on patient tolerance and his physical condition.

## Assist Mode of Ventilation

Ventilators may also be coordinated with the patient's inspiratory effort by adjusting the sensitivity control to allow the patient to "trigger" the mechanical ventilator to cycle to inspiration. It should be adjusted so that the inspiratory effort between –1 to –3 cm of water pressure is required to cycle on the ventilator. This mode of ventilator cycling allows the patient to create his own inspiratory effort and set his own respiratory rate, although he receives all breaths from the ventilator. An assist mode allows the patient to use his respiratory muscles for initial "cycling on" of the ventilator, but it requires passive acceptance of the volume once the ventilator is cycled on.

When using the assist mode, a back-up control rate should always be set on the mechanical ventilator. For example, if the patient is breathing on his own at a total respiratory rate of 16 breaths per minute, then a control rate should be set between 10 and 12 breaths per minute to act as a back-up rate in case of apnea or sedation. This control rate set lower than the patient's assisting rate will prevent respiratory embarrassment if apnea should occur. The reserve rate should be set 4–5 cycles per minute less than the total respiratory rate of the patient.

## CONTROLLING THE PATIENT
## ON MECHANICAL VENTILATION

1. *Reassurance.* The most important form of controlling or coordinating a patient on a mechanical ventilator is to reassure the patient of the temporary support of the mechanical ventilator and to instruct him in the reason for the use of the mechanical ventilator and its importance to his treatment. The patient should be encouraged to relax and allow the mechanical ventilator to move gas into his lungs.

2. *Hyperinflation.* Another method of coordinating patient effort and preventing or limiting the amount of "fighting" that the patient does on the ventilator is the use of a combination of a greater than predicted patient tidal volume (greater than 3-4 ml/lb) and a reduced respiratory rate. This is used to maintain the patient's predicted minute ventilation and also to reduce the inspiratory stimulus going to the central nervous system from the respiratory system. A reduction in inspiratory stimuli occurs with the stretching of alveoli with the larger than normal tidal volume. The Hering-Breuer stretch receptors in the alveoli are stimulated more by using large tidal volumes, therefore, reducing central nervous system inspiratory stimuli.

3. *Eliminate hypoxic drive.* Patients with chronic respiratory disease that have developed hypoxic drive as a respiratory stimuli may be controlled on a mechanical ventilator by increasing the inspired oxygen concentration until the patient's arterial oxygen tension levels rise above a point greater than his normal hypoxic drive oxygen level. This low oxygen stimulus to breathe is taken away by the increased $P_aO_2$ that is maintained above his physiological oxygen needs. For example, if the patient's $P_aO_2$ is normally 45 torr and a $P_aO_2$ of 60 torr is maintained in the blood, then his need to breathe will be reduced and he will better accept the mechanical ventilator. This method of control requires cautious application and can encourage patient dependence on the mechanical ventilator. Chronic lung disease patients very rapidly become psychologically and physically dependent on positive pressure ventilation; therefore, the use of this method should be limited in the amount of time that the patient is exposed to it. The $P_aO_2$ should be kept below 100 torr in the chronic lung patient to reduce the possibility of oxygen toxicity. This method of control will have little effect on the patient that has a normal $P_aCO_2$ drive.

4. *Reduced carbon dioxide levels.* With a patient who has a normal carbon dioxide respiratory drive, hyperventilation may be used. This reduces arterial carbon dioxide tension, and, therefore, reduces the respiratory stimulus to breathe. The $P_aCO_2$ should never be reduced below 25 torr under any circumstances. Use of this method of hypocapnea can cause tetany and coma and can lead to death if $P_aCO_2$ levels are

allowed to decrease less than 25 torr. This method of controlling the patient must be administered with great care and close monitoring of the patient through pulse, blood pressure, respiratory rate, and periodic measurement of arterial carbon-dioxide tension.

5. *Use of pharmacological agents.* If the patient must be "controlled" to synchronize him with the mechanical ventilator, drugs also may be used to relax and/or sedate the patient. Central nervous-system depressants and paralyzing agents can eliminate all patient inspiratory effort and patient movement, allowing passive mechanical ventilation of the patient's lungs. Their effect depends on the drug and the dosages. (see Chap. 4).

## WEANING FROM MECHANICAL VENTILATION

The process of removing a patient from mechanical ventilation is affected by the length of time the patient has been on the mechanical ventilator, his present physical condition, his disease process, and whether or not patient has developed any psychological dependence on the ventilator. When weaning a patient from a mechanical ventilator, the patient's readiness for removal from the ventilator must be evaluated. Weaning should always be started in the morning when the patient is rested and more alert and never late at night following a full day of activity. The following section describes guidelines for patient removal from mechanical ventilation.

1. *Observations.* As the patient is examined with each mechanical ventilator check, an increased effort by the patient to ventilate himself will be noted as his condition improves. Changes of awareness should also be noted. Improvement in physical condition and reduction of the disease process are indications of a decreasing need for mechanical ventilation. A reduction in the amount and viscosity of pulmonary secretion also will decrease the patient's work of breathing.

2. *Measured parameters.* Table 8-11 lists parameters to estimate the patient's ability to be removed from the ventilator and the chances of the patient's staying off the ventilator. The therapist or nurse must realize that these are estimates and that weaning requires close monitoring for the success of the process. As the measured parameters of the patient approach the normal ranges, the need for mechanical ventilation decreases. Patients within the range of the measured parameters on Table 8-10 will have the best chance of successful weaning from mechanical ventilation.

3. *Disease process.* For removal of mechanical ventilation to be successful, the initial cause that required the patient to be placed on mechanical ventilation system must be resolved. An example is severe pneumonia.

TABLE 8-11

**Weaning Parameters: Physiological Parameters to Estimate Patient Ventilatory Reserve**

| Parameter | Range |
|---|---|
| Respiratory rate | Less than 25 breaths per minute |
| Vital capacity* | Greater than 10 ml/kg or at least 3 $\times$ predicted normal tidal volume |
| Tidal volume* | 3–4 ml/lb. |
| Inspiratory effort | Greater than –30 mm Hg |
| $A\text{-}a$ $DO_2$ ($A\text{-}a$ gradient) | Less than 350 torr |
| $V_D/V_T$ ratio | Less than 0.5 |
| $F_IO_2$ | Less than 0.5 |
| PEEP (C.P.A.P.) | Less than +5 cm $H_2O$ |
| $P_aO_2/F_IO_2$ ratio | Greater than 150 |

*Measured during spontaneous ventilation after patient has been off mechanical ventilation for at least one half a minute.

This leads to respiratory failure and requires the reduction of the infection to provide the patient with adequate amounts of energy to ventilate his own lungs again. Therefore, the disease process must be considered before weaning takes place. The disease must be eliminated or reduced to the point that the patient can again support himself with his own ventilatory muscles without the assistance of a mechanical ventilator system.

## Methods of Weaning

**Patient Triggering of Mechanical Ventilation**: By allowing the patient to create his own inspiratory effort to cycle on the mechanical ventilator, the patient can use his own neuromuscular system to initiate inspiration. This is limited, but can benefit the patient who has been totally controlled on the mechanical ventilator. It also allows him to take an active part in coordinating his ventilatory pattern and to become accustomed to initiating ventilation. This is especially needed in patients that have been on long-term mechanical ventilatory support. It is recommended that patients not be placed on totally controlled ventilation. They should be allowed to assist as much as possible so that the central nervous sytem, respiratory coordination, and respiratory muscle tone will not be altered any more than necessary on the mechanical ventilator system.

**Periodic Removal of Mechanical Ventilation**: The following is a procedure for periodic removal from mechanical ventilation after the measured parameters (see Table 8-11) have been evaluated and satisfactorily met:

1. *Preparation and explanation.* The therapist or nurse should explain to the patient the procedure that is to be followed. During the entire process,

the patient is to be encouraged. A high-flow gas system should be set up with humidified oxygen at the same oxygen concentration or higher than that of the ventilator to assure adequate oxygen delivery during removal. If possible, the patient should be positioned in a semi-Fowler's position to allow for more effective use of his respiratory muscles. The patient should understand the possibility of feeling "tightness" in his chest and the need for an increased effort to breathe. It should be reinforced that these are normal. A therapist or nurse should be present at all times to make sure that the patient is ventilating himself adequately. Periodic weaning from mechanical ventilation often requires a series of trials to be successful. The patient should be informed that it may require several trials.

2. *Removal from the ventilator.* When the patient is removed from the mechanical ventilator, he should be connected to the humidified oxygen source immediately. He also may be ventilated with a resuscitating bag as he is removed from the mechanical ventilator, reducing the trauma of removal and gradually changing him from a system of total mechanical ventilation to one of spontaneous ventilation. This may be done over a $\frac{1}{2}$-1 minute period of time as needed. The therapist or nurse must closely monitor the patient's reactions and reassure the patient's efforts during this initial removal from the ventilator.

3. *Cardiopulmonary monitoring.* As the patient is removed from the ventilator, his electrocardiogram and arterial pressure should be monitored. If premature ventricular contractions (PVCs) or other arrythmias appear, the patient should be returned to mechanical ventilation immediately. Normally, there will be a slight increase in cardiac rate and blood pressure to compensate for the cardiovascular changes that accompany mechanical ventilation. In addition, the patient's respiratory rate is usually more rapid and the depth of respirations more shallow because of the past effects of the mechanical ventilator.

4. *Length of removal.* The length of removal from mechanical ventilation may be only 3-5 minutes initially, depending on the patient's tolerance. Vital signs must remain stable or the patient should be placed back on the mechanical ventilator immediately. As the patient continues to remain stable, the length of removal of the mechanical ventilator can be lengthened. For example, intervals prescribed for removal of mechanical ventilation can be from 3-5 min every $\frac{1}{2}$-1 hr. The patient no longer requires mechanical support when he can maintain his normal arterial blood gas values.

5. *Cardiopulmonary evaluation.* During initial weaning time, the patient's pulse, respiratory rate, and blood pressure should be measured every five minutes. Once the patient has been off the ventilator for at least 15 minutes with stable vital signs, arterial blood gases should be measured. The vital capacity should be measured after the patient has been removed from the ventilator for three minutes and then every five minutes there-

after until the patient is stable. This will estimate the ventilatory reserve that the patient can maintain. The ability of the patient to maintain himself depends on his physical condition and his psychological readiness for removal.

Weaning the patient from a ventilator also may be a process of decreasing drug therapy that has prevented him from using his own respiratory muscles. This type of weaning may require only initial evaluation of his cardiopulmonary parameters, as described in Table 8-10, followed by removal from the ventilator to a humidified oxygen source. This situation often occurs with post-operative patients. As the "controlling" drugs are stopped, the patient's ventilatory abilities return. In patients such as the chronic obstructive lung disease patient or the severe multiple-trauma patient suffering from flail chest, the gradual removal of long-term mechanical ventilator support may require days to weeks.

**Intermittent Mandatory Ventilation (IMV):** IMV allows the patient to use his own respiratory muscles and coordinate his own inspiratory effort and depth of ventilation with only minimum support by mechanical ventilator. Care must be taken to assure that the patient coordinates his efforts with the mandatory ventilator tidal volume and that the patient is not struggling against the ventilator. Patients are weaned gradually by reducing the ventilator rate. The following are therapeutic considerations of IMV:

1.  Using an IMV system the patient can use his own respiratory muscles and central nervous system respiratory centers to regulate respiration. The IMV can be used to wean patients from long-term mechanical ventilatory support, providing gradual strengthening of muscular function. It is also considered a mode of mechanical ventilation and is used as initial ventilatory support as described in an earlier section of this chapter.

2.  The ventilator rate of the IMV system is initially set lower than the patient's respiratory rate to act as reinforcement of the patient's ventilatory effort. The correct IMV rate is determined by the arterial $PCO_2$. If the $P_aCO_2$ is less than 35, then the rate set may be reduced to bring the arterial $P_aCO_2$ within normal range. If it is greater than 45, it should be increased to reduce the $P_aCO_2$ within normal range. If the patient is a chronic obstructive lung disease patient, the rate should be adjusted to bring the $P_aCO_2$ within the "normal" range of the patient receiving the therapy. The rate of the IMV system should be reduced in increments of 1–3 cycles per minute.

3.  The IMV high-flow gas system should have a flow at least two times the patient's peak inspiratory flowrate or 3–4 times their minute ventilation. (See section on *High-Flow Gas Systems* in Chap. 1.) Inadequate flow is indicated by a pull of greater than 2 cm of negative water pressure during spontaneous breathing on the IMV system.

## POST-VENTILATORY CARE

1. *Observation.* It is critical that the patient receive close monitoring of his cardiopulmonary status following mechanical ventilation discontinuance. Continual measurement of electrocardiogram and arterial pressure should be done. The EKG, arterial pressure, and arterial blood gases should remain stable or continue to improve as the patient's disease is resolved.

2. *Breathing exercises.* Cough training, chest percussion, and postural drainage should be prescribed as necessary to assist the patient with removal of secretions, and breathing exercises and general muscle exercise should be used to return respiratory muscle tone and coordinate efficient breathing patterns.

3. *Airway removal.* The artificial airway should be removed as soon as possible to reduce the presence of this artificial airway restriction and the hazards of the artificial airway. If the mechanical ventilator system was the only purpose of the artificial airway, then extubation may follow immediately.

## EMERGENCY CARDIOPULMONARY CARE (CPR)

Emergency cardiopulmonary care is an essential part of critical patient care. It is necessary to immediately intervene in life-threatening situations to prevent death from cardiac or respiratory arrest. The therapist and nurse must be fully trained to provide this emergency care. Basic life support is an emergency first-aid procedure that consists of recognizing respiratory and cardiac arrest and initiating the proper application of cardiopulmonary resuscitation to maintain life until advanced support systems may be instituted. Cardiopulmonary resuscitation is indicated in the presence of respiratory and cardiac arrest.

*Clinical Death* occurs immediately. The therapist or nurse must be able to identify respiratory and cardiac arrest. The signs of clinical and biological death are listed on Table 8-12. Clinical death is recognized by

**TABLE 8-12**

**Signs of Clinical and Biological Death**

| Clinical Death | Biological Death |
|---|---|
| Occurs immediately | Occurs 4–6 minutes after clinical death |
| Heartbeat not audible | Irreversible damage to heart and brain tissue |
| Pulse not palpable | Nonreactive, fixed, dilated pupils |
| Breathing not detectable | |

the absence of audible heartbeat and the absence of breathing. Pulse will not be palpable apically or at the carotid artery. *Biological Death* occurs within 4-6 minutes after clinical death; if it is not resolved, irreversible brain damage and heart damage will occur. Patients that suffer biological death will have nonreactive fixed and dilated pupils within one minute after anoxia within the body.

## Steps in Cardiopulmonary Resuscitation

The steps below are followed in cardiopulmonary resuscitation.

1. Evaluate unresponsiveness (shout and shake patient)
2. Open the airway (head tilt maneuver)
3. Check for and identify the absence of breathing
4. Initial ventilation given if necessary (four rapid, deep breaths)
5. Remove any airway obstruction
6. Check for and identify the absence of pulse (carotid or apical pulse)
7. Initiate cardiac compression if necessary (60 compressions per per minute)
8. Continue cardiopulmonary resuscitation (adult ratio one ventilation for each five cardiac compressions with two rescuers)
9. Assessment of patient's response to CPR

Figure 8-3 is a systematic approach to this CPR procedure. The following describes the steps of CPR:

1. *Evaluate responsiveness.* Upon the initial recognition of a patient who is thought to have suffered a cardiopulmonary arrest, the therapist or nurse must make sure that the patient has suffered an arrest. When approaching the victim, they should grab him by the shoulders and shake him shouting, "Are you okay?" and turn him onto his back. Cardiopulmonary resuscitation should never be performed on a patient who is alert and who has not suffered a cardiopulmonary arrest. If the patient is asleep, unconscious, or has fainted, the initial step is to determine his present consciousness and his responsiveness.

2. *Opening the airway.* If the patient does not respond to tactile and verbal stimulation, then the patient should be placed so that his airway is open by tilting the head backward as far as it will go. With the patient on his back, one hand should be placed beneath the patient's neck and the other hand on his forehead. The therapist or nurse should be kneeling beside the patient and the hand under the neck should be lifted up to extend the neck and bring the patient's head into an extended position. The patient's head should be maintained in this position at all times. Opening the airway in this manner may be all that is required for the

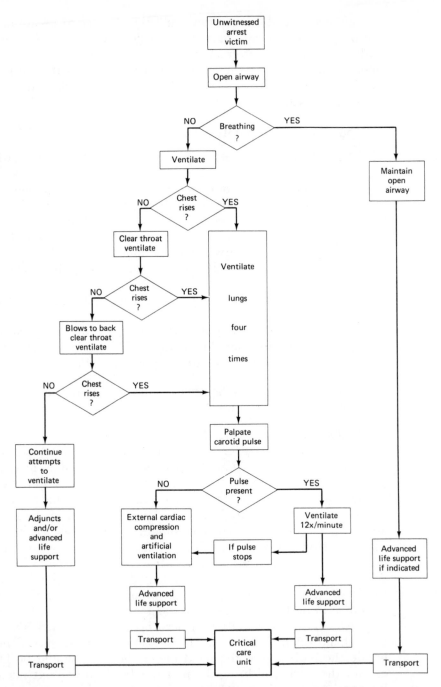

**FIG. 8-3.** System approach to the CPR. (*Adapted from "Standards for Cardiopulmonary Resuscitation and Emergency Cardiac Care," JAMA, 227:7, Feb. 1974, p. 833, with permission.*)

patient. This maneuver is described as the head-tilt maneuver which is illustrated in Fig. 8-4.

3. *Check for absence of breathing.* At this time, initial assessment of the absence of breathing must be done. The rescuer places his ear over the patient's mouth and nose, looking toward the patient's chest and stomach. He should listen and feel for breathing, which will be indicated by either the movement of air or the warmth that is felt by the rescuer's ear. It is important to remember that the patient may be able to make respiratory efforts and still have his upper airway obstructed.

4. *Initiate ventilation.* If the patient is not breathing, then the patient should immediately be given four rapid, deep breaths, not allowing exhalation to take place between the breaths. This may be done with either a manual resuscitating bag or by mouth-to-mouth, mouth-to-stoma, or mouth-to-artificial airway. With resuscitation the rescuer should pinch off the nostrils of the victim with his left hand, using his right hand to lift the neck, maintaining a patent airway.

5. *Removal of airway obstruction.* When attempting to ventilate the patient's lungs, if no air can be forced in, then it must be assumed that the upper airway is obstructed. If this is true, the airway must be cleared immediately. Removal of obstruction should be done by turning the patient on his side, using the thumb and forefinger to hold the mouth open, clearing the mouth using the opposite hand. No time should be taken to clear the airway prior to initiation of ventilation. This would be a waste of time if the airway was clear and identification of the airway obstruction will be evident when initial ventilation is attempted.

6. *Check and identify for the absence of pulse.* Immediately following the four-breath ventilation of the lungs, the rescuer should place his hand on the patient's carotid artery and palpate the pulse. If more than one rescuer is available, which will be true under normal circumstances in the hospital setting, the apical pulse may be taken by the second rescuer as initial ventilation is taking place. The pulse should be taken at the carotid or apical sites to better assure adequate oxygenation of the brain and the cardiac muscle.

7. *Initiate compression.* If pulse is absent cardiac compression can be initiated. Cardiac compressions should be performed by placing the right hand on the chest and identifying the position of the xiphoid process or the notch where the ribs join. Using his right hand, the rescuer should

**FIG. 8-4.** Head tilt method of opening airway. (*Adapted from "Standards for Cardiopulmonary Resuscitation and Emergency Cardiac Care,"* JAMA, 227:7, Feb. 1974, p. 833, with permission.)

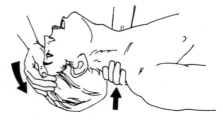

place three fingers in the mid-portion of the lower sternum. The heel of the left hand should be on top of the sternum above the fingers and the second hand placed on top of the first hand to prevent any pressure during compression being placed on the rib cage. Compression is performed by rolling forward so that the shoulders are over the patient's midline, locking elbows and directing the pressure straight down on the sternum. During cardiac compression the sternum is depressed $1\frac{1}{2}$ to 2 inches. This will compress the heart between the sternum and the vertebral column, causing a systolic action reduced but similar to the normal ejection of the heart. Compression of the sternum using approximately 90 lb of pressure for an adult will create a cardiac output of approximately 25–35% of normal.

Effective cardiac compression is indicated by the presence of a palpable carotid and/or femoral pulse. The efficiency of the total cardiopulmonary resuscitation technique is determined by the examination of the patient's pupils. The pupils of the eye should be small and not dilated. They should also be reactive to light. A small pupil indicates that appropriate oxygen is reaching the cerebral tissue, and it may be used as a reference for the effectiveness of the procedure.

8. *Precordial thump.* The only time that a blow is struck to the chest is when a monitored cardiac arrest has taken place. The rescuer should open the airway of the patient that has just arrested and feel for 10 sec. for the pulse. If a pulse is not present, with the patient in a supine position, a single blow should be delivered with the fleshy part of the fist to the mid-portion of the patient's chest. This precordial thump should be delivered directly at the patient's sternum. It must be a sharp blow delivered by first placing the fist on the patient's chest and then lifting it 8–12 in. off the chest wall and striking downward (see Fig. 8-5). The patient's pulse should be palpated and if it is not present, cardiac compressions should be started. If the patient does not respond to the initial precordial thump, additional precordial thumps throughout the cardiopulmonary resuscitation procedures will have little physiological effect and will be a waste of time and effort, interrupting the cardiopulmonary resuscitation technique. The precordial thump should never be used in an unmonitored cardiopulmonary arrest whether or not it is witnessed or unwitnessed.

## Ventilation:

1. The most important factor of successful artificial ventilation of the lung is the immediate opening of the airway. Initially time should not be taken to clear the airway of unknown obstructions. Once the airway is open using the head-tilt method, the initial effort is to ventilate the patient's lungs. In many situations this may be all that is required to resuscitate the patient. The head-tilt method will be effective in most cases.

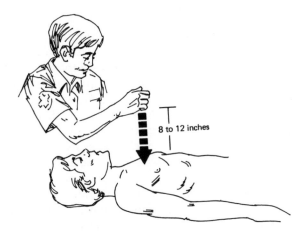

8 to 12 inches

**FIG. 8-5.** Precordial thump. (*Adapted from "Standards for Cardiopulmonary Resuscitation and Emergency Cardiac Care,"* JAMA, *227:7, Feb. 1974, p. 833, with permission.*)

If it is not effective, additional forward movement of the lower jaw may be required to more greatly hyperextend the patient's neck, moving the tongue from the airway.

2. Artificial ventilations of the patient's lungs should be repeated as long as the patient is not ventilating his own lungs. Adequate ventilation is assured with each breath if the following is observed by the rescuer: observing the chest rise and fall, feeling resistance in his own airway to the exhaling of gas into the patient's lungs to expand them, and hearing and feeling the gas escape during exhalation.

3. The initial ventilatory maneuver of four quick full breaths into the patient's lungs should be done without allowing full lung deflation between breaths. This will allow the build-up of a residual volume of gas and an increased oxygen concentration to provide diffusion for more effective circulation of oxygen during cardiac compression. The exhaled gas of the rescuer contains about 18 percent $O_2$. As soon as possible, the patient should be given as much supplemental oxygen as can be delivered to him during the resuscitation technique. The goal should be 100 percent $O_2$ with each lung inflation.

4. Artificial airways and manual resuscitating equipment should be available for use during artificial ventilation with the CPR technique. An oropharyngeal or nasopharyngeal airway should be placed to assure adequate tongue displacement to provide an open airway. A resuscitation bag and mask that will deliver 100 percent $O_2$ should be used as soon as it is available to assure an adequate seal around the patient's nose and mouth and the highest oxygen concentration. Intubation of the patient should be

completed when the patient is stable to guarantee a sealed lower airway to prevent aspirations if vomiting should occur. The likelihood of vomiting is increased because of gastric distention during artificial ventilation. Artificial ventilation by the mouth-to-mouth method should be initiated when no equipment is available. Mouth-to-mouth resuscitation is performed by closing off the patient's nose using the thumb and index finger while holding the patient's head and neck in an extended position with the hand (see Fig. 8-6) on the forehead. The rescuer seals his mouth over the patient's to provide a closed system for exhalation. Resuscitation effort can also be made with the seal of the mouth over any type of artificial airway that is in place or the stoma of a tracheostomy or laryngostomy patients. It is important to remember that patients who have had a laryngectomy cannot have mouth-to-mouth resuscitation performed on them since the upper airway is no longer connected to the lower respiratory tract. Therefore, only mouth-to-stoma resuscitation will be effective.

5. Resuscitation effort should never be interrupted for more than 5 seconds except for two procedures. Those are intubation and the movement of the patient to a more appropriate position for delivering cardiopulmonary resuscitation. These interruptions must not be longer than 15 seconds. Any interruption greater than 5 sec other than the two described will lead to an increase in tissue damage and a decrease in the effectiveness of the total cardiopulmonary resuscitation effort.

6. Artificial ventilation often causes stomach distention with air from the ventilatory efforts of the rescuer. This is most common in children but can also occur in adults. Marked distention of the stomach inhibits the ventilation of the lungs because of the elevation of the diaphragm as the stomach expands. It can also lead to regurgitation and vomiting, increasing the possibility of aspiration. A nasogastric tube should be placed in the stomach as soon as possible to help prevent this situation. Gastric rupture may also result from overdistention if it is not resolved.

7. If vomiting occurs during the cardiopulmonary resuscitation procedure, the victim's head and shoulders should be turned to one side to

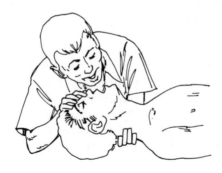

**FIG. 8-6.** Mouth to mouth resuscitation. (*Adapted from "Standards for Cardiopulmonary Resuscitation and Emergency Cardiac Care,"* JAMA, 227:7, Feb. 1974, p. 833, *with permission.*)

prevent aspiration of gastric contents during this maneuver. This change of position must not interrupt the CPR technique.

**Circulation (External Cardiac Compression):** Cardiopulmonary arrest is recognized by a lack of pulse in the large arteries of the unconscious patient who has a deathlike appearance and lacks breathing. The carotid artery pulse should be checked rapidly as soon as a cardiac arrest is suspected and ventilation has been established. It is essential in the presence of the cardiopulmonary arrest that both effective artificial ventilation and artificial circulation be delivered to the patient. The following are therapeutic considerations of artificial circulation:

1. The patient must have a residual volume of gas in the lung before cardiac compressions begin. If a volume of fresh inhaled gas is not in the lung, then there is no need to circulate unoxygenated blood. Therefore, before delivering cardiac compressions, the patient should be placed using the head-tilt method to open the airway and given four rapid deep breaths followed by a checking of the carotid pulse.

2. Artificial circulation is produced by the external compression of the heart with a rhythmic application of pressure over the lower $\frac{1}{2}$ of the sternum. The heart lays slightly left of the middle of the chest between the lower sternum and the spine. By compressing the sternum $1\frac{1}{2}$-2 in. the external cardiac compression can produce a systolic blood pressure peak of about 100 mm Hg. The diastolic pressure still remains at zero and the mean pressure seldom exceeds 40 mm Hg in the carotid artery. The return of artificial circulation in the body produces about 25–30 percent of the normal circulatory blood flow.

3. Effective external cardiac compressions require sufficient pressure to depress the patient's lower sternum a minimum of $1\frac{1}{2}$-2 in. The patient must be placed on a firm surface such as the ground, the floor, or an emergency resuscitation board. A resuscitation board should be kept on every emergency cart and these carts should be distributed throughout the hospital so that there is one for each nursing and laboratory unit. Cardiac compressions should be started immediately if needed. Cardiac compressions must be regular, smooth, and uninterrupted, and pressure must be removed from the chest immediately after it is compressed to allow ejection and filling of blood in the heart.

4. Appropriate hand positions for cardiac compressions is found by the rescuer's feeling the tip of the xiphoid process and using two to three fingers as a reference placing the heel of the hand on the lower $\frac{1}{2}$ of the sternum, about $1$-$1\frac{1}{2}$ in. from the xiphoid process toward the patient's head.

5. The compression rate for artificial circulation for two rescuers is 60 compressions per minute (see Fig. 8-7). Artificial ventilation should be interposed between every fifth compression without any pause. It may be

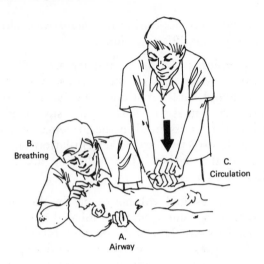

B.
Breathing

C.
Circulation

A.
Airway

**FIG. 8-7.** Two-rescuer cardiopulmonary resuscitation. (*Adapted from "Standards for Cardiopulmonary Resuscitation and Emergency Cardiac Care,"* JAMA, *227:7, Feb. 1974, p. 833, with permission.*)

effectively performed by beginning the artificial ventilation just as the chest is compressed. Any interruption in cardiac compression will result in a drop in blood pressure to zero.

6. In the hospital setting normally more than one person will be available to perform cardiopulmonary resuscitation, but if there is only one rescuer, cardiac compressions must be followed by two very quick lung inflations. This creates a ratio of 15 compressions to two lung inflations. The two lung inflations must be delivered without allowing full exhalation between breaths (see Fig. 8-8).

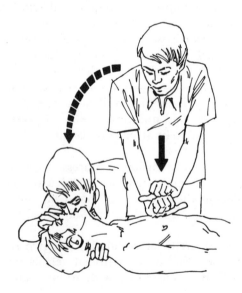

**FIG. 8-8.** One-rescuer cardiopulmonary resuscitation. (*Adapted from "Standards for Cardiopulmonary Resuscitation and Emergency Cardiac Care,"* JAMA, *227:7, Feb. 1974, p. 833, with permission.*)

**Evaluating CPR:** The effectiveness of CPR is checked periodically during cardio-pulmonary resuscitation by examining the pupil reactivity of the patient. When exposed to light, the pupils' reacting by constricting indicates that adequate oxygenation and blood flow is being received by the brain. If pupils do not react to light and remain widely dilated, serious brain damage may have occurred. Dilated but reactive pupils do not clearly indicate cerebral damage. Consideration must be given to the fact that age and the administration of drugs also affect the dilation and constriction of the pupils and their reactibility to light. The carotid pulse should be palpated at least once within the first minute of the initiation of CPR, and every few minutes thereafter. It should be checked particularly when there is a change of rescuers performing CPR.

**Considerations of Cardiopulmonary Resuscitation:** If CPR is performed improperly or inadequately, artificial ventilation and circulation may be ineffective in providing basic life support to the patient suffering from cardiopulmonary arrest. The following are therapeutic considerations that should be followed to deliver effective external cardiac compression and artificial ventilation:

1. Cardiopulmonary resuscitation should not be interrupted for more than 5 sec for any reason. If qualified persons are present and the patient is properly positioned and all preparations are made, then CPR may be interrupted for the endotracheal intubation of the patient or for moving the patient into a position where more effective cardiopulmonary resuscitation can be performed. These two exceptions should never exceed 15 seconds.

2. The major cause of complications in cardiopulmonary resuscitation is the improper placement of the hand on the sternum. Cardiac compression performed with the hand in the wrong position can lead to fractured and broken ribs, a fractured sternum, laceration of the liver by the xiphoid process, and an increased potential of pneumothorax. Never compress the xiphoid process at the tip of the sternum. The process extends downward over the abdomen and the pressure can cause laceration of internal organs leading to internal bleeding. Between compressions, the heel of the hand must be kept completely free of pressure but should remain in constant contact with the chest wall over the lower half of the sternum to maintain proper position. Also the rescuer's fingers should never rest over the victim's ribs during cardiac compression.

3. All physicians, respiratory therapy personnel, and nursing personnel and adjunct personnel should be trained in the effective delivery of CPR within the hospital. The ability of a person to deliver cardiopulmonary resuscitation should be evaluated at least annually and the procedures should be reviewed using a mannequin at that time. It is the responsibility

of the medical environment in the hospital to provide an adequate number of effectively trained persons in effective CPR.

**Termination of CPR:** Cardiopulmonary resuscitation is not indicated for patients who are known to be in the terminal stages of an incurable condition. This is a medical decision that must be made by a licensed physician. When resuscitation is indicated and started in the absence of a physician, it should be continued until one of the following occurs:

1. The patient recovers and effective spontaneous circulation and ventilation is restored.
2. Resuscitation efforts are transferred to other responsible trained individuals who can continue the CPR support.
3. The patient is transferred to a properly trained and designated area charged with the responsibility of emergency medical services and/or continued cardiopulmonary support of the patient.
4. A physician assumes responsibility and through evaluation of the patient determines that the resuscitation efforts should be stopped.
5. If you are not in a medical facility, CPR efforts may be stopped once the resuscitating person has become exhausted and can no longer continue with the resuscitation efforts.

## CARDIAC DEFIBRILLATION

One of the major needs for cardiopulmonary resuscitation is ventricular defibrillation of the heart. If the cardiac tissue is fibrillating, this may be identified by a rapid or slow oscillation of varying amplitudes creating a wavy picture on the oscilloscope screen on the EKG monitor. (See Chap. 11.) Cardiac standstill in comparison to ventricular fibrillation will be identified by a straight line showing no cardiac activity on the EKG oscilloscope. Ventricular fibrillation is a condition of diffuse erratic, and totally insufficient myocardial electrical and functional activity. Ventricular fibrillation produces no useful cardiac output. The heart is rapidly contracting and cardiac metabolism is occurring at a high rate. Just as with cardiac standstill, if ventricular fibrillation is not immediately treated, the patient will expire.

The treatment for fibrillation is to defibrillate the heart using an electrical shock. This causes complete depolarization of the heart in one rapid instant. Following this complete depolarization the heart is required to become repolarized in a more uniform manner berfore any cardiac activity can occur. This allows the myocardial tissue an opportunity to return to normal rhythm and contraction.

The external method of electrical defibrillation of the heart is performed by placing electrodes in a position along the axis of the cardiac silhouette with one paddle at the apices and one paddle at the base of the heart. Electrodes are applied firmly with a pressure equivalent of 8-10 lb by the resuscitator and an electrical voltage of 200–400 J (watt-seconds or joules) is delivered. The actual duration of the shock is approximately 4 msec (miliseconds). Following defibrillation of the heart, the patient's EKG should be observed to determine whether defibrillation is effective. When the electrical shock is delivered, no one must be touching the patient or any equipment attached to the patient.

## PHARMACOLOGICAL SUPPORT

It may be necessary to administer specific drugs to maintain cardio-vascular integrity and tone to provide adequate arterial circulation. (See Chap. 4) Drugs may also be given to increase the heart's contractility and to decrease its myocardial irritability. Antacids such as sodium bicar-bonate (1 ampule equaling 44.6 meq) should be given initially and re-peated at 8-10 minute intervals to reduce the acidity that develops because of hypoxia and the build-up of carbon-dioxide tension. EKG monitoring should continue for at least 48 hr following resuscitation to assure the clearance of arrhythmias.

Within their legal structure, many states provide a "good samaritan" law that frees anyone from legal liability who offers to stop and help someone in an emergency situation. This would legally free the individual from liability in performing cardiopulmonary resuscitation in an emer-gency situation or anyone whether within the hospital or in the com-munity. This actually has more relevance to community emergency situations. Within the hospital, the therapists and nurses should perform all procedures and follow all policies authorized by the medical staff and the department medical director within that hospital.

## BIBLIOGRAPHY

Bendixen, H.H., *et al.*, *Respiratory Care*, C.V. Mosby, St. Louis, 1965.

Brunner, L.S., and D.S. Suddarth, *Lippincott Manual of Nursing Practice*, J.B. Lippin-cott, Philadelphia, 1974.

Burton, G., Gee, G., and J. Hodgkins, *Respiratory Care: A Guide to Clinical Practice*, J.B. Lippincott, 1977.

Bushnell, S.S., *Respiratory Intensive Care Nursing*, Little, Brown, Boston, 1973.

Campbell, E.J.M., "Respiratory Failure," *British Medical Journal*, June, 1965, pages 1451-1460.

Cherniack, R.M., Cherniack, L. and A. Naimark, *Respiration in Health and Disease,* 2nd edition, W.B. Saunders, Philadelphia, 1972.

Comroe, J.H., *et al., The Lung,* 2nd edition, Year Book Medical Publishers, Chicago, 1962.

Dammann, J. Frances, *et al.,* "Assessment of Continuous Monitoring in the Critically Ill Patient," *Diseases of the Chest,* 55:33, pages 240–244.

Demers, R.H. and M. Sakland, "Respiratory Mechanics: A Theoretical and Empirical Approach," *Respiratory Care,* 20:8, pages 727–744.

Downs, J.B. *et al.,* "Intermittent Mandatory Ventilation," *Chest,* 64:3, pages 331–335.

Egan, D.F., *Fundamentals of Respiratory Therapy,* 3rd edition, C.V. Mosby, St. Louis, 1977.

Gilbert, R., *et al.,* "The First Few Hours Off of a Respirator," *Chest,* 65:1974, page 152.

Grenard, S., *et al., Advanced Study in Respiratory Therapy,* Glenn Educational Medical Services, New York, 1971.

Hedley-White, J., *Applied Physiology of Respiratory Care,* Little, Brown, Boston, 1976.

Hessell, E.A., "Monitoring the Patient in Acute Respiratory Failure." *Respiratory Therapy,* 6:4, page 27, 1976.

Hunsinger, D.L., *et al., Respiratory Technology: A Procedure Manual,* 2nd edition, Reston, Reston, Virginia, 1976.

Jude, J.R. and J.O. Elam, *Fundamentals of Cardiopulmonary Resuscitation,* F.A. Davis, Philadelphia, 1975.

Kamen, J.D. and C.J. Wilkinson, "A New Low Pressure Cuff for Endotracheal Tubes," *Anesthesiology,* 34:482, 1971.

Kirimili, B., King, J.E., and H.H. Pfaeffle, "Evaluation of Tracheobronchial Suction Techniques, *Journal of Thorac Cardiovasc Surgery,* 59:340–344, 1970.

Krugman, M.E., "Tracheostomy," *Respiratory Therapy,* July-August, 1974, page 21.

Modell, J.H., "Use and Abuse of Aerosol Therapy," *Respiratory Care.* 20:4, page 356, 1975.

Modell, J.H., "Weaning Patients for Mechanical Ventilation," *Respiratory Care,* 20:4, pages 373–376.

Powaser, M.M., *et al.,* "The Effectiveness of Hourly Cuff Deflation in Minimizing Tracheal Damage," *Heart and Lung,* 5:5, p 734, 1976.

Safar, P., *Respiratory Therapy,* F.A. Davis, Philadelphia, 1965.

Shapiro, B.A., Harrison, R.A. and C.A. Trout, *Clinical Application of Respiratory Care,* 2nd edition, Year Book Medical Publishers, Chicago, 1979.

Shenkin, Henry, "Clinical Methods of Reducing Intercranial Pressure, *New England Journal of Medicine,* 282:26, pp. 1465–1471.

Shin, Chang, "Volume Cycles vs. Pressure Cycled Respirators Ventilatory Failure Due to Chronic Obstruction Pulmonary Disease," *Diseases of the Chest*, 55:6, pages 500–502.

Sladen, Arnold, "Pulmonary Complications and Water Retention in Prolonged Ventilation," *New England Journal of Medicine*, 279:9, pp 448–453.

"Standards for Cardiopulmonary Resuscitation and Emergency Cardiac Care," *Journal of American Medical Association*, 227, February 7, 1974, pp 833–867.

Young, J.A. and D. Crocker, *Principles and Practices of Respiratory Therapy*, 2nd edition, Year Book Medical Publishers, Chicago, 1976.

# CHAPTER
# 9

# Mechanical
# Ventilation
# Equipment

The purpose of this chapter is to provide a description of the functional analysis of major types of mechanical ventilators on the market today. There is a very definite relationship between the physical characteristics of a given mechanical ventilator and the physiological consequences that results with its use. For example, high intrathoracic pressures that can result from positive-pressure ventilation produce a reduction of venous return and therefore subsequent reduction of the cardiac output. Also the I:E ratios that are possible with given mechanical ventilators have an effect on determining the mean intrathoracic pressure. The goal is to support the vital life-support systems of a patient with minimal harmful effects on the physiological processes. A basic understanding of the relationship between physical characteristics of mechanical ventilators and their potential physiologic effect is necessary. The respiratory therapist must have an understanding of the physical principles behind a given ventilator and how these relate to the patient and to other mechanical ventilators.

# USE OF SPECIFIC VENTILATORS

Mechanical ventilation is affected by the knowledge of the different types of mechanical ventilators. It is the purpose of this chapter to provide general and classifying information so that effective decisions in choosing a mechanical ventilator for patient use can be made.

One of the major problems in the area of mechanical ventilation has been the lack of consistency in the classification of ventilators. Most ventilators today exert a positive pressure on the upper airway that establishes the necessary pressure gradient needed to move a volume of air into the patient's lungs. When discussing the mode of operation of the ventilator, it becomes evident that all mechanical ventilators must accomplish four functions:

1. The ventilator must be able to inflate the patient's lungs. This is called the *inspiratory phase* of the ventilator.
2. The ventilator must be able to deflate the patient's lungs or must be able to allow for passive expiration. This is called the *expiratory phase.*
3. The ventilator must have some mechanism by which it stops the process of inspiration and allows for the process of expiration. This is called the *changeover* from inspiratory to expiratory phase.
4. The ventilator must have another mechanism by which the process of expiration comes to an end and the process of inspiration begins. This is called the *changeover* from expiratory to inspiratory phase.

The two changeover phases occur during the ventilatory cycle: the changeover from inspiratory to expiratory phase and the changeover from expiratory to inspiratory phase. When a mechanical ventilator possesses these four functions, it is capable of providing a controlled life-support system to the patient. The ability of a ventilator to perform all of these functions differentiates it from a nebulization unit used for a routine IPPB or aerosol treatment.

## CLASSIFICATION SYSTEMS

**By Cycling:** The most common system of classification today is that system developed by Mushin[1]. In this system, ventilators are classified by the cycling mechanism. By cycling, we mean the change from inspiratory phase to expiratory phase of the machine.

1. Mushin, William W., "Automatic Ventilation of the Lungs", *Blackwell Scientific Publications,* Oxford and Edinburgh, 1969.

1.  A pressure-cycled machine, therefore, means that the changeover from inspiratory to expiratory phase occurs when a set pressure is reached. Volume, time, and/or flow may all vary as a result of airway resistance and system or lung compliance. Examples of pressure-cycled machines include the Bird Mark 7, 8, and 10; and the Bennett PR-1 and PR-2.

2.  A volume-cycled machine is one where the changeover from inspiratory to expiratory phases occurs when a preset volume is reached or delivered. In such ventilators, pressure, time, I:E ratio, and flow may all be variables. Examples of volume-cycled machines are the Bennett MA-1, MA-2; the Ohio Critical Care; the Bourns LS104-150 and the Bourns Bear 1.

3.  Ventilators that are classified as time-cycled are those where the changeover from the inspiratory to the expiratory phase occurs after a set period of time elapses. In such ventilators the volume, flow, and pressure may all be variables. Generally an I:E ratio is set on these units. Examples of time-cycled ventilators include the Emerson, the Baby Bird, and the Foregger 210. It should be noted that the Bennett PR-1 and PR-2 may also be time cycled. Table 9-1 shows the relationship between variables and constants in the three types of ventilators described.

**By Displacement:** Another mechanism used in the classification of mechanical ventilators has been the type of displacement that occurs to a given volume of air. For example, when ventilation is caused by positive pressure (volume-cycled, pressure-cycled, or time-cycled) at the airway forcing gas into the lungs, this has been called positive displacement. All the ventilators mentioned previously are examples of positive-displacement ventilators. When ventilation occurs as a result of the creation of a negative pressure around the lungs caused by a negative pressure (subatmospheric) around the chest, this is called negative displacement. Examples of nega-

TABLE 9-1

**Relationship Between Classification System and Ventilator Variables**

| Variable | Classification System | | |
| | Pressure Cycled | Volume Cycled | Time Cycled |
|---|---|---|---|
| Inspiratory Pressure | Constant | Vary | Vary |
| Delivered Tidal Volume | Vary | Constant | Vary |
| Inspiratory Time | Vary | Vary (usually is set but can vary) | Constant |
| Inspiratory Flow Rate | Vary | Vary (usually set to a wave pattern) | Vary (usually set to a wave pattern) |

tive displacement ventilators include the Drinker Body Respirator (Iron Lung) and the Emerson Cuirass.

**By Flow Pattern:** A third mechanism for classification of ventilators describes the type of flow pattern that the ventilator creates during the inspiratory phase. If the ventilator delivers the inspiratory gas at a constant flowrate that has been set by the therapist, this ventilator is called a constant-flow ventilator. Generally flow will decrease more or less in a given ventilator in the face of increasing inspiratory pressure because of the compressibility of gas. The flow pattern of a constant flow ventilator is a square wave (see Fig. 9-1). Ventilators producing square-wave flow patterns include the MA-1, the Ohio Critical Care Ventilator, and the Gill Ventilator, among others.

When a mechanical ventilator delivers the gas to the patient in a non-constant flow pattern, the ventilator produces a variable flow wave. There are two types of variable flow patterns. One is called the irregular or modified square-wave flow pattern (see Fig. 9-2). Examples of ventilators that produce irregular or modified square-wave flow patterns include the Bird Pressure Ventilators (Mark 7 and Mark 8) on air dilution and the Bennett PR-1 and PR-2 ventilators. The variable flow pattern may be an unpredictable or regular flow pattern. Some ventilators produce the regular variable flow wave called a Sine Wave (see Fig. 9-3). The Emerson and the Engstrom ventilators produce sine waves.

**By Patient's Interaction:** Ventilators also may be classified by their mode of patient interaction.

1. A control ventilator is one that does not respond to a patient's inspiratory demand. For example, the Engstrom and the MA-1, with decreased sensitivity, are control ventilators. The term control has also been used to describe a ventilator when the patient is not making any inspiratory demand and the machine is setting the rate. Such a machine may not be considered a pure controller when the patient does have the ability to vary the mode of operation.

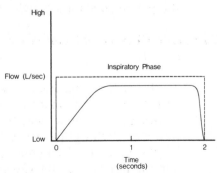

FIG. 9-1. Constant (square) wave flow pattern.

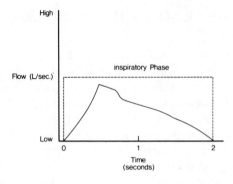

FIG. 9-2. Irregular (modified square) wave flow patterns.

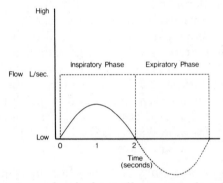

FIG. 9-3. Regular (sine) wave flow pattern.

2.   A mechanical ventilator may be classified as an assistor when the machine ventilates the patient on an inspiratory demand. The MA-1 with normal sensitivity and rate control turned off will operate as an assistor. The Bennett PR-2 and the Bird Mark 7 and 8 are also assist ventilators when the rate control is turned off.

3.   Most of the mechanical ventilators fall under the classification of assist-control machines. In such a machine, a back-up or minimal rate is set on the ventilator. Although the patient is able to trigger the machine upon demand, if the patient fails to create a sufficient inspiratory effort or if the patient becomes apneic, the machine will cycle at a given preset rate.

**By Pneumatic Circuits:**  Machines can also be classified on the basis of their gas circuits.

1.   A machine classified as a single-circuit ventilator is one where the gas used to power the machine is also the gas used to ventilate the patient. In addition, a machine may be considered a single-circuit machine if the power of the machine is exerted directly on the gas, which is then inspired by the patient. The Bennett PR-2, the Emerson, the Bird Mark 7 and 8, and the Bourns LS-104-150 can be considered single-circuit machines.

2. A double-circuit machine is one with separate pneumatic circuits: one for power and the other for patient ventilation. Generally in such ventilators, one gas is used to compress a bellows or a bag containing a separate gas going to the patient. Examples of double-circuit machines include the MA-1 and the Ohio Critical Care Ventilator.

At least five classification systems can exist and one ventilator may fall into several of these categories. It is recommended that when studying the ventilators one simply describe the action of the ventilator. The physical description of a ventilator would have two components:

A simple classification and a functional analysis. The following classification of ventilators includes:

1. Pressure ventilator: This type of ventilator moves air by exerting a pressure, the magnitude of which is chosen by the operator;
2. Volume ventilator: This type of ventilator moves a preset volume of air, the magnitude of which is determined by the operator.

The functional analysis of the ventilator consists of six characteristics:

the cycling factor or process
the flow pattern created
the flow rates which are possible
the modes of operation (assist, control
assist-control)
the power source
the pressure limitation of the ventilator

This classification and functional analysis of given ventilators allows the therapist to evaluate, compare, and make a responsible decision on the choice of ventilators for patient use based on the advantages, disadvantages, and limitations of given mechanical ventilators. Figure 9-4 describes the relationships between flow, volume, and airway pressure for the constant-flow wave pattern, the variable-flow pattern and the sine-wave flow pattern.

In the constant-flow wave pattern the flow maintains a relatively constant pattern during the inspiratory phase. The volume continually increases until the end of the inspiratory phase, and the airway pressure increases to a sharp peak at the end of the inspiratory phase. In the variable-flow pattern or modified square-wave flow pattern, the flow is not consistent during the inspiratory phase. The airway pressure does not come to a sharp a peak as is observed in the constant-wave flow pattern, where the sine-wave flow pattern best represents the normal ventilator

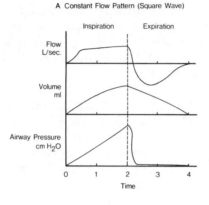

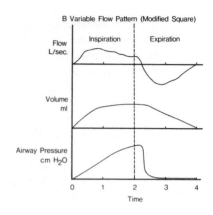

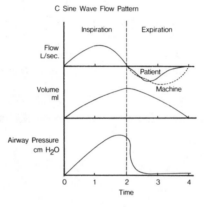

FIG. 9-4. Flow, volume, and pressure curves.

pattern of an individual. It should be noted here that some mechanical ventilators have the ability to change or adjust the type of flow pattern. For example, the Foregger 210 and the Searle ventilators can give either a sine-wave or a constant-flow pattern.

### BENNETT MA-1 RESPIRATION UNIT

The Bennett MA-1 ventilator is an electrically powered, positive displacement, volume-limited ventilator that can function in the control, assist, and assist-control modes. The MA-1 is a double-circuit machine using a bellows to separate the driving circuit from the patient delivery system. The driving pneumatic circuit is powered by an air compressor, which supplies a jet-venturi flow augmentation device and is flow-limited by a peak flow-control valve. The characteristic flow output to the bellows chamber is responsive to the resistance and compliance of the patient and delivery tube system, so that flow will tend to reduce as patient and system pressures increase; however, the shape of the flow curve is most nearly represented by a square wave for most operating conditions. Thus, it can be considered a constant flow generator. The primary gas is room air that is drawn into the unit during the expiratory phase and delivered to the patient during inspiration. This room air may be enriched with oxygen to an infinitely adjustable percentage up to 100 percent. The oxygen is supplied from a standard 50-psi pressure source.

As a controller, inspiration is begun by a timer. As an assistor, inspiration is begun by patient effort, attuned to an adjustable sensitivity control. As an assistor-controller, inspiration may be controlled or assisted; when patient effort starts inspiration, the timer is rephased, so that there is no conflict between control and assist. Inspiration is ended by volume or pressure limits. In standard use, the unit is operated to deliver a fixed volume in each inspiration, unless the pressure limit is reached earlier. The volume limit is determined by the permitted excursion of the bellows.

The ventilator has an internal pressure-relief valve set at 85 cm $H_2O$ that serves as the safety control mechanism against excessively high pressures in the patient circuit. In the event that the normal or sigh pressure limits should fail, the safety relief valve will vent the excess gas to the outside of the machine. In normal use, whenever the normal pressure limit or the sigh pressure limit is exceeded, the inspiratory phase of the unit is terminated; the excess gas is not vented to the outside. This is an important differentiation between the MA-1 and some other volume ventilators. For example, in the Emerson Post Operative Ventilator, when the pressure-relief valve is activated, the excess gas is routed to the outside of the machine and the inspiratory phase continues. Specifications for the MA-1 volume ventilator are:

| | |
|---|---|
| *Normal Tidal Volume:* | Calibrated 0–2200 ml. |
| *Normal Pressure Limit:* | Calibrated 20–80 cm $H_2O$, limits maximum pressure during normal inspiration. |
| *Normal Rate:* | Calibrated 1–60 BPM and uncalibrated to 90 BPM. Earlier units were calibrated 6 to 60 BPM and uncalibrated to 90 BPM. |
| *Sigh Volume:* | Calibrated 0–2200 ml. |
| *Sigh-Pressure Limit:* | Calibrated 20–80 cm $H_2O$, limits maximum pressure during sigh inspiration. |
| *Sigh Rate:* | Calibrated intervals between sigh cycles of 4, 6, 8, 10, or 15 times per hour. |
| *Sigh Multiples:* | For each sigh cycle, a choice of 1, 2, or 3 sigh breaths is available. |
| *Peak Flow:* | Calibrated, approximately 15–100 lpm, controls inspirator flow. |
| *Sensitivity:* | Adjustable to set degree of patient effort to trigger inspiration, from off through approximately minus 10 to minus 0.1 cm $H_2O$ and |

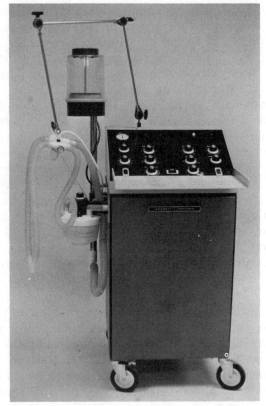

**FIG. 9-5.** Bennett MA-1. (*Courtesy of Bennett Respiration Products, Inc., Santa Monica, California.*)

| | to an oversensitive, or self-cycling condition. |
| --- | --- |
| *Oxygen Percentage:* | Calibrated and infinitely adjustable, sets oxygen concentration in delivered gas from 21 percent (air) to 100 percent. |
| *Nebulizer:* | Supplies nebulization gas flow in inspiration only. |
| *Expiratory Resistance:* | Retards expiratory flow and may be adjusted to provide a plateau effect. |
| *Manual Normal Inspiration:* | Push button to initiate normal inspiration manually. |
| *Manual Sigh Inspiration:* | Push button to initiate sigh inspiration manually. |
| *Pressure Gauge:* | Indicates system pressure from $-10-+80$ cm $H_2O$. |
| *Indicators:* | Colored lights indicate the status of the ventilator: |

1. *Assist (amber).* Lights when patient effort triggers inspiration, or if the sensitivity control is set oversensitive so that the unit self-cycles.
2. *Sigh (white).* Lights during the sigh breathing cycle.
3. *Oxygen (green).* Lights when oxygen percentage has been set to enrichment.

# Model MA-1 Pneumatic System

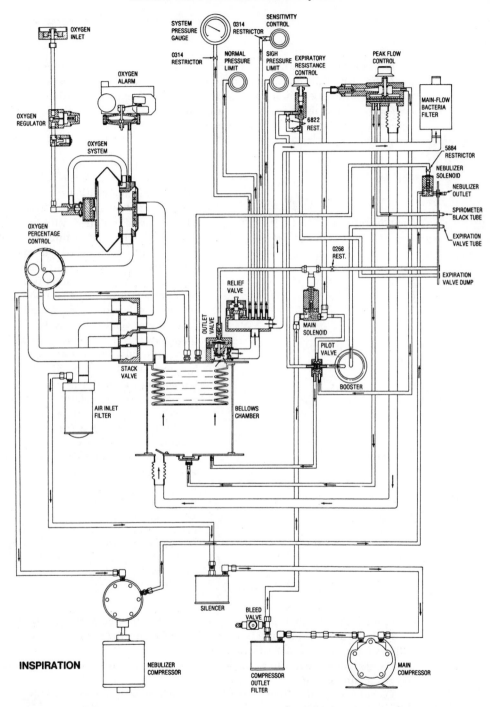

**FIG. 9-6.** Schematic of MA-1 circuit. (*Courtesy of Bennett Respiration Products, Inc., Santa Monica, California.*)

*Alarms:*                          Colored lights and a buzzer warn of unsafe
                                   operation.

1. *Pressure limit.* Red light and buzzer warn that normal or sigh pressure is reached.
2. *Ratio.* Red light during controlled inspiration warns that inspiration is longer than
will be the following expiration; that is, an inspiration/expiration ratio of less than 1:1.
3. *Oxygen.* Red light and buzzer warn that oxygen percentage is less than setting
because of inadequate source pressure.

*Fail Safe:*                       In the event of a power failure, a fail-safe
                                   valve within the ventilator operates to allow
                                   the patient to breathe to the atmosphere.

*Humidification:*                  The MA-1 is supplied with a Cascade II
                                   humidifier. The temperature of the delivered
                                   gas is monitored at the patient manifold and
                                   the water heater is proportionally controlled
                                   to ensure optimum humidification. Tem-
                                   perature at the patient manifold may be pre-
                                   set by a calibrated control and the actual
                                   temperature achieved is displayed. An alarm
                                   temperature may be preset, which if ex-
                                   ceeded, results in a blinking visible and
                                   beeping audible alarm. Should the water
                                   temperature exceed a safe limit, a continu-
                                   ous audible-visible alarm is given. Earlier
                                   MA-1's were supplied with the Cascade
                                   humidifier, which has adjustable thermosta-
                                   tic control of the heater.

*Spirometry:*                      The monitoring spirometer gives a visible
                                   and audible warning when it does not receive
                                   a set tidal volume within a preset time. This
                                   preset time is adjustable from 5–20 sec.

*Filters:*                         Ultra-high efficiency bacteria filters inter-
                                   cept mainflow and flow to the nebulizer, to
                                   reduce the possibilities of cross-infection or
                                   reinfection. The pneumatic system is pro-
                                   tected by four filters:

1. Cooling air filter that filters room air drawn into the compressor compartment.
2. Patient air filter that filters room air drawn into the oxygen-mixing system and
bellows for subsequent delivery to the patient.
3. Oxygen filter that filters oxygen from the gas source before admitting to the
oxygen-mixing system.
4. Compressor outlet filter that filters air delivered by the main compressor to the
driving pneumatic circuit.

*Compliance:* The tube system compliance is approximately 3 ml of volume for each cm of water pressure.

*IMV Accessory:* The IMV regulator accessory extends the capabilities of the MA-1 to include both IMV and CPAP modes of operation. With this device, the patient receives a tidal volume in proportion to his demand. In the IMV mode of operation, mandatory, volume-limited breaths are delivered intermittently at the set MA-1 cycle rate. A unique feature is that spirometer and alarm are fully operational during IMV regulator operation.

*PEEP Accessory:* PEEP/CPAP pressure level is adjustable from 0–15 cm $H_2O$ normal; by optional repositioning of the control knob, pressures to 30 cm $H_2O$ are available.

The control provides uncalibrated adjustable positive-end expiratory pressure from 0 to 15 cm $H_2O$. Readout is on the system pressure gauge.

*Negative Accessory:* The control provides uncalibrated adjustable negative expiratory pressure from –1 to –9 cm $H_2O$. Readout is on the system pressure gauge. When negative pressure is used, the spirometer cannot be used. Figures 9-5 and 9-6 show the Bennett MA-1 respiration unit and system schematic respectively.

## BENNETT MA-2 VOLUME VENTILATOR

The Bennett MA-2 Volume Ventilator (Fig. 9-7) represents a second-generation volume ventilator for Puritan-Bennett. The MA-2 uses the basic design and function of the MA-1, but has added features and refinements. The major changes over the MA-1 include continuous mandatory ventilation (CMV) mode, intermittent mandatory ventilatory mode (IMV), and a more comprehensive alarm system. In addition, the maximum system pressure has been increased to 120 cm $H_2O$ with a peak flow increase to 125 LPM. Pressures up to 45 cm $H_2O$ are possible now for PEEP and CPAP. An optional feature is a continuous oxygen-monitoring system using a polarographic electrode for sensing $O_2$. Major improvements in the alarm system include a fail-to-cycle alarm, high and low pressure alarm, and a temperature display and alarm system.

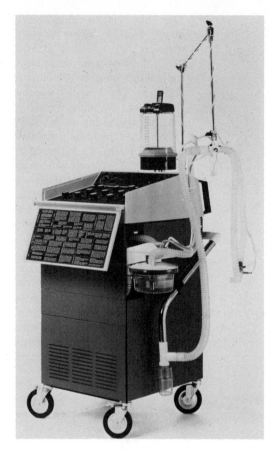

**FIG. 9-7.** Bennett MA-2. (*Courtesy of Bennett Respiration Products, Inc., Santa Monica, California.*)

## EMERSON VOLUME VENTILATOR

The Emerson volume ventilator is an electrically powered, time-cycled (simultaneous volume limited), flow-variable, pressure-variable, pressure-limited ventilator. The Emerson volume ventilator can be used in the control, assist, or assist/control mode of operation. The ventilator uses a rotary drive piston in a single gas circuit. It is a positive displacement ventilator that produces sine-wave flow pattern (see Fig. 9-8).

The changeover from the inspiratory phase to the expiratory phase is both time cycled and volume cycled. The therapist can set both the inspiratory time and the tidal volume that is to be delivered. The preset volume will always be delivered at whatever time has been set on the inspiratory phase control, if the pop-off pressure isn't reached. The only variable is the inspiratory flowrate. For example, if a given volume is delivered in a shortened inspiratory time, then the inspiratory flowrate must be high; likewise, for the same set tidal volume, if the inspiratory

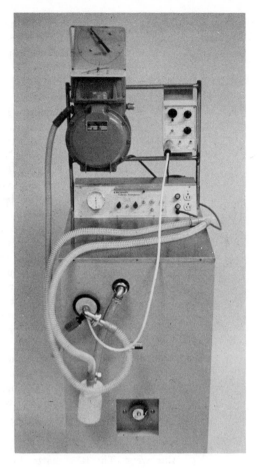

**FIG. 9-8.** Emerson 3-PV.

phase is increased, then the inspiratory flowrate will go down. Because of operator's control over the inspiratory time, we choose to use the general classification as a time-cycled ventilator; however, it must be remembered that the preset volume and preset time occur concurrently. Specifications of the Emerson volume ventilator include:

| | |
|---|---|
| *Tidal Volume:* | 0–2,000 ml (adult cylinder) |
| | 0–1,000 ml (pediatric cylinder) |
| | 0–500 ml (infant cylinder) |
| *Sigh:* | The sigh or deep-breath module on the ventilator is comprised of a separate compressor that adds additional volume to the preset tidal volume. The sigh mechanism works in cycles or intervals of every 7 min. A control is set for a percentage of each 7-min interval, |

during which time every breath will be a sigh breath. This percentage can be increased up to a maximum of 50 percent; therefore, out of every 7-min interval, $3\frac{1}{2}$ min can be comprised of sigh volumes. Sigh-volume mechanism is a blower that automatically adds additional volume during the inspiratory phase. The sigh mechanism runs continuously when activated, but the additional volume is added to the patient's circuit only during the inspiratory phase. The only way to determine the actual sigh volume is by direct measurement of exhaled tidal volumes. There is no sigh volume indicator as is found in most other ventilators.

*Pressure Limits:*

The Emerson uses a simple pressure popoff located on the humidifier. This pressure popoff is variable and can be adjusted by the operator. When the pressure limit is reached, the excess volume is routed to the outside, but the inspiratory phase is not interrupted; therefore, a pressure plateau exists until the expiratory phase begins.

*Rate:*

The rate on the Emerson volume ventilator is determined by the inhalation time setting and the exhalation time setting. With these settings, it is possible to get a wide range of rates from 4 to approximately 55 breaths/min.

*Flow:*

The pattern of inspiratory flow is that of a sine wave. The flow starts slowly, becomes rapid during the middle phase of the inspiratory cycle and slows down again towards the end of inspiration. This type of flow pattern most closely approximates the normal inspiratory flow pattern. The difference in the sine waves produced by a mechanical ventilator and that found normally during the respiratory cycle, is the displacement. Mechanical ventilators use a positive displacement, while during normal inspiration, a negative displacement situation exists.

*Oxygen:*

A supplementary oxygen supply may be added to the single circuit via a flow meter that can be connected to the back of the ventilator and attached to a trombone accumulator near the piston chamber. The supplementary oxygen collects in the accumulator and is drawn into the cylinder at the beginning of the subsequent piston stroke. There are no direct oxygen setting controls on the Emerson ventilator. It is necessary to calculate the oxygen concentration (the manufacturer provides a table for this purpose—see Fig. 9-9). The formula used for determination of oxygen percentage is as follows:

$$O_2\% = \frac{S + 0.2\ (MV - S)}{MV}$$

$S$ = supplementary oxygen flow rate in LPM

$MV$ = minute volume (set tidal volume $\times$ actual patient rate)

*Alarms:*

The Emerson volume ventilator has no alarms built into the system; however, accessory alarms for $O_2$, pressure, and apnea are available from the manufacturer.

*Humidification:*

The humidification of the Emerson ventilator is exceptional. The unit uses a humidifier kettle (hot pot) that is heated above body

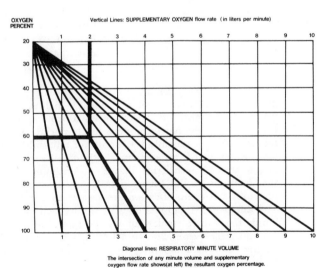

FIG. 9-9. Oxygen concentration table for 3-PV. (*Modified from Operation Manual. J.H. Emerson Co., Cambridge, Massachusetts.*)

temperature. The gas delivered to the patient enters the humidification kettle and uses a passover principle and leaves the kettle by way of a delivery hose that is filled with copper wool. The copper wool in the delivery tubing has several functions:

It serves as a coarse filter
It greatly increases the surface area
It reduces the heat loss from the inspiratory gas

In addition, when the copper oxide is warm and wet it is an active bacteriostatic agent. Thus the patient gas is purified as it passes through the copper mesh, and bacteria are rapidly destroyed by the copper oxide. The humidification system does not produce an aerosol. The temperature of the gas delivered to the patient is within safe temperature ranges.

*Compliance:*

The volume of the humidification kettle is a significant factor in changes of machine compliance. As the water level drops in the kettle, the compliance of the machine increases. This needs to be taken into consideration by the therapist when checking the ventilator.

*NOTE: The early Emerson volume ventilators were sensitive to decreases in line voltage that occur occasionally in hospitals. When the line voltage dropped, the motor that slowed down prolonged each phase of the ventilatory cycle. In the newer models, this has been corrected. Positive-end expiratory pressure is possible by the use of adjustable spring-loaded valves or an underwater PEEP attachment, both of which are available. Emerson also makes an IMV ventilator that is a continuous-flow system. Many of the specifications of the Emerson IMV ventilator such as flow, timing, volume, pressure, and humidification are similar to the Emerson volume ventilator. The Emerson IMV model does use an oxygen analyzer (galvanic fuel cell), a humidifier control which allows the humidifier to be set at a variable temperature range from 30° to 40°C, and the basic IMV control module that determines ventilatory rate, the system pressure gauge, and the stroke-volume indicator.

The Emerson ventilators have several connections inside the cabinet that serve as potential sources of air leak and should be checked routinely by the therapist. The Emerson is considered a stable and reliable mechanical ventilator (see Fig. 9-10).

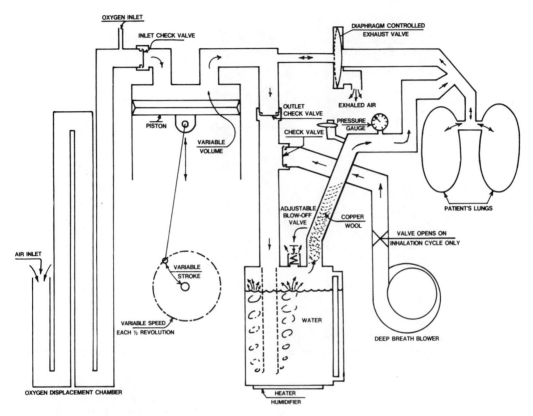

**FIG. 9-10.** Emerson post-operative ventilator, Model #3-PV flow schematic. (*Modified from Operation Manual. J.H. Emerson Co., Cambridge, Massachusetts.*)

## ENGSTROM VENTILATOR

The Engstrom ventilator is an electrically powered, positive-displacement, time-cycled, flow-variable, control ventilator. The Engstrom uses a double circuit that is piston driven and produces a sine-wave flow pattern. The mode of operation is controlled with a set I:E ratio of 1:2. The Engstrom ventilator is a minute-volume ventilator in which the frequency in minute-volume is set. The Engstrom ventilator has the following specifications:

| | |
|---|---|
| *Tidal Volume:* | Tidal volume cannot be set directly. The desired minute volume must be set and |

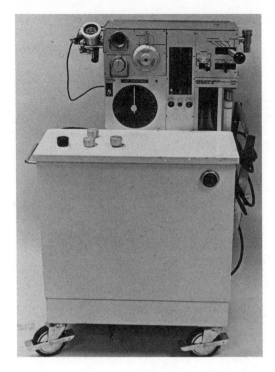

**FIG. 9-11.** Engström respirator 300.

*Sigh:*

*Pressure Limit:*

*Rate:*

*Flow:*

frequency is chosen with a "frequency regulator." The result of these two will determine the set tidal volume.

There is no automatic sigh control on the Engstrom ventilator.

The Engstrom unit is equipped with an adjustable pressure relief valve and airway pressures are adjustable to a maximum of 70 cm water pressure.

The frequency is controllable from 10 to 35 breaths per minute during which time the same I : E ratio is maintained.

The inspiratory flow rate may not be controlled directly but rather is a result of pressure in the reservoir bag. The ventilator uses a double-circuit system in which a bag is suspended in a rigid cylinder. The inspiratory flowrate will be determined by the pressure in the primary system that compresses the respiratory bag, thus delivering the gas to the patient. Excess pressures

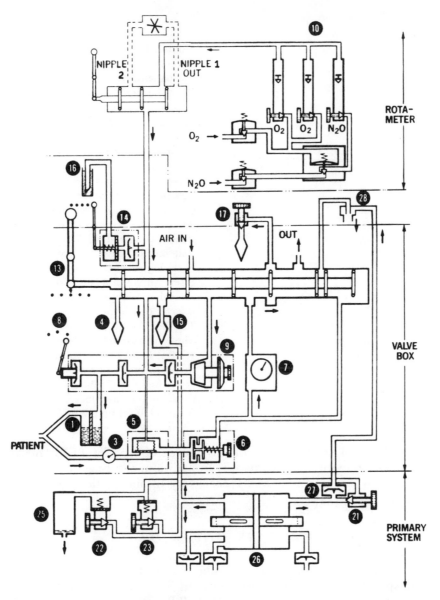

FIG. 9-12. Schematic of Engström Circuit. The numbers on the figure indicate the following: 1. Humidifier. 3. Precision manometer in the patient circuit. 4. Bag for manual ventilation. 5. Plug-in unit for expiration valve. 6. Plug-in unit for expiratory resistance and control of end-expiratory pressure. 7. Gas meter. 9. Plug-in unit for air and gas-mixture dosage valve. 10. Rotameters with reducing valves. 13. Multifunction valve and function control. 14. Plug-in unit for pressure limit control. 15. Patient breathing bag. 16. Water safety lock. 26. Compressor-force generator. 28. Venturi. *Place for Holothane vaporizer. *The following breathing systems may be used:* Nonrebreathing, circular absorption—closed or semiclosed, manual or mechanical ventilation. (*Courtesy of Acta Anaesthesiologica Scandinavica Norlander, O.P., et al.: 1968, 12, 213-223.*)

around the respiratory bag will increase the inspiratory flowrate but is not delivered to the patient. The Engstrom ventilators use a short inspiratory pause at the end of the inspiratory phase. As the inspiratory flowrate increases, a longer pressure plateau is maintained at the end of inspiration. The inspiratory flowrates vary with changes in compliance.

*Oxygen:*    Oxygen concentrations from 21 percent to 100 percent are possible with the machine. On 21 percent, the ventilator entrains room air into the respiratory bag. The ventilator is also equipped with rotometer gauges so that medical gases or oxygen can be added. A dosing valve calibrator is used for mixing gases. An entrainment system is not used in achieving oxygen concentrations greater than 21 percent.

*Alarms:*    The unit has a built-in power failure alarm.

*Humidification:*    The ventilator uses a passover humidification system. It uses a reservoir (hot pot) in which the water may be heated.

*Compliance:*    Only Engstrom tubing systems should be used on the machines and the compliance for an adult set up is 5 ml/cm water pressure.

The Engstrom ventilator has the capability for PEEP, negative pressure, and expiratory resistance. In addition, the Engstrom ventilators can be used for anesthesia and the delivery of anesthetic gases (see Figs. 9-11 and 9-12).

## OHIO CRITICAL-CARE VENTILATOR

The Ohio Critical-Care Ventilator is an electrically powered, positive-displacement, volume-cycled, constant-flow ventilator capable of operating in the control, assist-control, and IMV modes of operation. The Ohio Critical Care Ventilator is representative of a series of new ventilators on the market by various manufacturers that incorporate sophisticated alarm and warning detection systems. In addition, the Ohio Critical Care Ventilator uses a double circuit that is made up of a bellows filled with the patient gas suspended in a cannister, which is then pressurized by a compressor and thus causes the gas within the bellows to be delivered to the patient. The sigh mechanism within the machine is also a bellows driven system (see Figs. 9-13 and 9-14). Specifications of the Ohio Critical Care Ventilator include:

*Tidal Volume:*

The tidal volume is adjustable from 200 to 2000 ml.

*Sigh:*

The sigh volume is adjustable from 200 to 2000 ml. It is important to note here that the sigh volume set on the ventilator is additive to the tidal volume set; therefore, with both the tidal volume and deep breath bellows set at their maximum, it is possible to deliver 4000 ml of gas to the patient. This differs from the sigh volume setting on the Bennett MA-1 respiration unit. In that unit the two controls operate independently and are not additive. The sighs may be delivered in intervals of 3, 5, 7.5, and 15 min for 1, 2, or 3 deep consecutive breaths. The venti-

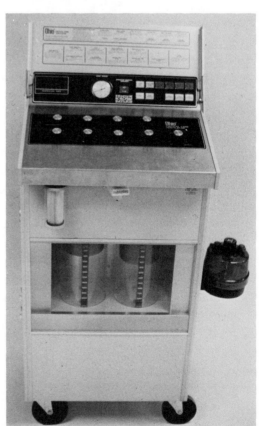

FIG. 9-13. Ohio critical care ventilator. (*Courtesy of Ohio Medical Products, Inc., Madison, Wisconsin.*)

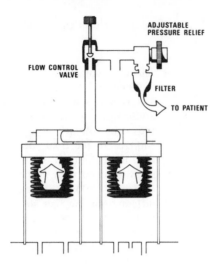

**ADJUSTABLE PRESSURE RELIEF**

**FLOW CONTROL VALVE**

**FILTER**

**TO PATIENT**

**FIG. 9-14.** Ohio critical care schematic during inspiratory phase. (*Courtesy of Ohio Medical Products, Inc., Madison, Wisconsin.*)

lator automatically doubles the expiratory time following each deep breath. The unit is also equipped with a manual deep breath switch.

*Pressure Limits:*

The high pressure alarm setting on the Ohio Critical Care Ventilator serves two functions:

1. It sets the maximum pressure capability of the machine;

2. It will activate the high-pressure alarm if the pressure reaches the preset setting for two consecutive breaths.

When the preset pressure is reached during any stage of the inspiratory phase, the machine will cycle to the expiratory phase, except during the deep breath cycle. In this way, the machine serves as a pressure-cycled ventilator. This feature of the Ohio Critical Care Ventilator differentiates it from the Ohio 560 which uses a similar type of pressure popoff, as does the Emerson Volume Ventilator.

*Rate:*

Three parameters in the Critical Care determine the respiratory rate. These are the tidal volume setting, the inspiratory flow setting, and the expiratory time. The rate is a function of these and in changing any one of these parameters will in fact change the respiratory rate. The Ohio Critical Care uses a digital readout for respiratory rate. The meter is updated after each breath. It is important at this point to differentiate this type of feature from that on other ventilators. In the Emerson Volume Ventilator, the rate is a function of the inspiratory time and expiratory time. On the Bennett MA-1 respiration unit, the rate is a direct setting. Therefore, the variable on the MA-1 will be the expiratory time since the rate, tidal volume and peak flow are preset. For this reason, the MA-1 is equipped with an I:E ratio alarm. The Ohio 560 volume ventilator uses the same type of rate control as the Ohio Critical Care.

*Flow:*

The inspiratory flow control is adjustable from a minimum to a maximum setting. This corresponds to an inspiratory flowrate of 10 l/min to approximately 200 l/min calibrated against 40 cm of water back pressure. The letters on the indicator dial are for reference and repeatability of ventilator settings and have no quantitative value in and of themselves.

*Expiratory Time Control:*

Expiratory time is calibrated in seconds and is continuously variable from 1 to 10 sec. Remember that the tidal volume, inspiratory flow, and expiratory time are infinitely adjustable to any position desired and thereby allow a tremendous variability in set breathing patterns.

*Inspiratory Hold Control:*

The Ohio Critical Care Ventilator has a control that allows the operator to hold and deliver tidal volume in the patient for up to 2 sec in increments of 0.5 sec. The Bennett MA-1 respiration unit does not have an inspiratory hold control as such; however, remember that when the expiratory resistence is at its maximum, an inspiratory plateau or hold effect will be created.

*Oxygen:*

On the Ohio Critical Care Ventilator, the $F_I O_2$ is continuously variable from 21 percent to 100 percent. These mixtures of gas will be constant regardless of the tidal volume or inspiratory flowrate. The control has an off position and, once set in this position, only room air will be drawn into the machine. If the control is in the on position and gas is not supplied to the unit, then the $O_2$ fail alarm will sound. The oxygen-concentration control on the Ohio Critical Care is not an oxygen analyzer; therefore, it is necessary that the unit be connected to a 100 percent $O_2$ source in order for the unit to function correctly. This type of oxygen-control setting is similar to that found in the Bennet MA-1 respiration unit. In each of these units, if the ventilator were attached to another gas source (50 psi) by mistake, and the percent oxygen control were set to some level greater than 21 percent, the unit would be unable to differentiate levels of oxygen concentration.

*Patient-Triggering Effort:*

The patient-triggering effort control is adjustable from a minimum effort to a full controller. As was true with the inspiratory flow control, the letters are for reference only. At the minimum setting, the patient cannot trigger the machine and will be ventilated only as it has been set. The patient triggering control automatically compensates for levels of PEEP. Thus it is not necessary for the patient to draw through the entire PEEP in order to trigger the machine.

*IMV:*

When the IMV control is activated, the IMV valve within the machine will open and allow the patient to begin breathing through the machine without any resistance. The patient will breathe at the $F_IO_2$ set on the control panel. The IMV frequency is adjusted by the expiratory time control and ranges from 1 IMV ventilation every 10 sec to one breath every 100 sec. The mandatory IMV breath is 10 times the indicated setting on the expiratory time control. For example, if the expiratory time control is set at 3, then the patient will receive one breath every 30 sec or two breaths per min; if set at 10 seconds, then the patient will receive one mandatory IMV breath every 100 sec. When the IMV unit is activated, the deep-breath control must be turned off and the patient triggering-effort control turned to the controller position. When IMV is in use, all machine alarms are deactivated and it is necessary to use alternative monitoring systems.

*Humidification:*

The humidifier used in the Ohio Critical Care Ventilator is a heated bubble-through type of humidifier with a large surface area. The maximum heater temperature is 160°F. The heater is adjustable from 90° to 160°F. The humidification system in the Ohio Critical Care is similar to that of the MA-1 Bennett Cascade. This humidification system differs from that used in the Emerson and Engstrom, which exemplifies the heated passover type of humidifier and is different from the humidification system in the Ohio 560 which used an ultrasonic nebulizer.

*Filters:*

The Ohio Critical Care Ventilator has two main filters affecting the cleanliness of gas being delivered to the patient. There is a long filter located on the front of the machine that filters the room air brought into the system and mixed with the oxygen source (which typically has an oxygen inlet filter). A disposable bacterial filter is also located on the front of the machine in the patient main-line tube.

*Alarm System:*

The Ohio Critical Care Ventilator has a sophisticated alarm and warning detection system:

1. *Fail-to-cycle.* The fail-to-cycle alarm will activate if inspiration takes longer than 5 sec or if the expiratory phase is longer than 22 sec. During the fail-to-cycle condition, the exhalation valve and the free-breathing valve will automatically open, allowing the patient to breathe to the atmosphere.

2. Oxygen-fail alarm. The oxygen-fail alarm will be activated whenever the $O_2$ control is on (22 percent–100 percent) and there is a drop in the source gas supply (less than 50 psi).

3. *Low-pressure alarm.* The low-pressure alarm will activate when the pressure within the patient's circuit does not reach 12 cm $H_2O$ on inspiration at least once every 15 sec.

4. *High-pressure alarm.* The high-pressure alarm activates when the circuit pressure has exceeded the pressure setting for two consecutive breaths. Exhalation will automatically occur when pressure reaches a set point, except during the deep breath cycle.

5. *Audio-alarm silence.* The audio portion of the alarm system may be silenced by activating this switch; however, the audio will automatically turn on in 2 min if the alarm has not been "reset." The audio-alarm volume may be adjusted by the control under the front edge of the ventilator.

6. *Power loss.* A battery operated alarm will emit an audible sound if there is a power failure or electrical malfunction within the ventilator. In the event of a power failure of the ventilator to cycle, the patient's circuit will automatically open. The premixed gas source will continue to be channeled to the patient and the exhalation valve will remain open.

| | |
|---|---|
| *Manual Controls:* | The Ohio Critical Care Ventilator has a manual deep-breath control, a manual inspiration control, and a manual expiration control. When held down continuously, the manual inspiration control will prevent expiration for up to 5 sec, thus facilitating X-ray or compliance procedures. |
| *Compliance:* | The compliance of the Ohio Ventilator tubing system is approximately 2.5 ml/cm $H_2O$. |

The Ohio Critical Care Ventilator-2 (CCV2) represents a refinement of the Critical Care Ventilator. The alarm system has been elaborated over the initial critical-care ventilators, although the basic mode of operation for the ventilator remains essentially unchanged. One of the unique features on the control panel of the CCV-2 is what Ohio calls the "Optic Manometer." This is a single pressure gauge that can monitor pressure change, the high pressure limit, and the patient triggering threshold.

## OHIO 550

The Ohio 550 Ventilator is a pneumatically powered, positive displacement, volume cycled, constant flow ventilator that can be operated in the assist, control, and assist/control modes. The Ohio 550 is an example of a pneumatic fluid control ventilator. The power for the Unit is from a 50 psig gas source. The specifications of the Ohio 550 fluidic ventilator include:

| | |
|---|---|
| *Tidal Volume:* | The tidal volume is adjustable from 200 to 2000 ml graduated in 200 ml increments. |
| *Sigh:* | The Ohio 550 Ventilator does not have a deep-breath or sigh mechanism. |
| *Inspiratory Flow Rate:* | The inspiratory flowrate on the Ohio 550 Ventilator even though theoretically considered to be a constant flow generator, the flow will vary depending upon bag pressure and the psig power supply. At 45 to 50 psig, the flowrate will be relatively constant until approximately 20 cm $H_2O$ bag pressure is reached. At that time, there |

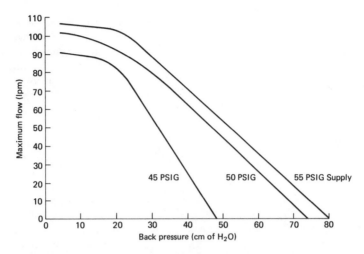

**FIG. 9-15.** Effect of back pressure on flow rate of Ohio 550. (*Courtesy of Ohio Medical Products, Inc., Madison, Wisconsin.*)

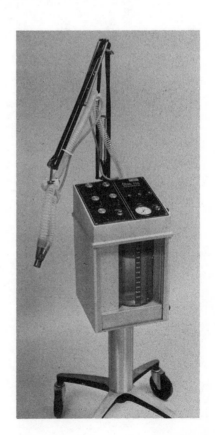

**FIG. 9-16.** Ohio 550 ventilator.

is a significant decrease in the maximum flowrate against increasing back pressures. The maximum flowrate between 45 psig and 55 psig will range from 90 to nearly 110 l/min, respectively (see Fig. 9-15).

*Pressure Limits:* The maximum pressure limits within the machine are 70 cm $H_2O$. An optional pressure-relief valve can be adjusted down to 10 cm $H_2O$ pressure. If the pressure-relief valve is used, and the pressure is reached, the excess volume will not be delivered to the patient but rather to the atmosphere.

*Rate:* The respiratory rate will be a function of tidal volume, inspiratory flowrate, and expiratory time. The expiratory time is variable and adjustable from 1 to 15 sec. This is the same mechanism that is used in the Ohio critical care ventilator.

*Oxygen:* Oxygen concentrations are adjustable from 21 percent to 100 percent. The unit does not have an oxygen alarm system.

*Alarms:* The ventilator has a low pressure visual and audible alarm that is activated if airway pressure of 8 cm $H_2O$ or greater is not achieved within a 15-sec interval.

*Failure to Cycle:* Visual and audible alarms will be activated if inspiration takes longer than 5 sec or expiration longer than 15 sec. The unit does have an emergency exhalation valve that permits the patient to exhale to the atmosphere should the ventilator valve malfunction.

*Humidification:* The ventilator uses a heated bubble-through humidifier with large surface area.

*Rate:* The unit does not have a rate control nor a rate indicator. Rate will be a function of inspiratory flow, set tidal volume, and expiratory time. Against relatively high-back pressures, the inspiratory flowrate will drop significantly and this will alter ventilation rate.

*Compliance:* The compliance of the tubing system of the Ohio 550 ventilator is approximately 2.5 ml/cm $H_2O$ pressure using Ohio tubing (see Figs. 9-16 and 9-17).

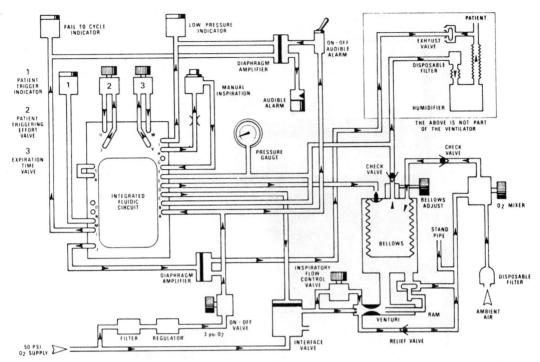

**FIG. 9-17.** Ohio 550 schematic. (*Courtesy of Ohio Medical Products, Inc., Madison, Wisconsin.*)

## OHIO 560

The Ohio model 560 respirator is an electrically operated, positive-displacement, volume-cycled, constant-flow ventilator capable of operating in the control and assist/control modes. The Ohio 560 uses a double circuit system (see Figs. 9-18 and 9-19). The specifications of the ventilator include:

| | |
|---|---|
| *Tidal Volume:* | The tidal volume is adjustable from 100 ml to 2000 ml. |
| *Sigh:* | The Ohio 560 uses the sigh or deep-breath mode of operation. The deep-breath volume is adjustable from 100 to 2000 ml. The deep-breath control volume is additive to the tidal volume, thus allowing for a maximum of 5000 ml. Note that this is the same as the Ohio Critical Care Ventilator. The |

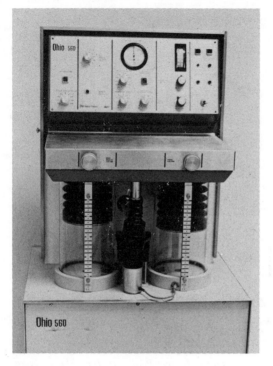

**FIG. 9-18.** Ohio 560 ventilator.

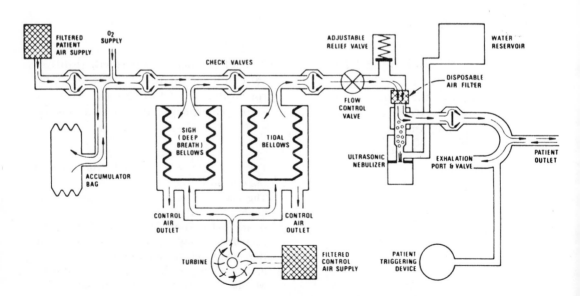

**FIG. 9-19.** Ohio 560 schematic. (*Courtesy of Ohio Medical Products, Inc., Madison, Wisconsin.*)

deep breath intervals are timed for 2, 4, 6, 8, and 10 minute intervals between deep-breath cycles. Note again that there are no multiple deep breaths possible. This is not true in the Ohio Critical Care Ventilator nor the Bennett MA-1 respiration unit. The expiratory time is doubled following a deep breath.

*Pressure Limits:* An adjustable pressure limiting valve provides a maximum patient pressure from 10 to 100 cm $H_2O$ pressure. This valve is located under the table top of the ventilator. When the pressure limit has been reached, the excess volume is routed out through the pressure popoff and does not interrupt the inspiratory phase. Note again that this differs from the pressure-limit mechanism in the Bennett MA-1 respiration unit and the Ohio Critical Care Ventilator. In each of these ventilators, the inspiratory phase ends when the pressure limit has been reached.

*Rate:* The rate is a function of the inspiratory flow, the tidal-volume set, and the expiratory time. A rate indicator is on the front of the machine. The inspiratory flow control is calibrated and adjustable from the minimum to maximum settings which correlates to approximately 10 to 250 l/minute. Maximum flow depends on back pressure. The expiratory time control is adjustable from 0.5 to 7 sec.

*Oxygen:* The ventilator is capable of providing oxygen concentrations from 21 percent to 100 percent. An oxygen control switch on the front of the ventilator allows the operator to set the desired $F_IO_2$. The ventilator does not use an oxygen analyzer in determining the oxygen concentration. Although the unit allows oxygen concentrations from 21 to 100 percent, the unit is only calibrated from 30 to 100 percent.

*Sensitivity:* The ventilator may be adjustable to different sensitivities for patient triggering, using the patient triggering control. To operate the unit in the controller mode, the patient triggering effort control should be set to approximately 7 or greater on the scale. To operate in the assist-control mode, the pa-

*Humidification:*

tient triggering effort control must be less than 7 and can be adjusted as necessary in this range.

The Ohio 560 Ventilator uses an ultrasonic nebulizer with a variable output from 0 to 3 ccs per minute. In most clinical situations however, the Ohio 560 has been adapted to use a heated bubble-through type of nebulizer, such as the Bennett Cascade. In clinical practice, this is found to be a more reliable method providing accurate and constant humidification.

*Alarms:*

The Ohio 560 has several alarm systems:

1. *Oxygen alarm.* A red warning light indicates a gas source supply failure or a gross leak in the accumulator bag. It is important to remember that the alarm system does not monitor actual oxygen concentration.

2. *Low-pressure alarm.* The low pressure alarm will operate when pressure fails to reach 8 cm $H_2O$ on inspiration. This alarm uses a visible light and an audible "beep."

3. *Failure-to-cycle.* The failure-to-cycle alarm will operate when expiratory time exceeds 15 sec or when the inspiratory time exceeds 8 sec. A visible and audio beep are used.

4. *Power loss.* A battery-operated power-failure alarm that provides an audible beep is incorporated into the unit and is activated when the power to the ventilator fails.

5. *High-pressure alarm.* A visible light and audible beep alarm are activated when the patient's circuit exceeds the preset alarm pressure on two consecutive cycles. The high-pressure alarms are variable from 20 cm to 100 cm $H_2O$ pressure.

6. *Emergency exhalation valve.* The ventilator is equipped with an emergency exhalation valve that opens and allows the patient to breathe to the atmosphere. However, this emergency exhalation feature of the ventilator is inoperative when a negative end expiratory pressure system is used.

*Expiratory Resistance:*

Expiratory resistance is possible with this ventilator by use of a retard cap placed on the respirator valve. This differs from the Bennett MA-1 respiration unit in which the expiratory resistance can be dialed in.

*Inflation Hold:*

The Ohio 560 uses an inflation hold that is adjustable from 0 to 2 sec in increments of 0.20 sec. This inflation hold is similar to that of the Ohio Critical Care Ventilator, where the increments of adjustment are 0.5 seconds.

*Manual Operation:*

The unit is equipped with a manual inspiration, manual expiration, and a deep-breath control.

The Ohio 560 is no longer manufactured. Its inclusion in this chapter is felt to be necessary because many units are still used in clinical practice.

## BENNETT PR-1 AND PR-2 RESPIRATION UNITS

Both the Bennett PR-1 and PR-2 respiration units are pneumatically powered (40–70 psi), positive displacement, pressure-cycled (can be time-cycled) variable flow ventilators that can funciton in the control, assist and assist-control modes. They are single circuit ventilators that use a flow-sensitive valve (Bennett Valve) and a variable control pressure, so that the flow pattern adapts to patient resistance and compliance. The Bennett PR-1 and PR-2 units can be used for IPPB therapy, respiratory assistance and controlled ventilation. (See Figs. 9-20 and 9-22.)

The changeover from the inspiratory phase to the expiratory phase can be either pressure-cycled or time-cycled. When pressure-cycled, towards the end of the inspiratory phase, the patient pressure has increased almost to the value of the system pressure and patient flow drops to a low terminal point. At between 1 and 2 l/min terminal flow, the Bennett Valve closes, thereby ending the inspiration and starting the expiration phase. When the unit is time-cycled, inspiration is ended by the rate control that serves as the ventilator's timing control. Expiration is similarly timed in a preset ratio to inspiration time. Thus, these ventilators can be either pressure-cycled or time-cycled, depending on the control settings. Inspiration can begin by either the patient creating an inspiratory effort or by means of the rate control. (See Figs 9-21 and 9-23.)

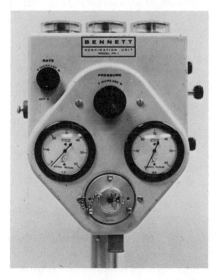

**FIG. 9-20.** Bennett PR-1.

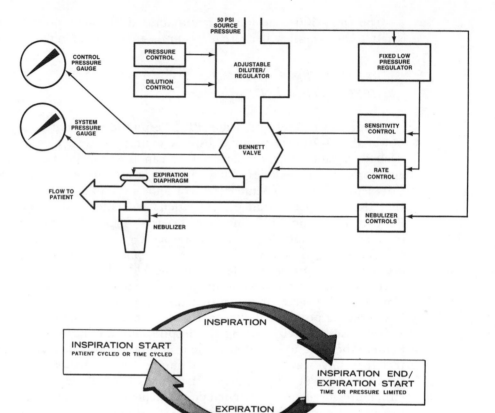

FIG. 9-21. Conceptual representation of Bennett PR-1. (*Courtesy of Bennett Respiration Products, Inc., Santa Monica, California*).

## Specifications— Controls common to both PR-1 and PR-2:

| | |
|---|---|
| *Tidal Volume:* | The tidal volume is a function of the pressure set for the control system and the compliance of the patient's lungs, during pressure-cycled ventilation. Volume will be delivered to the patient until either the preset pressure has almost been reached, thereby reducing flow through the Bennett Valve to the cut-off point, or the ventilator is time-cycled by the rate control circuit (see Fig. 9-24). |
| *Control Pressure:* | The control pressure of the pneumatic system is adjustable from 0 to 50 cm $H_2O$ and is indicated on the control pressure gauge. |

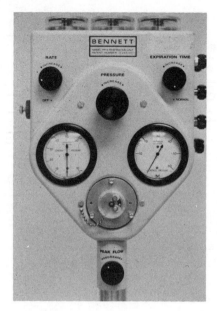

**FIG. 9-22.** Bennett PR-2.

*System Pressure:* The system pressure gauge indicates pressure in the delivery tube system.

*Rate:* The rate control is adjustable from 0 to approximately 70 cycles per minute. The rate control is not calibrated. When the rate control is used and the unit is being time-cycled, an I:E ratio of $1:1\frac{1}{2}$ is automatically maintained (or greater for the PR-2). If the unit is being pressure-cycled, the I:E ratio will be greater because of the shorter inspiratory time.

*Sigh:* There is no separate control for sigh, but a simulated sigh may be induced by increasing the control pressure for one or more inspirations.

*Flow:* Inspiratory flowrate will vary with the control pressure set and the resistance of the patient and tubing system. Maximum inspiratory flowrates up to 90 l/min are possible. Towards the end of the inspiratory phase when system pressure approaches control pressure, flowrate will fall to 2–4 LPM, at which time the Bennett Valve will close and end the inspiratory phase.

*Sensitivity:* The assist sensitivity is adjustable through a full range, from totally locked-out through

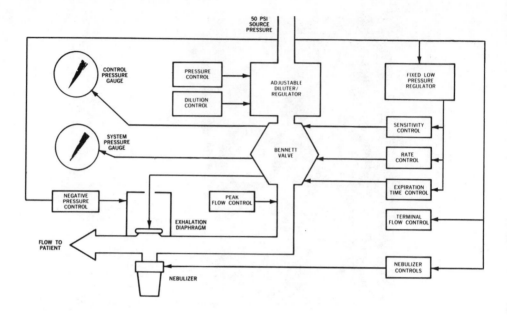

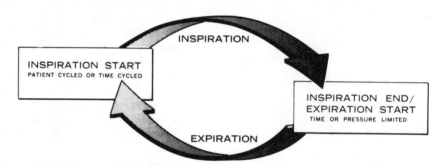

**FIG. 9-23.** Conceptual representation of Bennett PR-2. (*Courtesy of Bennett Respiration Products, Inc., Santa Monica, California.*)

*Oxygen:*

extreme sensitivity to a self-cycling condition.

A dilution control is provided for varying the oxygen concentration; when pushed in, the ventilator supplies 100 percent $O_2$, unless the terminal flow control on PR-2 is in use, in which case the concentration will be slightly reduced. When the dilution control is pulled out, the concentration of oxygen delivered to the patient will be greater than

**SCHEMATIC**

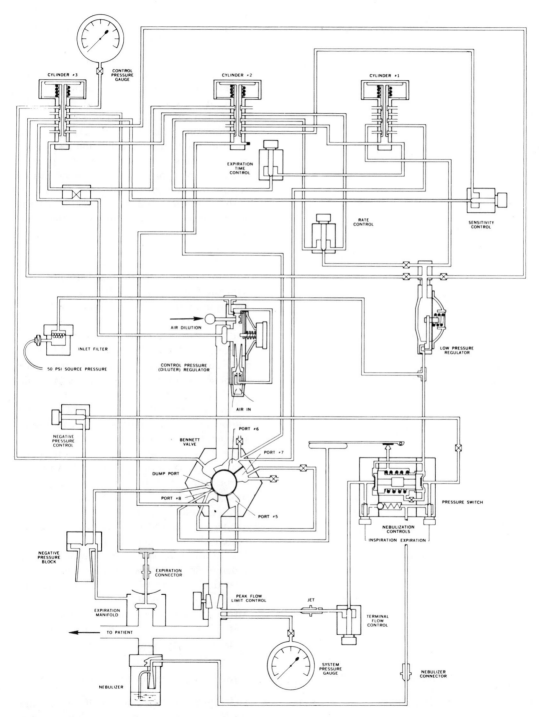

**FIG. 9-24.** Bennett PR-2 schematic. (*Courtesy of Bennett Respiration Products, Inc., Santa Monica, California.*)

40 percent. Since the degree of dilution depends on system flowrate and also is affected by nebulization setting and the terminal flow control (PR-2 only), accurate control of oxygen concentration is best achieved by supplying the respiration unit from an oxygen blender and setting the respiration unit on 100 percent.

*Nebulizer:*

Two nebulization controls are provided for the PR-1. The nebulization-inspiration control allows the nebulizer to operate during inspiration only. The nebulization-continuous control provides nebulization in both inspiration and expiration. When the ventilator is set on dilution, use of the nebulizer tends to increase delivered oxygen concentrations.

*Alarms:*

The PR-1 and PR-2 respiration units have no built-in alarms, but they are usually used with the Cascade II humidifier and monitoring spirometer, which provide additional patient safeguards.

*Humidification:*

The ventilators are used with the Bennett Cascade II humidifier, for humidification and comprehensive safety features. The temperature of the delivered gas is monitored at the patient manifold and the water heater proportionally controlled for response to changing patient flow conditions. Temperature at the patient manifold may be preset by a calibrated control, and the actual temperature achieved is displayed. An alarm temperature may be preset, which, if exceeded, results in a blinking visible and beeping audible alarm. Should the water temperature exceed a safe limit, a continuous audible-visible alarm is given.

*Spirometry:*

The monitoring spirometer gives a visible and audible warning when it does not receive a set tidal volume within a preset time. This preset time is adjustable from 5 to 20 sec.

*Filters:*

An air-dilution filter on the left side of the unit filters room air and a high pressure filter intercepts flow from the oxygen supply source.

The Bennett PR-2 has additional controls which include:

*Expiration Time:*

The expiration time control allows the time available for expiration to be extended, thus

| | |
|---|---|
| | reducing the cycling rate. When the expiration time control is not used (normal position), the ventilator operates at a $1:1\frac{1}{2}$ I : E ratio. |
| *Peak Flow:* | The peak-flow control adds a variable resistance to the delivery-tubing system, allowing for lower inspiratory flow rates. |
| *Terminal Flow:* | The terminal flow control provides for cut-off at higher terminal flows up to 10–15 l/min, compensating for leaks in the system. It provides an additional flow below the level of the Bennett Valve, thus increasing the patient flow at which inspiration ends. Because the terminal flow circuit uses an injector system separate from the main dilution system, the additional flow will tend to increase oxygen concentration when the ventilator is set on 100 percent. |
| *Nebulization:* | Separate controls are provided for nebulization during inspiration or expiration. When the ventilator is set on dilution, use of the nebulizer will tend to increase delivered oxygen concentration. |
| *Negative Pressure:* | The negative pressure control is adjustable from 0 to −6 cm $H_2O$. |

## BIRD VENTILATORS: BIRD MARK 7 AND MARK 8

The Bird Mark 7 and Mark 8 ventilators are pneumatically powered, positive-displacement, pressure-cycled, variable flow on air mix and constant flow on 100 percent source gas ventilators that are capable of operating in the assist, assist/control, and control modes. The Bird Mark 7 and Mark 8 ventilators represent a single-circuit machine that can operate at source pressures between 25 and 100 psi. The change-over from the inspiratory phase to the expiratory phase is pressure-cycled only. The change-over from the expiratory phase to the inspiratory phase can be achieved by:

1. The inspiratory effort of the patient,
2. The "expiratory time" control that determines the length of time the machine will stay in the expiratory phase.

Specifications of the Bird Mark 7 ventilator include (see Figs. 9-25 and 9-26):

| | |
|---|---|
| *Tidal Volume Control:* | The Bird Mark 7 does not have a tidal volume control. The tidal volume is a function |

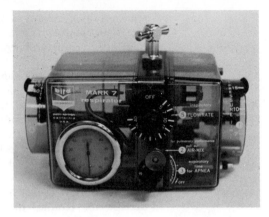

**FIG. 9-25.** Bird Mark 7.

of the inspiratory pressure set on the machine and the patient's compliance and/or resistance.

*Sigh:*

The Bird Mark 7 ventilator does not have a sigh control. In most pressure ventilators such as the Bird Mark 7, Mark 8, or the Bennett Respiration Units, sighs can be achieved by increasing the inspiratory pressure setting.

*Rate:*

The rate will be a function of several variables: the pressure setting, the inspiratory flowrate, the expiratory time control, the compliance and/or resistance of the patient, and the ability of the patient to cycle the machine. Those variables controlling the inspiratory time include the flowrate, the pressure setting, and the patient compliance and/or resistance. Those variables affecting the expiratory time are the expiratory time control or the patient's own inspiratory effort. Because of the numerous variables that can control the rate, ventilatory rates from 0 to 80 are possible. The primary difference of the Bird Mark 7 and the PR-2 units, with regard to rate, is that the Bird Mark 7 cannot be time-cycled. If a leak occurs in the patient's system, the inspiratory pressure is not reached, and the machine will remain in the inspiratory phase indefinitely.

*Pressure Limits:*

The pressure limits are adjustable between 5 and 60 cm $H_2O$.

*Flow:*

The flowrate is controlled by the (inspiratory time) flowrate control and flow rates

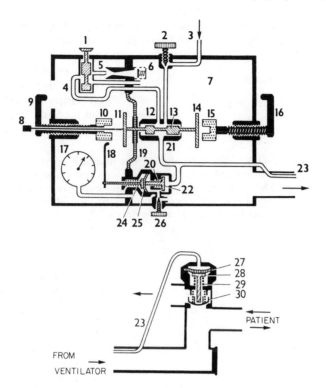

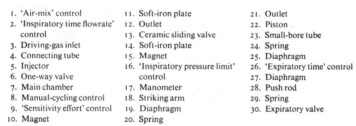

Diagrams of the Bird Mark 7 ventilator and expiratory-valve assembly.

| | | |
|---|---|---|
| 1. 'Air-mix' control | 11. Soft-iron plate | 21. Outlet |
| 2. 'Inspiratory time flowrate' control | 12. Outlet | 22. Piston |
| | 13. Ceramic sliding valve | 23. Small-bore tube |
| 3. Driving-gas inlet | 14. Soft-iron plate | 24. Diaphragm |
| 4. Connecting tube | 15. Magnet | 25. Diaphragm |
| 5. Injector | 16. 'Inspiratory pressure limit' control | 26. 'Expiratory time' control |
| 6. One-way valve | | 27. Diaphragm |
| 7. Main chamber | 17. Manometer | 28. Push rod |
| 8. Manual-cycling control | 18. Striking arm | 29. Spring |
| 9. 'Sensitivity effort' control | 19. Diaphragm | 30. Expiratory valve |
| 10. Magnet | 20. Spring | |

**FIG. 9-26.** Bird Mark 7 schematic. (*Mushin, W.W., et. al., "Automatic Ventilation of the Lungs".* Blackwell Scientific Publications, Oxford and Edinburgh, 1969, with permission.)

ranging to approximately 80 l/min are possible. Changes in the inspiratory flowrate on the Bird Mark 7 can affect other variables in the system:

1. Increasing inspiratory flowrate will decrease the inspiratory time. By delivering the inspiratory gas at a higher flowrate, the preset pressure will be met sooner.
2. Increasing the inspiratory flowrate can enable the therapist to compensate for minor leaks in the system.

3. The inspiratory flowrate will experience a major decrease when the machine is switched from air mix to 100 percent $O_2$ (see Fig. 9-27).

*Sensitivity:*

The sensitivity control on the Bird Mark 7 controls the inspiratory effort necessary for the patient to cycle the ventilator. The control is adjustable to self-cycle or lock out the patient and allow for controlled ventilation.

NOTE: The Bird Mark 7 has numbers on the inspiratory time flowrate control and the sensitivity effort control. These numbers are for reference only. The inspiratory pressure-setting numbers reflect the actual inspiratory pressure being set when the machine is calibrated. The expiratory time-control numbers are for reference only.

*Oxygen:*

When connected to a source gas of 100 percent $O_2$ the Bird Mark 7 is capable of delivering from approximately 60 to 100 percent $O_2$. The oxygen concentration is achieved by use of the *air-mix* control. When the machine is operating in the air-mix mode, room air and oxygen are mixed and provide approximately 60 percent $O_2$ to the patient. When the machine is being run on 100 percent $O_2$, and the air-mix control is pushed in all the way, the machine will deliver 100 percent of the source gas. It is important to remember, however, that the inspiratory flowrate will be significantly reduced when this is done. (See Fig. 9-27.)

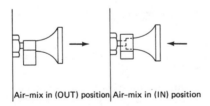

Air-mix in (OUT) position | Air-mix in (IN) position

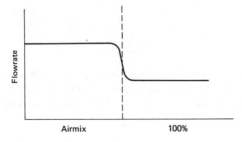

FIG. 9-27. Effect of air-mix control on flow rate.

*Alarms:*

*Compliance:*

*Humidification:*

The Bird Mark 7 ventilator has no inherent alarm system.

When using Bird tubing, the compliance of the system is approximately 1–2 ml/cm $H_2O$. When the machine is being operated on 100 percent source gas, a square-wave flow pattern is generated (see Fig. 9-1). When the machine is switched to the air-mix mode, and modified square-wave or irregular-wave flow pattern is created (see Fig. 9-2). When the Bird ventilator is operating on 100 percent source gas, essentially the patient's lungs are connected to the gas source immediately only by a flow control. In such a situation, the flow to the patient will, for all practical purposes, be held constant and uninfluenced by changes in compliance or resistance of the patient's lungs.

Humidification in the Bird Mark 7 is achieved via a 500 cc mainstream nebulizer. A heating jacket can be used to increase the humidification and is available from the manufacturer. The Bird Mark 7 can be used for IPPB, assisted ventilation, and controlled ventilation.

### Bird Mark 8

The only difference between the Bird Mark 7 and the Bird Mark 8 is that the Bird Mark 8 is capable of creating negative pressure during the expiratory phase (see Figs. 9-28 and 9-29). The negative pressure is created at the expiratory valve assembly. The Bird Mark 7 and Mark 8

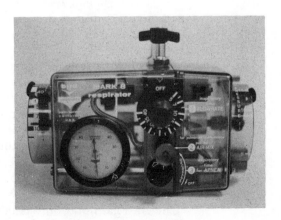

**FIG. 9-28.** Bird Mark 8.

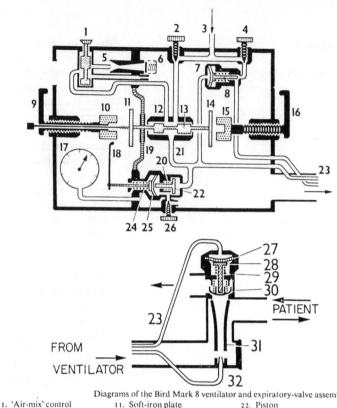

Diagrams of the Bird Mark 8 ventilator and expiratory-valve assembly.

| | | |
|---|---|---|
| 1. 'Air-mix' control | 11. Soft-iron plate | 22. Piston |
| 2. 'Inspiratory time flowrate' control | 12. Outlet | 23. Small-bore tube |
| | 13. Ceramic sliding valve | 24. Spring |
| 3. Driving-gas inlet | 14. Soft-iron plate | 25. Diaphragm |
| 4. 'Negative pressure generator' control | 15. Magnet | 26. 'Expiratory time' control |
| | 16. 'Inspiratory pressure limit' control | 27. Diaphragm |
| 5. Injector | | 28. Push rod |
| 6. One-way valve | 17. Manometer | 29. Spring |
| 7. Diaphragm | 18. Striking arm | 30. Expiratory valve |
| 8. Piston | 19. Diaphragm | 31. Injector |
| 9. 'Inspiratory effort' control | 20. Spring | 32. Small-bore tube |
| 10. Magnet | 21. Outlet | |

FIG. 9-29. Bird Mark 8 schematic. (*Mushin, W.W., et. al., "Automatic Ventilation of the Lungs".* Blackwell Scientific Publications, *Oxford and Edinburgh, 1969, with permission.*)

ventilators have a fail-safe mechanism via the venturi gate. The exhalation valve on the Bird set-up serves as a spring loaded one-way valve. Therefore, an inspiratory effort of a negative 2 cm $H_2O$ would be transferred to the venturi gate and the patient would be able to breathe through the system. In the PR-1 and PR-2 units, if the gas source were to fail, the patient would be able to breathe around the exhalation valve. If the exhalation valve (actually a balloon) were to occlude the expirator port (which is highly unlikely), the patient would be able to breathe through the Bennett Valve; however, the resistance would be extremely high.

The Bird Corporation has introduced a new series for the Mark 7 and

Mark 8. This new series has several modifications and changes over the units just described. The inspiratory time flowrate control has been changed with the deletion of the numerical control. The new control merely shows an increase or decrease setting. The air-mix control has been removed, thus allowing the unit to function always in the air-mix mode. An external ambient filter has been placed on the respirator for the entrained air. The unit now has a pressure pop-off on the pressure side. The unit, in addition, now has an automatic inspiratory nebulizer that is independent of the flowrate setting. The unit also allows for the development of PEEP via the expiratory flowrate control. The new series of Bird Mark 8 also includes these changes.

Also, a Mark 7A and 8A have been introduced. These units have the addition of apneustic flowtime that allows for time-cycling capabilities. They are pressure or pressure/time-cycled.

### BOURNS INFANT VENTILATOR: LS 104

The Bourns Infant Ventilator is an electrically displacement, volume-cycled, constant-flow ventilator that can operate in the assist, assist/control, and control modes of operation. The Bourns Infant Ventilator is a single circuit machine that uses a motor-driven piston to deliver the inspiratory flow at a constant rate. Unlike the Emerson Volume Ventilator that uses a rotary piston, the Bourns Ventilator uses a linear drive shaft on the piston.

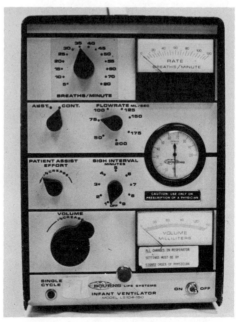

**FIG. 9-30.** Bourns LS-104. (*Courtesy of Bourns, Inc., Life Systems Division, Riverside, California.*)

## Specifications of the Bourns Infant Ventilator are:

*Tidal Volume:*      Adjustable from 10–150 ml.

*Sigh Volumes:*      The sigh is equivalent to double the preset tidal volume. The sighs are adjustable from 1-min to 9-min intervals.

*Pressure Limits:*      A high pressure limit is adjustable from 0–100 cm $H_2O$. When the preset pressure is reached, the ventilator ends the inspiratory phase immediately, sounds an audible alarm and illuminates the high pressure alarm light on the front of the ventilator. A low-pressure alarm that is adjustable from 0–50 cm $H_2O$ establishes the minimum pressure that must be reached during the inspiratory phase. If the low pressure is sustained for 15 sec, a continuous audible and visual alarm is activated. The ventilator also has a pressure relief valve at the rear of the ventilator that serves as a back-up pressure pop-off for the system.

*Pressure Limit Time Cycle:*      Since the Bourns is a constant volume and constant flow ventilator, once the controls are set, a constant inspiratory time will prevail. By adjusting the pressure relief valve at the rear of the ventilator, a maximum system pressure can be created. As the pressure in the patient breathing circuit meets the preset pressure relief level (which has been set at the rear of the machine), the excess gas is vented out through the relief valve, thus creating an inspiratory plateau until the inspiratory time is completed. In this way, the machine becomes time-cycled since the ventilator will cycle when the piston has completed its forward stroke. Since in this mode, the volume is not delivered to the patient, it is more appropriately called a time-cycled ventilator.

*Rate:*      The breathing rate selector is adjustable from 5–80 breaths/min. The rate selector is utilized in the control, assist/control, and intermittent mandatory volume ventilation modes. Since the inspiratory flow and set tidal volume establish the inspiratory time, the rate selector establishes the expiratory or apnea time. The ventilator is equipped with a meter with a range from 0–120 breaths/min.

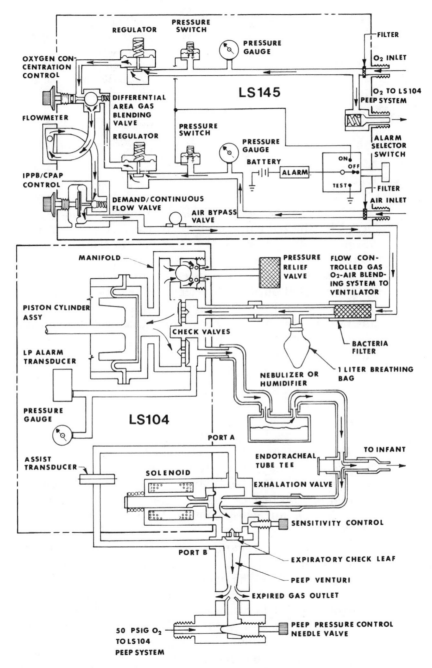

**FIG. 9-31.** Flow circuit for the LS-104. (*Courtesy of Bourns, Inc., Life Systems Division, Riverside, California.*)

*Flow:*

The flowrate selector is adjustable from 50–200 ml/sec. The inspiratory flowrate is set independently of volume or rate.

*Oxygen:*

The ventilator itself does not have an oxygen control setting, but must be used in conjunction with either: (1) the Bourns $O_2$ Blender Model LS 145; or (2) the Bourns Oxygen Controller Model LS 108-1 (no longer sold in U.S.A.)

## Modes of Operation

1. *Assist.* In the assist mode, the ventilator will only cycle when triggered by the patient. The patient assist effort (sensitivity) is adjustable from 0.05 to 1.0 cm $H_2O$. At maximum sensitivity, this requires an inspired volume of 0.05 ml and has a response time of 35 msec.
2. *Assist/Control.* In the assist/control mode, the minimum breathing rate is selected on the rate selector. The patient may trigger the ventilator and thus override the control timer. Should the respiratory rate fall below the rate selected, the ventilator will initiate the next breath.
3. *Control ventilation.* In the control mode, the patient cannot override the control breathing rate with patient effort nor can the control rate be changed with the single cycle button.

## Features

1. *Pressure manometer.* 0–100 cm $H_2O$.
2. *Pressure relief valve.* Adjustable pressure pop-off 25–100 cm $H_2O$.
3. *Sensitivity.* The sensitivity adjustment compensates for leaks and is located on the rear of the machine. This controls the sensitivity to the breathing circuit when compensating for minor leaks in the presence of PEEP.
4. *Divide-by-ten circuit.* A respiratory rate divide by ten circuit is included for this ventilator. It will work in the control mode only. To use this feature, place the mode switch in the divide-by-ten position. This automatically divides by ten the respiratory rate set on the breaths/minute control. A red light also will become immediately illuminated to indicate the ventilator is in a divide-by-ten respiratory rate situation. The visual rate meter will continue to display the breaths/minute set on the control and not the divide-by-ten rate.
5. *Inflation hold.* An inflation-hold control is also included in this ventilator. This function is achieved by holding the exhalation valve closed for a certain period of time. The inflation-hold control is calibrated in

1-sec increments from 0 to 2 sec. It will work in the assist, assist-control, control, and divide-by-ten modes. In addition, it will also function with or without PEEP. The alarms will not be affected in any manner by the use of inflation hold.

**6.** *PEEP assembly.* Positive-end expired pressure is available and adjustable from 0 to 18 cm $H_2O$ pressure. The PEEP assembly must be powered by a 50-psi unrestricted gas source.

I:E RATIO: The I:E ratio and the system compliance can be calculated using the Bourns slide rule.

Figures 9-30 and 9-31 show the Bourns infant ventilator model LS-104 and unit schematic respectively.

## BOURNS INFANT PRESSURE VENTILATOR MODEL BP200

The Bourns Infant Pressure Ventilator Model BP200 is a pneumatically powered, electronically controlled, positive displacement, time-cycled, continuous-flow ventilator that operates in the control mode. The ventilator can be used in the CPAP, IMV, and control modes of operation.

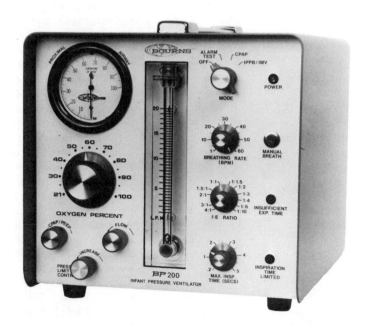

**FIG. 9-32.** Bourns BP200. (*Courtesy of Bourns, Inc., Life Systems Division, Riverside, California.*)

## Specifications of the Bourns BP 200 include:

| | |
|---|---|
| *Tidal Volume:* | The tidal volume delivered will depend on the inspiratory flowrate and the inspiratory time. |
| *I:E Ratio:* | The I:E ratio is adjustable from 4:1 to 1:10. |
| *Inspiratory Flowrate:* | This is 0–20 l/min as set on the flowmeter located on the front of the machine. |
| *Pressure Limit:* | The Bourns BP200 uses a pop-off valve that is adjustable from 10 to 80 cm $H_2O$. It is used to prevent excessive inspiratory pressures in the patient's system and can also be used to establish an inspiratory plateau. |
| *Rate:* | The rate is adjustable from 1 to 60 breaths per minute. The principle of operation of the Bourns BP200 is very simple. A continuous source of gas is delivered to the patient via the flowmeter, and at preset intervals (determined by the breathing rate selector), the expiratory line is occluded by an exhalation valve diaphragm which is pushed over secondary to a solenoid switch. This allows the pressure to build up in the patient circuit and thus inflate the infant. The time during which the exhalation port is occluded is determined by the I:E ratio and the selected rate. |
| *Oxygen:* | The BP200 uses an oxygen blender in the ventilator and is capable of delivering precise oxygen concentrations from 21 percent to 100 percent. |
| *Maximum Inspiration Time:* | A maximum inspiration time control is adjustable from 0.20 to 5.0 sec. This control is normally set just above the normal time it takes to deliver the patient inspiratory phase; therefore, excessive inspiratory times are prevented. |
| *Alarms:* | An audible alarm sounds if the air or oxygen inlet pressure is inadequate (for $O_2$, 30–75 psi; air 15–75 psi). There is also an audible alarm if there is a power failure or electrical disconnect. This alarm is powered by an alkaline battery. The system is also equipped with a patient fail-safe valve. |
| *Humidification:* | The BP200 is equipped with a heated water humidifier that uses a passover principle. The temperature of the humidifier is adjustable. |

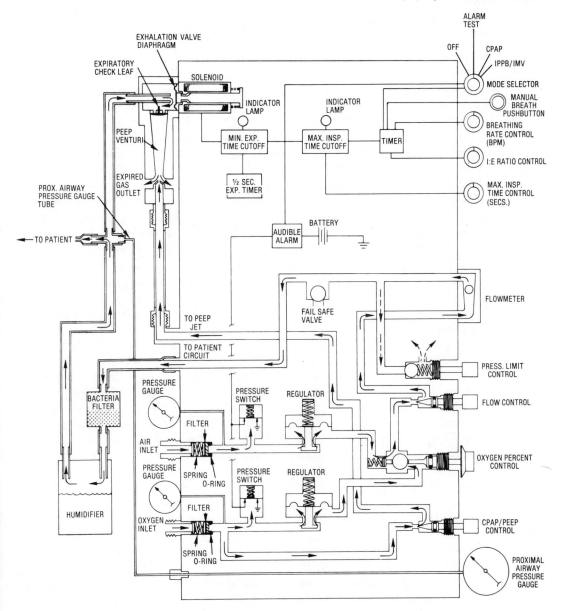

**FIG. 9-33.** Model BP200 infant pressure ventilator flow diagram. (*Courtesy of Bourns, Inc., Life Systems Division, Riverside, California.*)

The Bourns Model BP200 Infant Pressure Ventilator is a single circuit ventilator that is capable of reverse I:E ratios during the control mode. Figures 9-32 and 9-33 show the Bourns BP200 and schematic respectively.

## BOURNS ADULT VOLUME VENTILATOR: BEAR 1

The Bourns Bear 1 is an electrically powered, positive displacement, volume-cycled, flow-variable ventilator that is capable of operating in the control, assist/control, SIMV, and CPAP modes of operation. The Bear may be time-cycled if one turns the 1:1 ratio limit control to the off position. It can also be pressure-cycled if the pressure limit control is used (the audible alarm would be activated). The Bourns Ventilator is representative of a new concept in mechanical ventilation (see Fig 9-34). The traditional ventilators such as the MA-1, Ohio 560, and Emerson, use a bellows or piston system to deliver gas. The rate of excursion of the bellows or piston then determines the flowrate to the patient. The Bourns Bear 1 uses an electronic control system to deliver the gas mixture to the patient. The ventilator is attached to air and oxygen gas sources ranging from 30 to 100 psi. When a compressed air source is not available, the ventilator will automatically operate from an internal air compressor and only an oxygen hose needs to be connected. The gas sources connect to the air/oxygen blender inside the machine. This serves as the source of gas to the patient. During positive pressure breathing (control and assist/control), the gas flow to the patient is controlled by the main flow solenoid. During inspiration, the solenoid opens and allows the blended gas to flow from the air/oxygen blender, through the peak-flow and wave-form valve, and through the vortex flow sensor to the patient (see Fig 9-36). The volume of gas delivered to the patient is monitored by the vortex flow sensor. When the volume delivered reaches the value set on the tidal volume control, the main flow solenoid is closed. The Bourns uses the vortex principle as the primary control of the ventilator. Vortices are waves that are created in a fluid stream. Vortices are caused by air moving over a rod that has been placed in the path of the gas flow (see Fig. 9-35). As the flow of air moves over the strut, vibrations are created from side to side in the tube. The faster the air stream flows around the strut, the faster the rate of vibration. These vibrations or wave forms are detected by an ultrasonic beam. The vibrating airstream changes this ultrasonic beam and provides an electronic signal directly proportional to the flow. The electronic circuit of the Bourns then processes this signal and computes the tidal volume. The vortex concept is unaffected by the nature of the gas, temperature, or humidity. The Vortex Principle is used when the ventilator is functioning in the control and assist/control modes. During spontaneous breathing, the ventilator's second gas delivery system is used. This system allows the patient to breathe spontaneously via a demand valve connected to the air/oxygen blender. The tidal volume and inspiratory flowrate varies on the demands of the patient. Both of the gas systems used for control of spontaneous breathing are connected to the same air/oxygen blender;

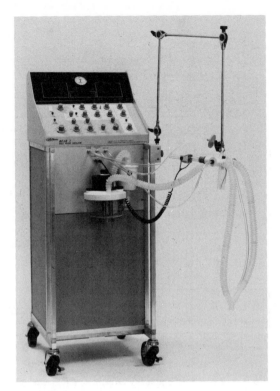

FIG. 9-34. Bourns Bear I. (*Courtesy of Bourns, Inc., Life Systems Division, Riverside, California.*)

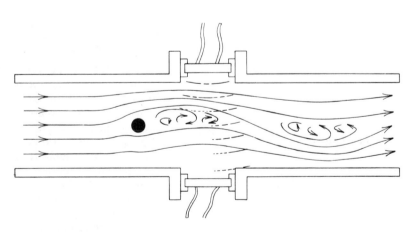

FIG. 9-35. The Vortex Principle. (*Courtesy of Bourns, Inc., Life Systems Division, Riverside, California.*)

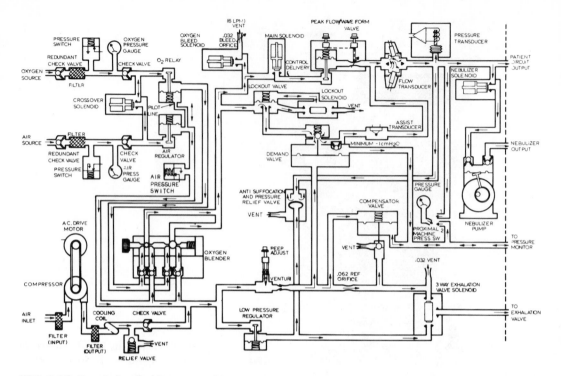

**FIG. 9-36.** Bear I circuit. (*Courtesy of Bourns, Inc., Life Systems Division, Riverside, California.*)

however, the gas circuits will differ in each of these modes (see Fig. 9-36). Specifications of the Bourns Adult Volume Ventilator Bear 1 are:

*Tidal Volume:* 100–2000 ml

*Respiratory Rate:* 5–60 breaths/min. The rate control has a division switch that can be used during IMV. This switch allows the operator to set a rate comparable to 1/10 the set rate. For example, with the respiratory rate set at 60 breaths/min and the switch set to a division marked 10, the ventilator will deliver 6 breaths/min.

*Sigh Volume:* The sigh volume varies from 150 to 3000 ml. The sigh volume is not additive to the set volume. The sigh rates are adjustable from 2 to 60 breaths/min and can provide multiple sighs of 1, 2, and 3 sighs/interval. The sigh control does not function in the SIMV or CPAP modes.

*Pressure Limits:* The ventilator has both a sigh pressure limit and a normal pressure limit. Both controls operate in a similar fashion and both are adjustable from 0 to 100 cm $H_2O$. When the preset pressure limit is reached, inspiration is terminated and an audible and visible alarm is activated.

*Flowrate:*

The peak flow is adjustable from 20 to 200 l/min. The peak flow adjusts the inspiratory flowrate only when the ventilator is operating in the control mode. During demand ventilation, gas is drawn from a separate system and peak flow control has no effect on the spontaneous inspiratory flowrate. The ventilator also has a waveform adjustment that allows flow patterns to be varied from a square-wave position to a tapered position with decelerating flows. The degree of taper is controlled by the pressure in the patient's circuit; however, the inspiratory flowrate will not taper below 40 l/min.

*Oxygen Concentration:*

Oxygen concentrations are continuously adjustable from 21 percent to 100 percent $O_2$. In order for the blender to operate accurately, the ventilator must be connected to a 30–100 psi oxygen source.

*Humidification:*

The Bourns uses a Bennett-Cascade humidifier for humidification. A nebulizer is also available for the delivery of medication.

*Response Time:*

In the assist/control mode, the ventilator has a 50 ml/sec response time.

*SIMV:*

Synchronized intermittent mandatory ventilation (SIMV) allows the patient to breathe via the ventilator's demand valve and receive a backup rate as set by the normal rate control. The IMV is not a continuous flow.

*CPAP:*

Is adjustable from 0 to 30 cm $H_2O$ pressure.

*PEEP:*

PEEP is adjustable from 0 to 30 cm $H_2O$ pressure. The PEEP circuit is a compensatory circuit able to maintain stable levels in the presence of minor leaks.

*I:E Ratio Limit:*

When the I:E ratio limit is activated, the ventilator will terminate the inspiration and provide an audible and visual alarm when a 1:1 inspiratory to expiratory ratio is achieved. When the I:E ratio limit control is in the off position, a visual indicator lights when the inspiratory period is prolonged while allowing inspiration to continue. In this way, reverse I:E ratios can be obtained.

*Alarms:*                    The Bourns Bear 1 ventilator has a sophisti-
                             cated display panel of ventilator status,
                             modes, and alarm systems.

## BABY BIRD VENTILATOR

The Baby Bird Ventilator is a pneumatically powered, positive displacement, time-cycled, continuous flow ventilator that operates in the
control mode. The ventilator can be used in the CPAP, IMV, and control
modes of operation. Specification of the Baby Bird include (see Figs. 9-
37 and 9-38):

| | |
|---|---|
| *Tidal Volume:* | The tidal volume delivered will depend upon the inspiratory flowrate and inspiratory time. |
| *Inspiratory Time Range:* | 0.4 or less–2.5 sec. |
| *Expiratory Time Range:* | 0.4 or less–10 sec. |
| *Frequency Range:* | 4.2–100/min. |
| *Peak Control Range:* | 13–81 cm $H_2O$ (10–60 mm Hg). |
| *Peak Inspiratory Flow Rate:* | 30 LPM. |
| *Maximum Safety Pressure:* | 88 cm $H_2O$ (65 mm Hg). |
| *Negative Pressure Range:* | 0--10 cm $H_2O$ (0--8 mm Hg). |
| *End Expiratory Positive Pressure Range:* | 0–20 cm $H_2O$ (0–15 mm Hg). |
| *Inspiratory Mixture:* | This is 21–100 percent $O_2$ by use of the Bird oxygen blender. |
| *Power Source:* | 50 psi oxygen in air. |
| *Inspiratory Time Limit:* | 0–infinity. |

The principle of operation of the Baby Bird Ventilator is very simple.
The ventilator operates in two modes: *Spontaneous breathing* and *ventilator on* mode. During the spontaneous breathing mode, the Baby Bird
Ventilator serves as a continuous flow gas source to the patient via the
breathing circuit. Gas enters the ventilator from the oxygen blender and
continues through the patient circuit and out the expiratory valve. During
this time, the infant may breathe at his own frequency and inspiratory
flowrates. The ventilator has no backup or assist mode when it is in the
spontaneous breathing phase. When the ventilator is switched to the
*ventilator on* phase, then the machine operates as an intermittent positive-
pressure ventilator. The operator sets an inspiratory time and expiratory
time on the ventilator that is achieved by a Bird Mark II Servo Unit inside
the ventilator itself. At predetermined periods of time, the expiratory
valve will be occluded and the air will be delivered to the patient. The
amount of time that the expiratory valve is occluded is determined by the
inspiratory time setting. At the end of the inspiratory time setting,
the pressure is relieved off the expiratory valve and the patient is able

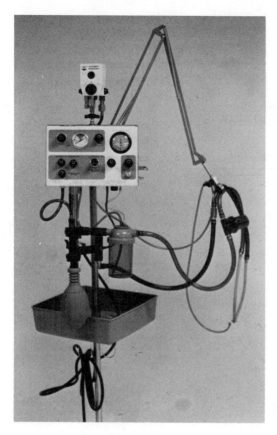

**FIG. 9-37.** Baby Bird. (*Courtesy of Bird Corporation, Palm Springs, California.*)

to exhale. The amount of time that the machine is in the expiratory phase is determined by the expiratory time control. At the end of the expiratory time, the expiratory valve will be pressurized again and the inspiratory phase will begin. This process is repeated and determines the ventilatory rate. Because of the continuously adjustable inspiratory and expiratory time rate, numerous I:E ratios (including reverse I:E ratios) can be achieved. The Baby Bird does not have a tidal volume setting. The delivered tidal volume will be a function of the inspiratory flowrate, the inspiratory time setting, and the resistance and/or compliance of the patient's lungs. Ventilation can be controlled manually with the Air Bird without delivering ambient air into the breathing circuit. When squeezed, the Air Bird occludes the outlet gasport and the flow from the gas source is delivered to the infant. If additional gas is required, it can be added to the system by further squeezing of the Air Bird. At the exhalation valve is a valve that serves to adjust the outflow of gas and thus maintain a constant positive breathing pressure within the circuit (CPAP). In addition, this valve limits the peak inspiratory pressures during con-

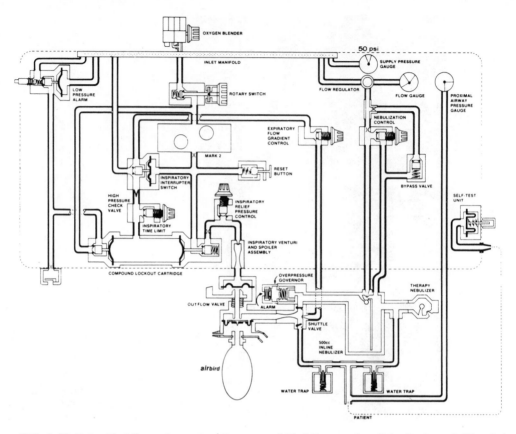

**FIG. 9-38.** Baby Bird flow schematic. (*Courtesy of Bird Corporation, Palm Springs, California.*)

trolled ventilation. There is also a peak inspiratory pressure limit that may be set on the ventilator to protect against excessive pressures during controlled ventilation.

The Baby Bird has several pneumatic alarms within the system. There is an inspiratory time limit alarm, a high pressure alarm, a low pressure alarm, and a maximum pressure alarm (65 mm Hg).

## BIBLIOGRAPHY

Egan, D.F., *Fundamentals of Respiratory Therapy*, 3rd edition, C.V. Mosby, St. Louis, 1977.

*Instruction Manual for Bird Mark 7, 8 Respirators, 7A & 8A, and Baby Bird Ventilator*, Bird Corporation, Palm Springs California.

*Instruction Manual For Bourns Infant Pressure Ventilator Model BP200, Model LS104-150, and Adult Volume Ventilator Bear I*, Bourns, Inc., Life Systems Division, Riverside, California.

Mushin, William W., *Automatic Ventilation of the Lungs*, Blackwell Scientfic Publications, Oxford and Edinburgh, 1969.

*Operation Manual for Ohio 550, Ohio 560, and Ohio Critical Care Ventilator*, Ohio Medical Products, Madison, Wisconsin.

*Operating Instructions, Bennett PR-1, PR-2, and MA-1 Models*, Bennett Respiration Products, Inc., Santa Monica, California.

*Technical Information Manual*, Bird Corporation, Palm Springs, California, 1977.

Young, J.A. and D. Crocker, *Principles and Practice of Respiratory Therapy*, 2nd edition, Yearbook Medical Publishers, Chicago, 1976.

# CHAPTER

# 10

# PULMONARY FUNCTION TESTING

Pulmonary function testing is prescribed to evaluate the lungs' ability to maintain ventilation and the effects of ventilation and oxygenation on the cardiopulmonary circulatory system. Pulmonary function tests are used to assist in patient care. Pulmonary function testing requires the following prescription:

> Date and time of test to be performed
> Specific test(s) to be performed
> Signature of physician

The overall evaluation of the lung requires multiple lung-function studies. Such studies measure lung volumes and capacities, flowrates, diffusion capacities, and distribution of ventilation. A combination of these tests are used to present a quantitative picture of lung function and to provide another source of data about the patient's condition.

## USES OF PULMONARY TESTING

1. *Screening of patients for pulmonary disease.* The measurement of ventilatory function is used to detect functional changes caused by disease in the general population at large. This has essentially developed in the area of industrial medicine in which such screening is used to detect the presence of pneumoconiosis. This screening includes defects such as diffusion capacities at rest and exercise and early asymptomatic emphysema and chronic bronchitis. Such use of pulmonary function testing has increased the possibility of preventive care for the patient. The development of the disease can be reduced by limiting air pollutants and environmental conditions such as cigarette smoking, industrial dusts, and other occupational inhalants.

2. *Preoperative evaluation of patients to identify increased risk of pulmonary complications.* If identified prior to surgery, hypoxemia or chronic carbon dioxide retention can be treated to prevent the possibility of additional complications resulting from surgery. Restrictive conditions involving thoracic and abdominal areas and chronic ventilatory dysfunction such as emphysema and bronchitis also can cause complications following surgery, during a time the patient may be bed ridden, immobilized by traction devices, and/or restricted by bandages or pain.

3. *Evaluation of the patient for diagnosis or assessment of pulmonary disease development.* Ventilatory tests are used to diagnose the presence of pulmonary dysfunction. A common symptom is breathlessness or dyspnea. Dyspnea is associated with a wide range of pulmonary diseases. It is a subjective complaint by the patient who experiences an increase in his awareness of his own breathing. These feelings of breathlessness are influenced by anxiety, excitement, the level of wakefulness, and pain. All of these stimuli to respiratory control alter the sensation of breathlessness in patients having normal and diseased lungs. Pulmonary function testing is used to identify the presence or absence of respiratory disease. Therefore, it acts to identify causes of breathlessness.

The patient who has been diagnosed with respiratory disease also is evaluated periodically to determine the stability or progression of the respiratory physiological dysfunction. The decisions made regarding treatment of his disease require that the patient be re-evaluated. Improvement in lung function can support a decision to continue or discontinue specific therapy.

## LUNG-VOLUME MEASUREMENT

There are four separate volumes of gas within the lung. These volumes are added together in different combinations that are called capacities. There are four basic volume measurements and four capacities. Static lung volumes are recorded and measured by a simple spirometer, except the residual volume. These volumes and capacities are identified in Fig. 10-1. The three volumes and two capacities that can be measured using simple spirometry include:

1. *The inspiratory reserve volume.* The maximum amount of gas that can be inhaled following a normal quiet inhalation of gas into the lung.
2. *The tidal volume.* The amount of gas that is inhaled and exhaled from the lung during quiet breathing.
3. *The expiratory reserve volume.* The amount of gas that can be exhaled from the lung following a quiet exhalation.
4. *The inspiratory capacity.* The inspiratory capacity is a combination of the tidal volume and the expiratory reserve volume. The inspiratory capacity is the maximum amount of gas that can be inhaled following a quiet exhalation.
5. *Vital capacity.* The vital capacity is a combination of the expiratory reserve volume, tidal volume, and inspiratory volume. It is the maximum amount of gas that can be inhaled following a maximum exhalation of air.

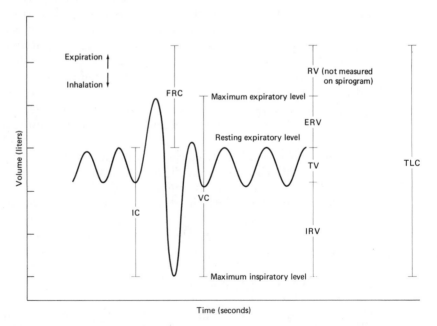

**FIG. 10-1.** Normal spirogram.

# VITAL CAPACITY

The vital capacity is routinely measured as a clinical indication of the ventilatory reserve. The vital capacity requires that the patient inhale as deeply as possible and then exhale fully, using as much time as needed to empty the gas from the lungs. A forced vital capacity requires that the patient inhale as deeply as possible and then exhale forcibly as fast and with as much force as he can (see Fig. 10-2). This maneuver is normally a single volume measurement. Tables 10-1 and 10-2 may be used to predict normal values of vital capacities for healthy men and women.

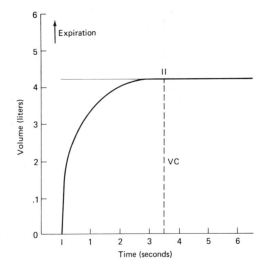

**FIG. 10-2.** Forced vital capacity curve (FVC)—normal curve; (I) initial point at maximum inspiratory level, (II) end point of maximum exhale volume.

Vital capacity can be reduced in two ways (see Figs. 10-3 and 10-4). The first is by a reduction in total lung capacity, and the second is by an increase in the residual volume. It is necessary to measure residual volume and calculate the total lung capacity to differentiate between these two causes in changes in the vital capacity. Significant elevation of residual volume is the cause of a reduced capacity in obstructive lung diseases such as chronic bronchitis, emphysema, and asthma. Diseases that restrict the lung, such as edema and infiltrates, cause a decrease in the vital capacity primarily by decreasing the total lung capacity. (Table 10-3 represents normal lung volumes and capacities.)

## TABLE 10-1

### Spirometric Standards for Normal MALES (BTPS)

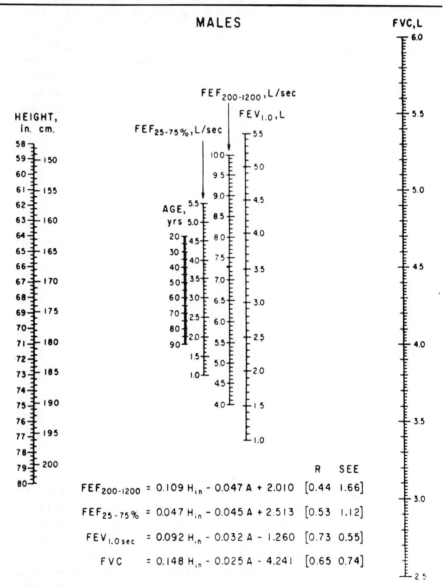

Prediction nomogram (BTPS), spirometric values in normal males. (From Morris, J.F., Koski, W.A., and Johnson, L.D.: Am. Rev. Resp. Dis. 103(1):57, 1971.)

TO USE NOMOGRAM: Lay a straight edge between the patient's height as read on the HEIGHT scale and his age as it appears on the AGE scale.

318

## TABLE 10-2

### Spirometric Standards for Normal FEMALES (BTPS)

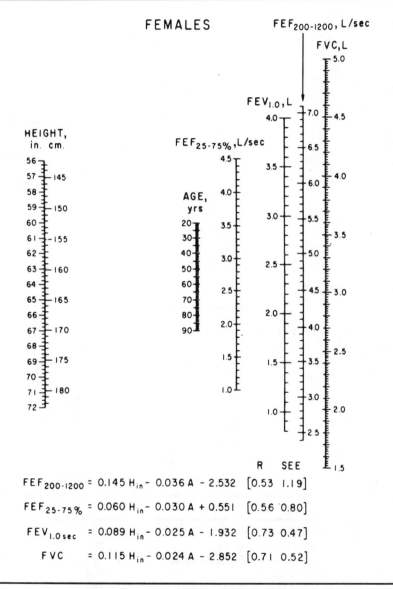

FEMALES

FEF$_{200-1200}$, L/sec

$$FEF_{200-1200} = 0.145\,H_{in} - 0.036\,A - 2.532 \quad [0.53 \;\; 1.19]$$

$$FEF_{25-75\%} = 0.060\,H_{in} - 0.030\,A + 0.551 \quad [0.56 \;\; 0.80]$$

$$FEV_{1.0\,sec} = 0.089\,H_{in} - 0.025\,A - 1.932 \quad [0.73 \;\; 0.47]$$

$$FVC = 0.115\,H_{in} - 0.024\,A - 2.852 \quad [0.71 \;\; 0.52]$$

Prediction nomogram (BTPS), spirometric values in normal females. (From Morris, J.F., Koski, W.A., and Johnson, L.C.: Am. Rev. Resp. Dis. 103(1):57, 1971.)

TO USE NOMOGRAM: Lay a straight edge between the patient's height as read on the HEIGHT scale, and his age as it appears on the AGE scale.

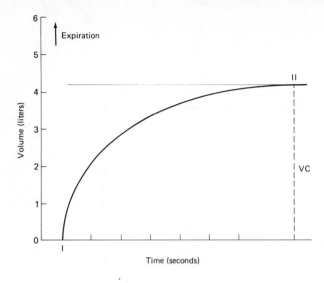

**FIG. 10-3.** Forced vital capacity (FVC) —obstructive pattern reflecting reduced expiratory flowrates.

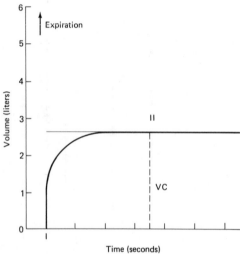

**FIG. 10-4.** Forced vital capacity (FVC)—restrictive pattern reflecting a reduced vital capacity.

**TABLE 10-3**

**Lung Volumes and Capacities\* (BTPS)**

| Names | Abbreviations | Volumes (ml) |
|---|---|---|
| Total Lung Capacity | TLC | 6000 |
| Inspiratory Capacity | IC | 3600 |
| Functional Residual Capacity | FRC | 2400 |
| Vital Capacity | VC | 4800 |
| Inspiratory Reserve Volume | IRV | 3100 |
| Expiratory Reserve Volume | ERV | 1200 |
| Tidal Volume | TV | 500 |
| Residual Volume | RV | 1200 |

\*Healthy, resting, recumbent, young males (1.7 M$^2$ surface area) Adapted from Comroe, J.H., Jr., *Physiology of Respiration.* Year Book Medical Publishers, Chicago, 1969.

# RESIDUAL VOLUME MEASUREMENT

Residual volume is the volume of gas remaining in the lungs at the end of a maximum exhalation. It can only be measured indirectly. Residual volume must be known in order to calculate the total lung capacity and functional residual capacity and to identify changes in the residual volume itself. Current indirect tests actually measure the functional residual capacity. Since $FRC = ERV + RV$, the residual volume can be calculated by subtracting the expiratory reserve volume from the functional residual capacity. The following methods are used for indirect measurement of residual volume:

1. *Helium dilution.* These measurements of functional residual capacity require the use of a closed spirometry system. It is performed by introducing a known volume and concentration of helium into the spirometry system following maximum exhalation by the patient. Carbon dioxide is removed by the use of an absorbant and oxygen is added at the rate that it is consumed. The helium concentration is continually monitored and the equilibration of helium within the system and patient's lungs is completed when the helium concentration stabilizes. This equilibration throughout the system is generally complete within seven minutes, although patients with chronic lung disease may take up to thirty minutes. Patients with chronic emphysema may not equilibrate because of poor ventilation of affected areas of the lung, and therefore, their residual volume will be erroneously calculated. Below is a basic formula for calculating the FRC using the helium dilution method.

EXAMPLE: Lung volume determination by helium dilution

$$FRC = \frac{V(He_1 - He_2)}{He_2} \ (BTPS)$$

$FRC$ = Functional residual capacity

$V$ = Volume of gas in the spirometry circuit

$He_1$ = Initial concentration of helium

$He_2$ = Final concentration of helium

BTPS = Body temperature pressure saturated

2. *Nitrogen washout* (see example below). Nitrogen and helium are both inert gases and therefore are harmless. The patient inhales pure oxygen from the spirometer system to wash the nitrogen from the lungs.

Nitrogen represents about 79 percent of the total gas atmospheric components, and therefore, the breathing of pure oxygen reduces the concentration. The patient's exhaled gas is monitored and its volume and nitrogen concentration are measured. The use of oxygen within the body and carbon dioxide reduction slightly alters the concentration within the lung but the functional residual capacity can be calculated accurately. The washout of nitrogen is begun following a quiet exhalation of the patient (see Fig. 10-5). The nitrogen washout normally requires less than seven minutes except in patients with obstructive diseases and abnormal distributions of ventilation. In these patients the process may require 20–30 minutes. Nitrogen washout must take place within a completely closed system since the addition of nitrogen to the system from room air would lead to an erroneous calculation.

EXAMPLE: Lung volume determination by nitrogen washout

$$V_1 N_1 = V_2 N_2$$

$$V_1 = \frac{V_2 N_2}{N_1}$$

$V_1$ = FRC (Volume of gas in the lungs at resting expiration, to be determined).

$V_2$ = Volume of gas in the spirometer at the end of the test (measured).

$N_1$ = Concentration of nitrogen in the lungs at the beginning of the test (assumed to be 79% as in room air).

$N_2$ = Concentration of nitrogen in the spirometer at the end of the test (measured).

3. *Plethysmography.* The plethysmograph uses the principles of Boyle's Law ($k = V \times P$) and the measurement of volume and pressure changes during ventilation against a closed shutter to measure functional residual capacity. The plethysmograph measures the total gas volume within the chest, including areas of poor ventilation. The functional residual capacity determined by inert gas techniques can be subtracted from the functional residual capacity determined by plethysmography prior to surgery to estimate the volume occupied by boli that are not functionally communicating with other airways within an emphysematous lung. Small airway disease and diffuse emphysema may create a discrepancy between the values because of the occlusion of certain air passages that limits the accuracy of inert gas measurement techniques. Plethysmography eliminates this inaccuracy.

Functional residual capacity by plethysmography is measured by placing an individual in a large sealed chamber. Pressure changes are measured under conditions of no air flow through a sensitive transducer at

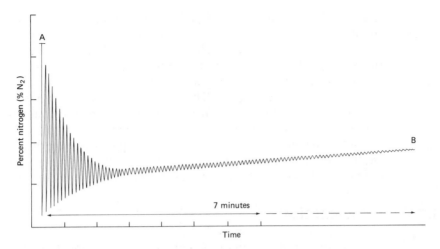

**FIG. 10-5.** Nitrogen washout test (nitrogen elimination)—test begins at end expiration (A) with the patient inhaling oxygen for a seven minute period while the nitrogen concentration of the exhaled gas is measured. The test ends also at end exhalation (B).

the mouth. The pressure measured is correlated as a reflection of the pressure within the thorax. At the same time the pressure within the chamber is measured. Volume changes within the thorax will create volume changes within the sealed chamber, and therefore, will reflect pressure changes within the chamber. Using Boyle's Law, the volume changes within the thorax are calculated representing the thoracic gas volume. Pressure and volume change within the chest are measured during attempted expiration and inspiration against the closed shutter of the mouthpiece within the plethysmograph. Two systems are available; the constant-volume variable-pressure plethysmograph and the constant-pressure variable-volume plethysmograph. Body plethysmographs are expensive and primarily limited to research in pulmonary medicine.

## RESIDUAL VOLUME CALCULATION

The residual volume is calculated by subtracting the expiratory reserve volume from the functional capacity ($FRC = RV + ERV$, therefore $FRC - ERV = RV$). The total lung capacity is calculated as follows: $IRV + TV + ERV + RV$. The functional residual capacity is used because it is the most independent effort and a more reproducible volume than the residual volume alone. The residual volume measurement alone would require exhaling fully, which would mean the patient would have to voluntarily create a maximal expiratory effort and be cooperative and completely understanding of the total technique. The test measuring functional residual capacity is initiated at the end of a normal breath simply by changing a valve to allow gas to enter the system of the patient's spirometry circuit. This conventional measurement of the functional residual capacity is used because of its accuracy and simplicity.

Residual volume is compared to total lung capacity in the form of a ratio described as $RV/TLC$. This ratio is recorded as a percentage. Therefore, changes in the percentage of this ratio indicate changes in the residual volume. The $RV/TLC$ ratio is evaluated for the development of restrictive or obstructive prostheses accompanying lung disease. In healthy adults the $RV/TLC$ ranges from 20% to 35%. With an increased total lung capacity ratios of greater than 35% may indicate chronic air trapping.

## FLOWRATE MEASUREMENT

The ability of the patient to exhale gas from the lung is evaluated by using a maneuver instructing the patient to exhale as much gas as possible. This maneuver is recorded on spirometry equipment as the forced vital capacity. The difference between the forced vital capacity and the spontaneous measurement of vital capacity is in the amount of effort and the speed of exhalation. If the end result of the test is only to measure the volume of gas that can be exhaled from the lungs following a maximal inhalation, then a spontaneous quiet vital capacity is measured. Forced vital capacity is used to calculate various flowrates that the patient is able to generate. Figure 10-2 represents the forced vital capacity recording. When this maneuver is performed with conventional spirometry equipment, volume is recorded on the vertical axis and time is recorded on the horizontal axis (see Fig. 10-2). Three measurements can be calculated from the forced vital capacity curve. These are the volume exhaled during a specific time interval (time forced expiratory volume), the ratio of the timed forced expiratory volume in relationship to the total forced vital volume capacity, and the average flowrate at specific portions of the curve. (Table 10-4 represents normal flowrate values.)

### TABLE 10-4

#### Forced Expiratory Flowrates

| | |
|---|---|
| Maximal expiratory flowrate ATPS, 1/min | 400 |
| Maximal inspiratory flowrate ATPS, 1/min | 300 |
| Forced expiratory volume, %, 1 sec | 83% |
| Forced expiratory volume, %, 3 sec | 97% |
| Maximal voluntary ventilation (BTPS), 1/min | 170 |

*Healthy, resting, recumbent, young males (1.7 $M_2$ surface area) Adapted from Comroe, *et al: The Lung.* Yearbook Medical Publishers, 2nd edition, 1962.

## FORCED EXPIRATORY FLOWRATES

These flowrates were originally described as maximal expiratory flow-rates. They are measured at two specific intervals on the forced expiratory flowrate curve. These measurements of average flowrate are calculated over the first 200–1200 ml exhaled by the patient ($FEF_{200-1200}$) and over the portion of the curve identified as 25 to 75 percent of the forced vital capacity ($FEF_{25-75}$ percent). (See Figs. 10-6 and 10-7.)

The forced expiratory flowrate is determined on a forced vital-capacity curve by marking the 200-ml and 1200-ml points on the shoulder of the curve and drawing a straight line connecting them (see Fig. 10-6). A flow-rate is calculated for 1 sec following correction of the volume exhaled between the 200- and 1200-ml point to BTPS.

The $FEF_{200-1200}$ is most affected by obstruction of the large airways and is most responsive to bronchodilator therapy. The first 200 ml are not used in this measurement because of the initiation of the respiratory maneuver by the patient and the equipment response time, both of which can be unstable. This first 1000 ml exhaled during the forced vital capacity initially will come from the larger airways as the diaphragm ascends forcing the air out of the lungs. Tables 10-1 and 10-2 may be used to compute normal values for $FEF_{200-1200}$ for healthy men and women. The $FEF_{200-1200}$ does not take into consideration the smaller airways. Decreased values for $FEF_{200-1200}$ indicate an abnormal condition in the mechanics of the lung-thorax structure or function. Restrictive disease affects this measurement less than obstructive disease. Flowrates may be as low as 1 l/sec or 60 l/min in patients with severe obstructive disease.

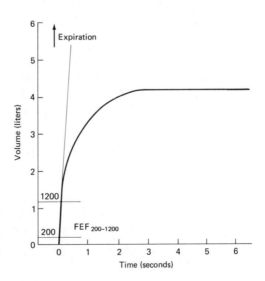

**FIG. 10-6.** Forced expiratory flow-rate ($FEF_{200-1200}$) between 200 and 1200 ml.

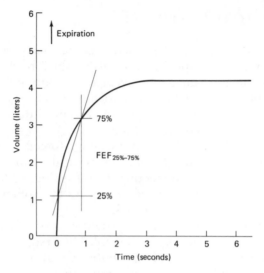

**FIG. 10-7.** Forced expiratory flow-rate between the middle 50% of the forced vital capacity ($FEF_{25-75}$).

$FEF_{25-75}$ represents that portion of the curve that is exhaled during the middle 50 percent of exhalation. The point of the curve representing 25 percent of the forced vital capacity and the point representing 75% of the vital capacity should be identified and a straight line drawn connecting these points (see Fig. 10-7). The flowrate is calculated in l/sec from the curve. Again, volumes must be corrected to BTPS.

The $FEF_{25-75}$ can be determined from Tables 10-1 and 10-2. It indicates changes in the small airways of the lung. Decreases in these flowrates can be an early indication of obstructive disease. The $FEF_{25-75}$ and the $FEF_{200-1200}$ continue to decrease with the severity of obstructive disease. The difference between the two measurements is the sensitivity of the $FEF_{25-75}$ to changes in small airway obstruction, which may not be apparent in the measurement of an $FEF_{200-1200}$ lung. The $FEF_{25-75}$ is intended to identify the more effort independent portion of the forced expiratory curve, and therefore, to increase the reliability and reproducability of the flowrate. Both the $FEF_{200-1200}$ and the $FEF_{25-75}$ demonstrate wide variation in normal population.

## TIMED FORCED EXPIRATORY VOLUMES

The forced expiratory volume and a specific amount of time is used to determine the maximum volume of gas that the patient can exhale over a specific interval of the forced vital capacity. These timed forced expiratory volumes are determined for 0.5 sec, 0.75 sec, (optional) 1.0 sec, 2.0 sec, and 3.0 sec (see Fig. 10-8). The timed force expiratory volume ($FEV_T$) is a dynamic measurement of volume (volume per unit of time

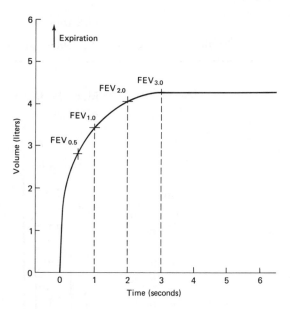

**FIG. 10-8.** Timed forced expiratory volumes (FEV)$_T$.

or flow). This measurement incorporates the early effort dependent portion of the vital capacity and enough of the midportion to make it reproducible and sensitive. The $FEV_T$ is calculated on the forced vital capacity curve by determining the time interval that is to be measured (for example, 0.5 sec, 1.0 sec) and by identifying the volume of gas that was exhaled during that time interval (see Fig. 10-8). The volume must be corrected to BTPS. Normal values for healthy men and women can be determined from Tables 10-5 and 10-6. The values are recorded as l/sec. The $FEV_T$, as a measurement of exhaled volume per unit time is used to estimate the presence of airway obstruction. The validity of the test depends on the cooperation of the patient.

**Timed Forced Expiratory Volume/Forced Vital Capacity Ratio** $(FEV_T/FVC)$: The forced expiratory volume is also expressed as a ratio in comparison to the forced vital capacity volume. This percentage of total forced vital capacity can be used as a crude indicator of airway obstruction. The limitation of this ratio is that a decrease in the ratio will reliably indicate airway obstruction but a normal ratio does not reliably exclude the possibility of airway obstruction if the forced vital capacity is also reduced. A reduction in the forced vital capacity would reflect a normal ratio and the percentage would then hide the presence of the obstructive process. The forced expiratory volume should be looked at both as a percentage of forced vital capacity and as an absolute value to reduce potential error in interpreta-

## TABLE 10-5

### Prediction Nomogram for Spirometry in Normal Females

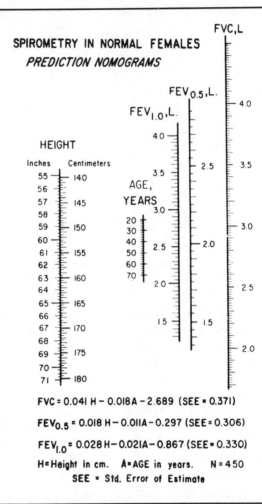

SPIROMETRY IN NORMAL FEMALES
PREDICTION NOMOGRAMS

FVC = 0.041 H − 0.018A − 2.689 (SEE = 0.371)

FEV$_{0.5}$ = 0.018 H − 0.011A − 0.297 (SEE = 0.306)

FEV$_{1.0}$ = 0.028 H − 0.021A − 0.867 (SEE = 0.330)

H = Height in cm.    A = AGE in years.    N = 450
SEE = Std. Error of Estimate

(Courtesy of Dr. Ross C. Kory, VA Hospital, Tampa, Fla. and Ruppel, G.: *Manual of Pulmonary Functions Testing*. C.V. Mosby Co., St. Louis, 1975).

tion. These normal values are $FEV_{0.5}$, > 75 percent; $FEV_{1.0}$, > 83 percent; $FEV_{3.0}$ > 97 percent.

## PEAK FLOWRATE

Peak expiratory flowrate (*PF*) is the maximum rate at which the patient can exhale gas from the lungs and the maximum flowrate produced during a forced expiratory maneuver. This expiratory volume is recorded

# TABLE 10-6

## Prediction Nomogram for Spirometry in Normal Men

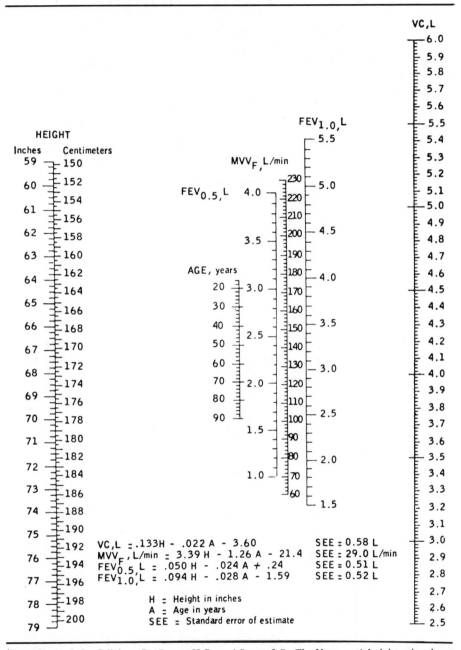

VC,L = .133H − .022 A − 3.60     SEE = 0.58 L
$MVV_F$, L/min = 3.39 H − 1.26 A − 21.4     SEE = 29.0 L/min
$FEV_{0.5}$ L = .050 H − .024 A + .24     SEE = 0.51 L
$FEV_{1.0}$ L = .094 H − .028 A − 1.59     SEE = 0.52 L

H = Height in inches
A = Age in years
SEE = Standard error of estimate

(From Kory, R.C., Callahan, R., Boren, H.G., and Syner, J.C.: The Veterans Administration Army Cooperative Study of Pulmonary Function. I. Clinical spirometry in normal men, Am. J. Med. 30:243; 1961.)

V.A. COOPERATIVE STUDY  Spirometry in Normal Males Prediction Nomograms

in 1/sec or 1/min. It is measured by drawing a line against the steepest portion of the forced vital capacity curve (see Fig. 10-9). The peak flow-rate is calculated by identifying the volume exhaled in a specific amount of time along this steepest portion of the curve. The peak flow can also be calculated from a flow-time curve (see Fig. 10-10).

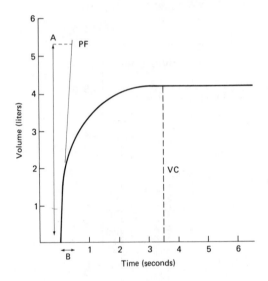

FIG. 10-9. Peak flowrate—volume (A) per unit time (B).

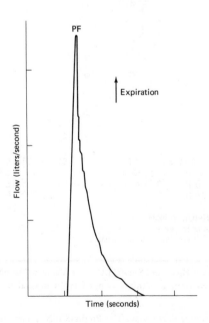

FIG. 10-10. Peak flow measurement (Flow Time Curve) used to compute peak expiratory flowrate.

Peak flowrates computed using a forced vital-capacity curve are very inaccurate. This method is erratic and its accuracy is limited, especially in normal individuals. Peak flow can be measured more accurately by using a pneumotachometer that employs the transducer to convert flow or pressure to an electronic pulse. Although the accuracy of measurement is increased, the reliability of this peak flowrate is limited because of the initial high flow that may occur with obstructive disease prior to airway closure. Decreased peak flow depends on patient effort and cooperation and only indicates nonspecific mechanical problems when it is decreased.

## MAXIMUM VOLUNTARY VENTILATION

Maximum voluntary ventilation (MVV) is the maximal volume of air in liters that can be moved with voluntary patient effort during one minute. It was previously called the maximal breathing capacity. The patient is instructed to breathe rapidly and deeply using the greatest effort possible for 12–30 sec. The patient's volumes are recorded on the spirogram as illustrated on Fig. 10-11. The results are expressed in l/min. The timed volume of 12–30 sec is used to calculate the maximal volume that could be moved in 1 minute (l/min).

The *MVV* is a performance test that depends on patient cooperation and effort. It is sensitive to the loss of muscular coordination in neurological disease, reconditioning from chronic illness, and musculoskeletal diseases of the chest wall. The *MVV* is reduced in patients with obstructive airway diseases and mildly reduced in patients with mild or moderate restrictive disease. It is a more satisfactory indication of the presence of

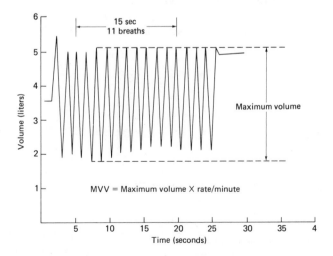

FIG. 10-11. Maximum voluntary ventilation.

obstructive disease because with restrictive disease, a more rapid shallow breathing pattern can be chosen that will compensate effectively for the mechanical defects of the restriction. Therefore, MVV is a simple and sensitive test to identify early obstructive small airway disease.

## CLOSING VOLUME MEASUREMENT

Closing volume is a measurement of the volume of gas, in addition to the residual volume, remaining in the lung when the small airways close during exhalation. Figure 10-12 represents the recording of a single-breath nitrogen test used to calculate the closing volume within the lung (see Fig. 10-12). The closing capacity is calculated by adding the residual volume to the closing volume $(CV + RV = CC)$. Closing volume is compared with vital capacity $(CV/VC)$ and closing capacity is compared with total lung capacity $(CC/TLC)$ and expressed as a percentage.

The single-breath nitrogen elimination test is performed by having the patient inhale a single breath of pure oxygen and exhaling slowly into a spirometry system with a nitrogen meter. As the patient exhales into the spirometry system, the larger airway empties first, followed by the distal smaller airways that tend to collapse after a point at which they are empty. At the point where these small airways in the basal regions of the lungs close, the nitrogen concentration will rise abruptly. The closing volume is the volume exhaled after the sudden increase in the nitrogen concentration (area labeled $CV$ in Fig. 10-12). Small-airway disease, age, and pulmonary edema will cause increases in closing volume. Closing volume measurement is used as a reliable indicator of obstructive small airway disease. The single-breath nitrogen elimination test is relatively independent of patient effort and is not dependent on the patient's individual functional residual capacity or residual volume.

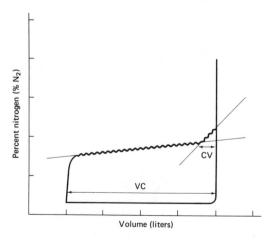

FIG. 10-12. Single breath nitrogen test is used to calculate closing volume.

## FLOW VOLUME MEASUREMENT

Flow-volume curves and loops have developed with electronic spirometry, which allows the plotting of flowrate against volume on a spirogram. The patient is instructed to inhale and exhale fully with maximum effort into an electronic spirometer capable of measuring flowrate and volume changes simultaneously (see Fig. 10-13). This curve gives the same information held in a conventional forced vital capacity and a graphic record of inspiratory flowrate and volume measurements. Figure 10-13 illustrates a display of ventilatory data that can be calculated on a flow-volume curve. Emphasis is on the dependence of maximal flow in determining lung volume. The flow-volume curve is used to measure a maximal expiratory and inspiratory maneuver producing a forced vital capacity.

The initial portion of the curve during the forced expiratory maneuver is basically effort-dependent but following expiration of the first 1/3 of the vital capacity, the curve is relatively effort-independent and reproducible. The effort-independent portion of the expiratory curve that follows the peak expiratory flowrate is reproducible and is altered in disease changes of restriction and obstruction.

Maximal effort flow-volume loops include both a maximal expiratory maneuver and a maximal inspiratory maneuver. The inspiratory curve of the maximal effort flow-volume loops is more sensitive to major central airway obstruction than is the expiratory portion. The expiratory portion

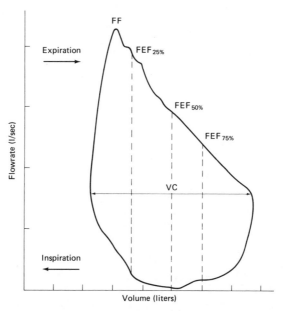

**FIG. 10-13.** Flow volume curve (loop)—normal.

is more sensitive to peripheral airway obstruction or restrictive disease. Flow-volume loops including a forced inspiratory maneuver are practical for identifying central airway obstruction and provide more specific data than conventional spirometry, which demonstrates only a nonspecific obstructive pattern. Figures 10-14 and 10-15 represent obstructive and restrictive maximal-effort flow volume curves.

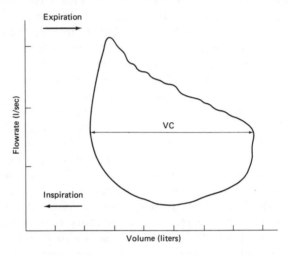

**FIG. 10-14.** Flow volume—obstructive pattern.

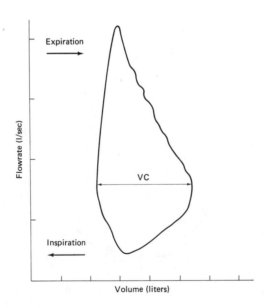

**FIG. 10-15.** Flow volume curve—restrictive pattern.

# DIFFUSION MEASUREMENTS

Diffusion testing is a method of evaluating the movement of gas across the alveolar capillary membrane into the alveolar blood. It will reflect the presence of changes in the diffusion rate of gas across the alveolar capillary membrane. Diffusion capacity is recorded in ml/min/mm Hg. When using a single-breath carbon monoxide diffusion capacity test, the patient is instructed to inhale a deep breath of a gas mixture containing a low concentration of carbon monoxide (CO) and 10 percent helium (He). Inhalation is begun following a maximal exhalation. At end exhalation, the patient is connected to the circuit containing carbon monoxide and asked to inhale to his inspiratory vital capacity (IVC). Following inhalation, the patient holds his breath for 10 sec. The amount of carbon monoxide that diffuses into the patient's lungs is the difference in the concentration of the carbon monoxide in the alveolar gas at the end of the 10-sec interval and the beginning concentration. Then, this is computed to determine the diffusion capacity of carbon monoxide in the lung. A closed breathing circuit is used containing carbon monoxide and helium analyzers.

Figure 10-16 demonstrates the curve characterized on the spirogram during a single-breath diffusion capacity test. Normal diffusion capacity of carbon monoxide is 25 ml/min/mm Hg. A rebreathing technique is also used to measure diffusion capacity of carbon monoxide. Samples of gas are analyzed at intervals of 10 to 30 sec and the total volume of the lung spirometer system is multiplied by the change in carbon-monoxide concentration to determine the volume of carbon-monoxide transferred. Table 10-7 describes diffusion changes with specific lung conditions.

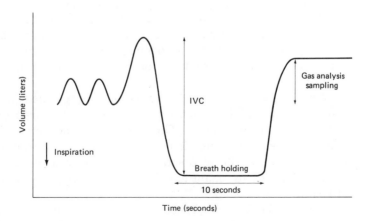

FIG. 10-16. Single breath diffusion capacity test.

**TABLE 10-7**

**Changes in Diffusing Capacity ($DL_{CO}$) With Lung Condition**

*Decreased Diffusion Capacity*

Anemia
Diffuse pulmonary fibrosis
Emphysema
Granulomatosis
Pulmonary embolism
Pulmonary hypertension

*Increased Diffusion Capacity*

Congestive heart disease with increased pulmonary blood flow
Exercise
Polycythemia

## GAS DISTRIBUTION MEASUREMENTS

Ventilation and perfusion studies by lung scan are used to assess gas distribution and blood flow in the lungs. The radioxenon method is used to measure regional distribution of ventilation. The patient is placed in a supine or sitting position. He is instructed to inhale a normal tidal volume from a closed system containing a measured dose of xeon (Xe133). The patient then holds his breath for 10–20 sec while photoscintograms are made over the lung field. Figures 10-17 and 10-18 represent normal and abnormal ventilation of a lung on photoscintograms. Serial photoscintograms may be made using a rebreathing technique over a 10–15-min interval to determine the rapidity and equilibration of the gas within the lung. Following the test, the patient is placed in a system to breathe atmospheric gas to wash out the xeon. Xeon, being a radioactive particle, is sent through a decontamination unit and vented to the atmosphere outside the hospital. Serial photoscintograms will indicate the areas in which xeon is trapped during the equilibration phase and unventilated areas the xeon did not reach.

Regional distribution of inspired gas is identified on the photoscintogram and provides a pictoral description for diagnosis of pulmonary distribution abnormalities. The half-life of radio-xeon is 5.27 days and must be monitored, since it is not metabolized by the body and remains in the gas phase. Body position and tidal volume should be controlled during testing to maintain constant testing parameters with each procedure.

Figures 10-19 and 10-20 show normal lung perfusion made with microaggragated albumin particles treated with radioactive iodine ($I_{131}$).

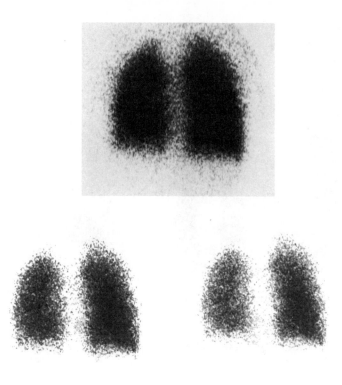

**FIG. 10-17.** Normal lung ventilation during lung scan, with posterior view.

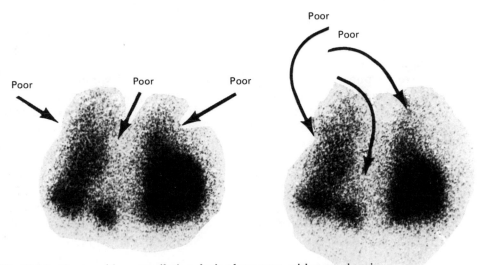

**FIG. 10-18.** Abnormal lung ventilation during lung scan, with posterior view.

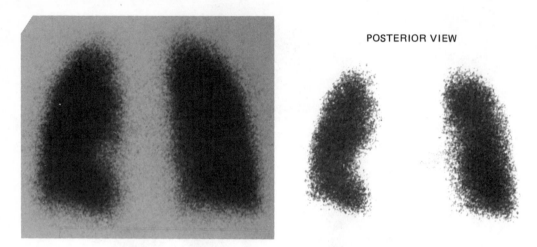

POSTERIOR VIEW

**FIG. 10-19.** Normal lung perfusion during lung scan, with posterior view.

This is an abnormal and normal perfusion scan of a patient with a pulmonary emboli.

## EXERCISE TESTING

Tidal breathing at rest requires less effort than a patient's normal maximum ability to ventilate; therefore, ventilatory impairments caused by disease must be extremely severe before a significant reduction in minute ventilation appears at rest. Exercise provided using steps, a multispeed treadmill, or a stationary bicycle stimulates an increase in ventilatory demand to measure the patient's ability to respond to increased metabolic activity. A baseline study of pulmonary functions is performed by the patient in a resting state, followed by exercise and retesting at a point where dyspnea occurs, or a predetermined minute volume or heart rate is achieved. The tests again are made following a recovery phase of the patient returning to a resting state. Ventilation, oxygen consumption, arterial gases, pulse, blood pressure, and EKG should be measured to determine the ability of the patient to meet metabolic demand through his cardiopulmonary system. With chronic obstructive lung disease, the patient may compensate during early stages by increasing his minute pulmonary ventilation to maintain arterial blood gases at a normal level during exercise. Exercise-test results can differentiate between cardiac and pulmonary disabilities and determine the relative importance of the two in a combined disease process.

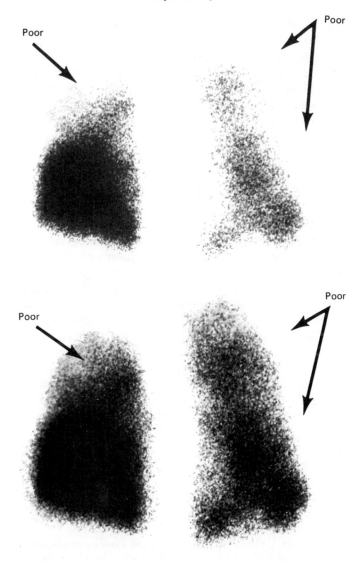

**FIG. 10-20.** Abnormal lung perfusion during lung scan, with posterior view.

# BEFORE AND AFTER BRONCHODILATOR MEASUREMENTS

Bronchodilator studies are used to determine a course of therapy for a patient with a potentially reversible disease process. An improvement of vital capacity greater than 15–20 percent is considered significant in the reversibility of airway obstruction. Asthma often shows an improvement of 50 percent. Pulmonary function studies are performed before a bronchodilator is administered to the patient, and then after the broncho-dilator therapy is administered. The follow-up pulmonary function test should be done at least 5–10 minutes after the bronchodilator therapy has been completed. Decreases in vital capacity sometimes observed after bronchodilator treatment are normally caused by a reduction in the residual volume that was previously increased by air trapping. This testing regime is very important in the decision to use bronchodilator therapy.

## THERAPEUTIC CONSIDERATIONS OF PFT

1. *Patient history.* Background information about the present condition and past development of the patient's pulmonary complaint can be identi-fied in an organized interview or questionnaire about the patient's pulmo-nary history. Such a questionnaire or interview should include a record of age, sex, height, weight, and weight gain or weight loss. The patient's and family's history of pulmonary disease, including both chronic and seasonal diseases such as colds, pneumonia, and allergy, should also be included. The history should identify the patient's present complaint and the com-plaint that originally brought him to the care of the physician. The pa-tient's professional and daily environment should also be described within such an outline. A pulmonary history acts as a data base for evaluation of the pulmonary test. The pulmonary history of the patient should be up-dated following the testing of the patient, as questions arise in regard to altered pulmonary test values.

2. *Percent of predicted.* Pulmonary function tests results are reported in relationship to predicted values based on the patient's age, sex, and height. The percentage is determined by dividing the measured value by the predicted value and multiplying times 100. The following is an exam-ple of a value recorded as percent of predicted:

> EXAMPLE: A patient's forced expiratory volume was measured after 1 sec, and had a $FEV_{1.0}$ of 450 ml/sec. The predicted normal value for this patient was 540 ml/sec. Therefore, the percent of predicted would be equal to 450 divided by 540 $\times$ 100, which equals 83 percent. Therefore, the percent of predicted $FEV_{1.0}$ for the patient is 83 percent.

3. *Predicted normal values.* Tables 10-1 and 10-2 and Tables 10-5 and 10-6 represent predicted normal values for adult healthy males and females. These graphs are based on predicted normal values of groups of patients of the same height, age, and sex. Such values are used for both computer programming and nomogram to identify predicted normal values.

4. *Disease changes.* Table 10-8 represents common test changes that occur with restrictive and obstructive pulmonary disease. Differential diagnosis of the two conditions is aided by specific pulmonary function changes that occur with each condition.

5. *Noseclips.* Noseclips should be used to assure that all the patient's exhaled volume enters the spirometer. Also the patient should be placed in the *same position* for each test. Table 10-9 lists positions of the patient for each test. The patient should not eat, smoke, or take any type of bronchodilator medication at least two hours prior to the tests. These factors may reduce the accuracy of the test results. Pulmonary function test results are not meant to be the only tool used in diagnosis of pulmonary disease, but as an information source to add to the accuracy of the diagnostic decision.

6. *Pulmonary function volumes.* These are measured at body temperature, ambient pressure and 100 percent saturated with water vapor (BTPS). Volumes, if they are recorded at room temperature and saturation (ATPS), must be adjusted to BTPS. Table 10-10 lists conversion factors to convert volumes to BTPS:

### TABLE 10-8

**Lung Changes with Obstructive and Restriction Disease**

| *Test* | *Obstructive Disease* | *Restrictive Disease* |
|--------|----------------------|----------------------|
| $VC$ | normal or decreased | decreased |
| $FRC$ | increased | decreased |
| $TLC$ | increased | decreased |
| $RV$ | increased | decreased |
| $FEV_{1.0}$ | decreased | normal or decreased |
| $MVV$ *(MBC)* | decreased | normal or decreased |
| $FEF$ | decreased | normal or decreased |

### TABLE 10-9

**Patient Position During Testing**

| *Test* | *Position* |
|--------|-----------|
| Spirogram (volume measurements) | sitting |
| Forced vital capacity (flowrate measurements) | standing |
| Maximum voluntary ventilation | standing |
| Residual volume measurement | sitting |
| Closing volume and capacity | sitting |
| Diffusion measurement | sitting |
| Lung scan | supine |

## TABLE 10-10

**Factors for Conversion of Gas Volumes for Room Temperature Saturated to 37°C. Saturated**

| When Gas Temperature is 0°C. | With Water Vapor Pressure (mm Hg) of | Factor to Convert Volume to 37°C Saturated (BTPS) |
|---|---|---|
| 20 | 17.5 | 1.102 |
| 21 | 18.7 | 1.096 |
| 22 | 19.8 | 1.091 |
| 23 | 21.1 | 1.085 |
| 24 | 22.4 | 1.080 |
| 25 | 23.8 | 1.075 |
| 26 | 25.2 | 1.068 |
| 27 | 26.7 | 1.063 |
| 28 | 28.3 | 1.057 |
| 29 | 30.0 | 1.051 |
| 30 | 31.8 | 1.045 |
| 31 | 33.7 | 1.039 |
| 32 | 35.7 | 1.032 |
| 33 | 37.7 | 1.026 |
| 34 | 39.9 | 1.020 |
| 35 | 42.2 | 1.014 |
| 36 | 44.6 | 1.007 |
| 37 | 47.0 | 1.000 |

Measured volume (ATPS) × conversion factor
= calculated volume (BTPS)

For example: a volume of 4 l is measured at a spirometer temperature of 25°C would be converted as:

$$4.0 \, l \times 1.075 = 4.3 \, l \, (BTPS)$$

## PULMONARY FUNCTION TESTING EQUIPMENT

### Spirometers

1. *Water-sealed spirometers.* Water-sealed spirometers consist of a large bell reservoir suspended in a large container of water. The bell, an open-end cylinder, is sealed by the water and carefully balanced to provide minimal resistance to gas flow. Figure 10-21 illustrates the water-sealed spirometer. The bell is counterbalanced by a weighted chain and, as it moves within the cylinder, it records the volume on a graph paper drum

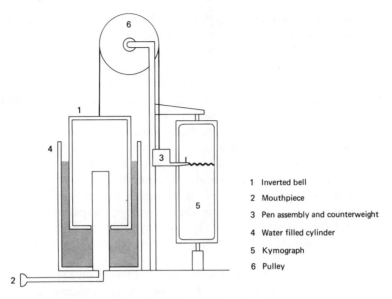

**FIG. 10-21.** Water seal spirometer.

1  Inverted bell
2  Mouthpiece
3  Pen assembly and counterweight
4  Water filled cylinder
5  Kymograph
6  Pulley

assembly called a *kymograph*. The kymograph provides a timing mechanism as it revolves. This volume/time relationship is used to calculate flowrates.

The water-sealed spirometer is commonly used to measure lung pulmonary flowrate and lung volume, including functional residual capacity, the appropriate gas analyzers to be used, and diffusion capacity. All measurements on the equipment should be corrected to BTPS. Water-sealed type spirometers include the Tissot, Stead-Wells, and Collins. The reliability of water-sealed spirometers depends on the resistance of the bell to movements and the correction of volumes to BTPS.

2. *Bellows spirometers (see Fig. 10-22).* Bellows spirometers are designed to work on a horizontal plain in which the expansion of the bellows responds to a volume of gas entering them. The expanding bellows is con-

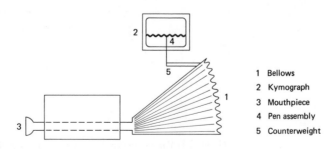

1  Bellows
2  Kymograph
3  Mouthpiece
4  Pen assembly
5  Counterweight

**FIG. 10-22.** Bellows spirometer.

nected to a recording pen and kymograph. The horizontal bellows can record both inspiration and expiration because it does not start in a totally collapsed position. The wedged bellows design offers less mechanical resistance than the water-sealed spirometer. The bellows spirometer measures vital capacity, timed vital capacities, flowrates, including inspiratory and expiratory flowrates, and maximal voluntary ventilation.

3. *Rolling seal spirometers (see Fig. 10-23).* A dry rolling-sealed spirometer incorporates a light weight piston moving on low-resistant, low-friction bearings along a horizontal plane. A flexible seal rolls outside of the piston, maintaining a tight fit along the piston wall. The rolling action reduces mechanical resistance to the flow and to the rolling piston. A pen or potentiometer, is attached to the pistons and connected to a kymograph, or electronic digital readout apparatus, for recording volume and flow changes. This type of dry sealed spirometer is used in measuring lung volumes, ventilation, diffusing capacity, and pulmonary flowrates. These types of spirometers also can be used with analoged functional computers with digital read-outs and hard copy recorders.

4. *Rotating vanes (see Fig. 10-24).* A rotating vane spirometer uses a vane connected to a series of gears so that the spirometer's flow through

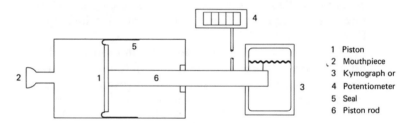

1 Piston
2 Mouthpiece
3 Kymograph or
4 Potentiometer
5 Seal
6 Piston rod

**FIG. 10-23.** Rolling seal spirometer.

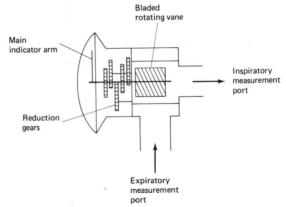

**FIG. 10-24.** Rotating vane spirometer (Wright respirometer).

the body rotates the vane and registers a volume. This type of spirometer measures lung volume such as vital capacity and tidal volume and minute ventilation. The Wright Respirometer functions on this principle and, because of its compact size, it may be used for bed-side spirometry. At very high and low flowrates, the vane within the spirometer becomes distorted and, therefore, its measurements are inaccurate.

## Pneumotachographs (see Fig. 10-25)

Pneumotachographs (pneumotachs) use physical and chemical principles to produce electrical flow that can be integrated for the measurement of volume and flowrate.

A *pressure drop* pneumotachograph uses a resistant element that causes a pressure drop as gas flows through the pneumotach tube. The pressure drop is proportional to the flow of the gas through the tube and, therefore, pressure-sensitive transducers can be used to measure the pressure before and after the resistance in the tube. This differential is converted into an electrical signal that varies as flow changes. Volume through pneumotachograph can be calculated by integrating the flow over the time interval during which the flow occurs.

A *heat transfer* pneumotachograph functions as a thermistor. This type of pneumotachograph uses a small heated element within the tube. This is usually a platinum wire. As the flow enters the tube of the pneumotach, the element cools. A greater current is required to maintain the constant temperature of the heated element. Current changes are correlated electronically and are proportional to gas flow. A constant signal is supplied to an integrated circuit to measure flow and volume changes through the pneumotachograph.

Pneumotachographs are suitable for measuring the following pulmonary function values when used with appropriate electronic outputs: lung volumes, ventilation measurements, distribution measurements, and flowrate measurements. A disadvantage of pneumotachographs is that at extreme high or low flows, signals generated may be nonproportional. The use of pneumotachographs offers precise testing with lightweight portable units and a limited amount of mechanical resistance due to the direct processing of the flowrate into an electronic output.

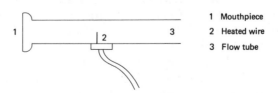

1 Mouthpiece
2 Heated wire
3 Flow tube

**FIG. 10-25.** Pneumotach (heat transfer type).

## ARTERIAL BLOOD GAS ASSESSMENT

Respiratory function may be evaluated by measuring arterial oxygen tension ($PaO_2$), carbon dioxide ($PaCO_2$), oxygen saturation ($SaO_2$), bicarbonate ($HCO_3^-$) and pH. This assessment is an estimate of the degree to which the lung is able to provide adequate oxygen and removal of carbon dioxide. The assessment of arterial blood values can also estimate the degree to which the kidneys are able to reabsorb and excrete bicarbonate ions to maintain a normal body pH. The physician prescribes arterial blood sampling whenever it is necessary to evaluate respiratory function.

Arterial blood gas assessment is indicated in the use of laboratory pulmonary function testing to determine a baseline prior to and following exercise. It is also indicated to determine a clinical baseline and evaluate changes with the delivery of specific respiratory care. For example, the drawing and analysis of arterial blood-gas values in the patient receiving mechanical ventilation following changes in ventilatory parameters or oxygenation techniques. It is also clinically indicated in patients who develop unexpected tachypnea and dyspnea, especially those with cardiopulmonary disease. Unexpected restlessness, anxiety, drowsiness, and confusion may require blood gas analysis to determine the extent to which these symptoms are attributed to hypoxia.

## ARTERIAL PUNCTURE PROCEDURE

The following is an arterial puncture procedure:

1. *Explanation.* The arterial puncture procedure should be explained to the patient to assure better patient cooperation and understanding. Explanation of the procedure should be simple and concise, emphasizing the importance of the gas analysis and the use of the analysis information.
2. *Equipment preparation.* The arterial puncture procedure should be handled as if sterile. Appropriate handling of the equipment will limit the potential hazard of infection to the patient. Table 10-11 lists the standard equipment used in the arterial puncture procedure. Prior to assembly of the equipment, the hands should be washed thoroughly with an antiseptic soap or solution. Following assembly of the equipment, the syringe that is used should be flushed with heparin. Heparin should be drawn up into the syringe through the needle, taking care to keep the heparin, syringe, and needle sterile. Only a few drops of heparin within the syringe are needed to prevent clotting of the blood during and following the arterial puncture procedure. Push all of the heparin out of the syringe once it has been rinsed. This will leave only a small amount of heparin filling the deadspace of the needle and the end of the syringe.

## TABLE 10-11

### Arterial Puncture Equipment

*Puncture Equipment*

5 or 10 ml glass syringe, luer lock
No. 22–25 gauge needle, 1½ in, bevel end
Syringe cap
1ml vial Sodium Heparin (1000 U.S.P. Units/ml)
Paper cup or plastic bag of crushed ice
Alcohol prep pads
1 rubber stopper
2 gauze sponges
1 adhesive bandage

*Anesthetic Equipment:*

3 ml plastic syringe
No. 25 gauge needle, 5/8 in
2 ml vial Procaine HCl 1%

**3.** *Puncture site.* Patient should be positioned so that the chosen arterial site is completely exposed and accessible for puncture. Figure 10-26 illustrates the common sites of arterial puncture. The most common site used for arterial punctures is the radial artery. This artery is used primarily because of its accessibility, the presence of collateral circulation through the ulnar artery, and its distance from the cardiopulmonary system.

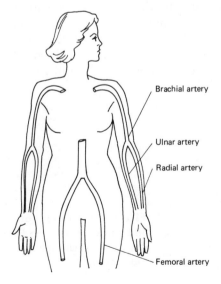

Brachial artery

Ulnar artery

Radial artery

Femoral artery

**FIG. 10-26.** Arteries used for obtaining blood gas samples (except ulnar artery which is only used for check of collateral circulation).

4. *The Allen Test.* The Allen Test is performed to check for collateral circulation through the ulnar artery. This collateral circulation is used to guarantee circulation to the hand if the radial artery becomes occluded by accident. When performing the Allen Test, both the ulnar and radial artery are compressed at the wrist to occlude circulation to the hand. The patient is then instructed to squeeze the fist and release using a pumping action to blanche the palm of the hand (creating a white blotchy condition in the palm caused by the absence of circulation). In the unconscious or uncooperative patient, the hand is elevated above the level of the heart and the hand is squeezed until this blanching occurs. With the radial artery still compressed, pressure is released from the ulnar artery, allowing circulation to return to the hand.

Rapid return of pinkness of the hand is an indication that the ulnar artery is functional and will act as collateral circulation in case of accidental occlusion of the radial artery. If pinkness fails to appear, collateral circulation must be assumed to be inadequate and the physician should be informed of such a condition. Another arterial puncture site for sample collection should be chosen. If the pinkness returns quickly, collateral circulation is assumed to be adequate.

5. *Arterial puncture.* Palpate the radial artery pulse and determine the point of maximal pulse. Once this is done the wrist should be stabilized so that the hand is flexed and should be rotated to extend the wrist puncture site and provide maximum exposure of the radial artery (see Fig. 10-27). Clean the puncture site with an alcohol or preferably a Betadine prep pad. Following this, adjust your position to place the needle at a 35–40 degree angle above the puncture site. Using a 22–25 gauge needle, insert the needle through the skin and into the artery. When inserting the needle into the arterial puncture site, make sure that the beveled edge of the needle is up. Inserting the needle into the arterial vessel so that the flow of blood is running against the open beveled edge of the needle. Advance the needle slowly, and as the artery is punctured, blood will enter the syringe.

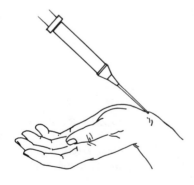

FIG. 10-27. Position of the hand and angle of the needle insertion during arterial puncture of the radial artery.

Using a glass syringe, it should not be necessary to aspirate the blood into the syringe because of the pulsating arterial pressure.

> NOTE: Prior to performing the arterial puncture, the punctured site may be anesthetized by using a 1 percent solution of Procaine applied to the subdermal area by pricking the skin with a needle and inserting the Procaine from the syringe. This will reduce part of the patient's initial pain with insertion of the larger gauge needle. For many patients this will cause as much discomfort as the arterial puncture itself. Table 10-11 lists the equipment used for preanesthesia.

6. *Compression.* Immediately following collection of the sample, the needle is withdrawn at the same angle as it was inserted and firm pressure should be maintained over the puncture site for at least 5 min. A 4 × 4 sterile pad may be used to compress the puncture site to absorb the small amount of bleeding that may occur and to maintain cleanliness in the area of the wound. Compression is vitally necessary to prevent the development of a hematoma and to aid in the development of clots within the arterial vessel. If the patient is on anticoagulant therapy, the direct pressure over the wound should be applied for at least 15 min, followed by a pressure dressing for 3–4 hours, as necessary.

7. *Handling the samples.* Follwing the removal of the needle from the puncture site, the syringe should be capped and placed in a container of ice. This will reduce the metabolic rate and oxygen consumption in the blood, preventing a significant fall of pH and $PaO_2$ within the blood. Also, care should be taken not to allow any gas bubbles within the syringe. Gas bubbles will cause a change in the oxygen tension, saturation, and $PaCO_2$ and, therefore, also lead to a change in pH. An air bubble will tend to cause an increase in $PaO_2$ and a decrease in $PaCO_2$. If any gas bubbles are visible within the syringe, the syringe should be inverted with the plunger end down and rotated in the hand until all the bubbles rise to the top of the syringe near the needle connection. Then the plunger may be pushed up, evacuating the air from the syringe. The blood sample should be transported in ice to the laboratory immediately after drawing. Ice is used to slow blood metabolism. Blood-gas analysis should be done as soon as possible after the blood is drawn because of the possibility of gas tension and pH changes if the sample is allowed to sit. Ideally, blood-gas analysis will occur within 15 min after the drawing of the blood.

8. *Follow-up.* The puncture site should be inspected and patient's condition assessed following arterial puncture. Damage to the artery, arterial thrombosis, and hematoma are all possible complications following the arterial blood-gas puncture. Examination of the puncture site is important to identify the complications and evaluate the puncture technique.

## THERAPEUTIC CONSIDERATIONS

1. *Use of an aseptic technique and sterile equipment.* This is necessary to prevent infection. Septicemia is a potential hazard of arterial puncture and can produce a life threatening condition for the patient; therefore, proper equipment handling is most important.

2. *Anticoagulation.* Heparin is used to coat the interior portion of the needle to prevent the natural clotting of blood that would occur as the blood leaves the body. Sodium heparin, in a concentration of 1000 units/ml, is mixed with a normal saline (0.9 percent sodium chloride) and flushed through the syringe prior to the procedure. Sodium heparin at 10,000 units/ml may be used but is not recommended. All but the heparin remaining in the needle and the needle connection should be flushed from the syringe prior to the arterial puncture. The coating of the syringe with heparin may be done by rolling the syringe between the palms of the hands.

3. *Puncture site.* Figure 10-26 illustrates the most common sites. The radial or brachial artery are commonly used because of the increased hazards of drawing arterial blood from the other sites. The radial artery is a superficial artery located just below the skin surface within the wrist. It is normally the easiest puncture site to locate by palpation of the pulse. Use of the radial artery for arterial puncture site rather than the brachial or femoral artery allows collateral circulation through the ulnar artery. The brachial and femoral arteries do not have a vessel of this size to provide collateral circulation to the extremities for which they supply arterial blood.

4. *The Allen Test.* The Allen Test is used to guarantee collateral circulation through the ulnar artery to the hand. It should be performed before *every* arterial blood-gas puncture of the radial artery.

5. *Test samples.* Analysis should never be delayed. Any delay in running the arterial samples will jeopardize the accuracy of the values measured. Blood gas values reflect the state of the patient at the time the sample is collected. As stated above, gas bubbles should be removed immediately from all samples to prevent changes in blood gas values. These changes are reduced by immersing the sample in ice immediately after the puncture and during transportation to the blood gas laboratory.

6. *Arterial sampling.* Arterial blood gas samples should be drawn whenever a change is made in medical gas therapy or mechanical ventilation of the critically ill patient. It is also valuable to follow up on the recovering patient with periodic blood gas evaluation. Also, any unexplained psychological or physical changes such as restlessness, anxiety, or drowsiness, confusion, or extreme vital sign changes may indicate a need for arterial blood gas assessment. If frequent arterial blood gas sampling is necessary it

**TABLE 10-12**

**Arterial Gas Values**

| | | | |
|---|---|---|---|
| pH | Concentration of free hydrogen ions in arterial blood | 7.35–7.45 | normal range |
| | | > 7.45 | alkemia |
| | | < 7.35 | acidemia |
| $PaCO_2$ | Partial pressure (tension) of carbon dioxide in arterial blood | 35–45 torr | normal |
| | | < 35 torr | alveolar hyperventilation |
| | | > 45 torr | alveolar hypoventilation |
| $PaO_2$ | Partial pressure (tension) of oxygen in arterial blood | 80–100 torr | normal breathing room air |
| | | > 600 torr | normal breathing 100% $O_2$ |
| | | < 60 torr | requires an increase in cardiac output to maintain adequate oxygen transport to the tissues. |

can be expediated by placement of an arterial line for drawing samples.

Arterial blood gas evaluation is an objective method of determining respiratory function. Clinical interpretation of arterial blood gases is impossible without knowing the patient's present respiratory rate, tidal volume, and oxygen concentration. Table 10-12 lists arterial blood gas values and interpretations.

## VARIABLES OF ARTERIAL BLOOD-GAS ANALYSIS

1. Blood gases are routinely analyzed at 37°C. When a patient is febrile or hypothermic, errors may be introduced into the blood-gas values if the blood is analyzed at the usual instrument temperature of 37°C.

An increase or decrease in temperature will cause a decrease or increase in oxygen saturation and hydrogen ion concentration at the varying temperatures. It is very important, then, that patients with a fever or hypothermia have their blood gas values corrected to their temperature. If this is not done, the $P_aO_2$ and pH will be incorrectly reflected in the blood gas value interpretation. This is an automatic function of a blood gas analyzer.

2. Care must be taken to assure that the blood sample is from an artery rather than a vein or area of hematoma. The analysis of venous blood will reflect venous blood-gas values which, if they were actually arterial samples, could require significant changes in therapy to correct them back to a normal arterial range. The misinterpretation may be a grave error. The

possibility of a blood gas value being from venous blood should always be considered when interpreting blood-gas values.

3. The use of arterial blood gas analysis instruments for measuring arterial blood, pH, $PO_2$, and $PCO_2$ creates the potential for analytical error. Faulty calibration of the equipment and/or mishandling of the instruments can lead to improper function of the analysis equipment. Quality control is very important. Blood gas analysis equipment should be calibrated before each blood gas analysis. Analytical error may also be the result of contamination of the specimen allowing air to enter the specimen, while injecting it into the instrument. In addition, manufacturer instructions concerning the calibration and maintenance of blood-gas equipment should be closely followed to limit the possibility of such errors.

## P.F.T. SYMBOLS AND ABBREVIATIONS

The following is a list of common symbols and abbreviations used in pulmonary function testing and respiratory care:

| | |
|---|---|
| ATPS | Ambient temperature and pressure saturated with water vapor |
| BTPS | Body temperature and pressure saturated with water vapor |
| $C_L$ | Lung compliance |
| $C_{LT}$ | Total lung compliance |
| $C_T$ | Thoracic compliance |
| $DL_{CO}$ | Diffusing capacity for carbon monoxide |
| $DLO_2$ | Diffusing capacity for oxygen |
| $ERV$ | Expiratory reserve volume |
| $f$ | Respiratory rate |
| $F$ | Fractional gas concentration |
| $FEF_{200-1200}$ | Forced expiratory flow rate over the 200–1200 ml points of an FEV maneuver (formerly MEFR) |
| $FEF_{25-75\%}$ | Forced expiratory flow rate over the middle 50% of an FEV maneuver (formerly $MMFR$) |
| $FEV_T$ | Forced expiratory volume for a specific interval of time ($T$) |
| $FEV_{T\%}$ | Forced expiratory volume for interval T as a percentage of $FVC$ |
| $FIO_2$ | Fractional concentration of inspired oxygen |

| | |
|---|---|
| *FRC* | Functional residual capacity |
| *FVC* | Forced vital capacity |
| *IC* | Inspiratory capacity |
| *IDI* | Inspired gas distribution index (for 7-min $N_2$ washout) |
| *IRV* | Inspiratory reserve volume |
| *MV* | Minute volume |
| *MVV* | Maximal voluntary ventilation (formerly *MBC*) |
| $\%N_{2\ 500}$ | Delta percent $N_2$ over the terminal 500 ml of an expired breath of 100% $O_2$ (sometimes over the closing volume) |
| $\%N_{2\ 750-1250}$ | Delta percent $N_2$ over 750 to 1250 ml portion of an expiration of a breath of 100% $O_2$ |
| *P* | Gas pressure |
| $PACO_2$ | Alveolar carbon dioxide tension |
| $PaCO_2$ | Arterial carbon dioxide tension |
| $PAO_2$ | Alveolar oxygen tension |
| $PaO_2$ | Arterial oxygen tension |
| *PF* | Peak flow, expiratory unless otherwise stated (sometimes *PEFR*) |
| pH | Negative logarithm of the H+ concentration used as a positive number (normally arterial) |
| $SaO_2$ | Percent of hemoglobin saturated with $O_2$ |
| *P/V* | Airway resistance |
| *Q* | Blood flow |
| *Q̃* | Blood flow/unit time (perfusion) |
| *RV* | Residual volume |
| *RV/TLC* × 100 | Residual volume to total lung capacity ratio |
| *STPD* | Zero degrees centigrade, 760 mm Hg, dry |
| *TLC* | Total lung capacity |
| *V* | Gas volume |
| *V̇* | Gas volume/unit time (flow) |
| $V_A$ | Alveolar ventilation |
| $V_D$ | Dead space volume |
| $V_T$ | Tidal volume |
| *VC* | Vital capacity |
| $V_A/Q_C$ | Ratio of alveolar ventilation to pulmonary capillary blood flow |

# BIBLIOGRAPHY

Brunner, L.S. and D.S. Suddarth, *Lippincott Manual of Nursing Practice*, Lippincott, Philadelphia, 1974.

Bushnell, S.S., *Respiratory Intensive Care Nursing*, Little, Brown, Boston, 1973.

Comroe, J.H., *et al.*, *The Lung*, 2nd edition, Year Book Medical Publishers, 1962.

Cotes, C.E., *Lung Function: Assessment and Application in Medicine*, 2nd edition, F.A. Davis, Philadelphia, 1979.

Garrett, D.F. and W.P. Donaldson, *Physical Principles of Respiratory Therapy Equipment*, Ohio Medical Products, Madison, Wisconsin, 1975.

Guenter, C.A. and M.H. Welch, *Pulmonary Medicine*, Lippincott, Philadelphia, 1977.

Hunsinger, D.L., *et al.*, *Respiratory Technology: A Procedure Manual*, 2nd edition, Reston, Reston, Virginia, 1976.

Johnson, R.F. *Pulmonary Care*, Gruene and Stratton, New York, 1973.

Kory, R.G., *et al.:* "The Veteran's Administration-Army Cooperative Study of Pulmonary Functions. I. Clinical Spirometry in Normal Men." *American Journal of Medicine.* 30:243, 1961.

Petty, T.L., *Pulmonary Diagnostic Techniques*, Lea and Febiger, Philadelphia, 1975.

Radford, E.P., *New England Journal of Medicine*, 251:877, 1954.

Ruppell, Greg, *Manual of Pulmonary Function Testing*, C.V. Mosby, St. Louis, 1975.

Shapiro, B.A., Harrison, R.A., and C.A. Trout, *Clinical Application of Respiratory Care*, 2nd edition, Year Book Medical Publishers, Chicago, 1979.

Slonim, N.B. and L.H. Hamilton, *Respiratory Physiology*, 2nd edition, C.V. Mosby, 1971.

West, J.B., *Ventilation/Blood Flow and Gas Exchange*, 2nd edition, Blackwell Scientific Publications, Oxford, 1970.

Young, J.A. and D. Crocker, *Principles and Practices of Respiratory Therapy*, 2nd edition, Year Book Medical Publishers, Chicago, 1976.

# CHAPTER
# 11
# Electrocardiogram (EKG) Testing

## CARDIAC PHYSIOLOGY

Cardiac cells have the property of automaticity, in that the heart will begin to beat automatically and rhythmically without necessarily being under hormonal or electrical control by the central nervous system. This inherent automatic rate mechanism of the heart is due to changes in the permeability of the cell membrane to certain ions, primarily sodium ions, in a specialized area of the right atrium called the sinoatrial ($S$-$A$) node (see Fig. 11-1). The $S$-$A$ Node is located in the right atrium near its junction with the superior vena cava and normally discharges an electrical charge approximately 75 times a minute. The $S$-$A$ Node is a mass of neuromuscular tissue that is highly vascularized and has lost its ability to contract. The $S$-$A$ node, because its inherent rate of discharge is greater than that of any other area of the heart during normal circumstances, has been called the pacemaker; however, all areas of the myocardium have the ability to serve in this capacity. If the pacemaker fails to discharge, or if the rate of discharge is too slow, then other areas of cardiac tissue will fire and thus

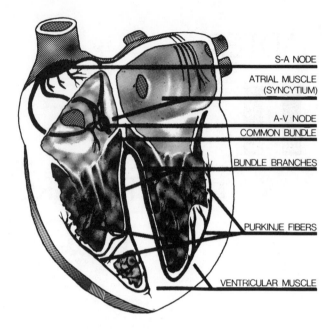

S-A NODE

ATRIAL MUSCLE
(SYNCYTIUM)

A-V NODE
COMMON BUNDLE

BUNDLE BRANCHES

PURKINJE FIBERS

VENTRICULAR MUSCLE

**FIG. 11-1.** Schematic representation of the conduction system in the heart.

become the new pacemaker for the heart. It is also possible for more than one pacemaker to be firing in the heart. This generally connotates a disease process and should be watched carefully. An electrical impulse that is generated at the *S-A* Node will follow a specific conduction pathway (see Fig. 11-1). It will send out an electrical impulse that moves across the *A-V* Node and passes down the Bundle of His (see Fig. 11-1). The atria and ventricles of the heart are separated by an electrically inert barrier called the *A-V* Fibrous Ring. The only communication electrically between the atria and the ventricles is through the atrio-ventricular (*A-V*) Node. The *A-V* Node, like the *S-A* Node, is highly specialized cardiac tissue that has lost its ability to contract. Since the *A-V* Node serves as the only means of connection between the atria and ventricles for the conduction of electrical impulses, in essence it controls the rhythm of cardiac contraction. The *A-V* Node lies in the upper portion of the interventricular septum and continues into the septum as the Bundle of His. The Bundle of His continues as the right and left bundle branches carrying the conduction impulse to the right and left ventricle muscle tissue simultaneously. The Bundle of His and the right and left bundle branches are structurally different. Their purpose is to serve as a conductor for the impulse. The right and left bundle branches terminate in the ventricular wall as the Purkinje fibers. The Purkinje fibers are located throughout the endocardial region of the ventricles and are the last point in cardiac excitation. Once the impulse has reached the ventricular mass, contraction occurs and the volume of blood is expelled from each ventricle. The right ventricle empties its volume into the pulmonary artery, while the left ventricle ejects its volume (stroke volume) into the highly elastic aorta. After contraction, the cardiac muscle is in a period of rest during which time the ventricles refill with blood. The subsequent impulse will occur when filling is complete and ventricular contraction will occur again. This sequence of events of contraction (depolarization) and rest (repolarization) make up the normal cardiac cycle.

The sinus node sends out electrical impulses at a faster rate than any other muscle tissue of the heart and, therefore, is the primary pacemaker of the heart. When the impulse from the *S-A* Node is depressed or stops completely, a new pacemaker will form. Several different regions of the heart have their own inherent rate of automaticity. The natural rate of automaticity is as follows:

> *S-A* Node, 70–90 beats/min;
> Atrial wall, approximately 60 beats/min;
> *A-V* Node, approximately 40–60 beats/min;
> Ventrical walls, approximately 20–40 beats/min

Whenever a higher rate of automaticity is depressed, the next lower level will take over as the pacemaker. During myocardial ischemia and hypoxia, several areas may become pacemakers and this hierarchial structure will not be maintained. When another area of the cardiac muscle originates an electrical impulse, this is called an *ectopic focus*. The presence of ectopic foci on an EKG generally signifies cardiac disease.

## EKG MONITORING

Figure 11-2 shows the relation of these electrical events within the heart to the deflections of the electrocardiogram (ECG or EKG). The *P*-wave represents depolarization of the atria. For all practical purposes, the electrical activity of the heart and the muscular activity of the heart occur simultaneously. Thus, when the electrical impulse is moving across the atrial wall and the *P*-wave is showing the depolarization, the atria are contracting at that time. The width of the *P*-wave is a function of the time required for activation. When the electrical impulse is at the *A-V* Node and upper portion of the Bundle of His, no electrical activity is noted on the electrocardiogram. This is represented by the flat segment at the end of the *P*-wave. The *QRS* complex begins when the electrical impulse leaves the Bundle of His and begins in the bundle branch systems (both right and left). The flat period at the end of the *QRS* complex signifies that the

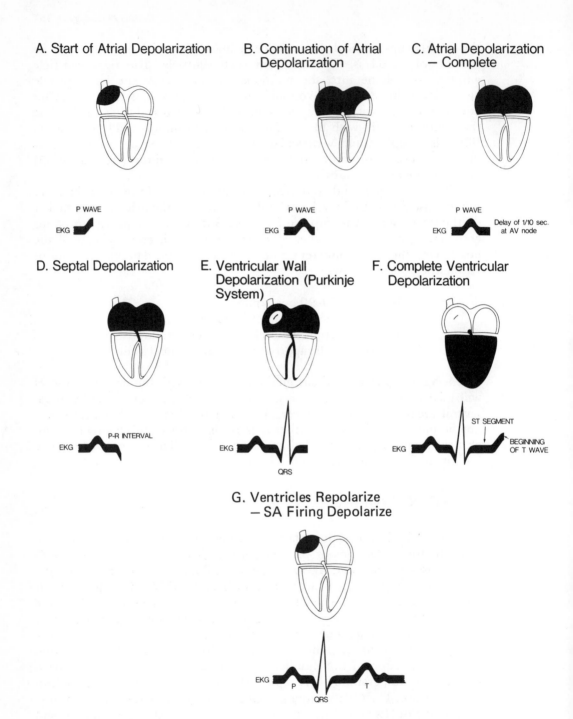

**FIG. 11-2.** Conduction pathway in the heart and the related EKG activity.

electrical impulse has passed through the ventricle wall and cardiac contraction has occurred. The *T*-wave represents the repolarization of the ventricles and signifies that no mechanical cardiac activity is occurring.

Figure 11-2 demonstrates one complete cardiac cycle with all waves and segments identified. Two things should be noticeable:

1. There is a pause between the *P*-wave and the *QRS* complex. This pause is normally about one tenth of a second and signifies the transmission through the *A-V* Node and Bundle of His.
2. A segment is noted between the QRS complex and the *T*-wave. This segment represents the time interval between depolarization of the ventricle walls and the beginning of repolarization.

The *S-T* segment becomes extremely important for identifying the presence of a myocardial infarction. Elevation of the *S-T* segment suggests injury to the ventricular wall. In other disease situations, the *S-T* segment may be depressed, and this suggests other cardiac disturbances such as coronary ischemia.

Prior to discussing the various cardiac arrhythmias that respiratory personnel should be familiar with, it is necessary to have a basic understanding of how EKGs are measured and what the various lines on an EKG recording represent. The EKG is recorded on ruled paper (see Fig. 11-3). The smallest squares on the paper are 1-ml squares. With the EKG recorder running at the normal paper speed of 2.5 cm/sec, each small square on the electrocardiogram equals 0.04 sec and each large square containing five of the smaller squares represents 0.2 sec in time. The period of time during which a cardiac event will occur, may be calculated by measuring along the horizontal line of the EKG paper. Figure 11-3 also shows the duration of the cardiac cycle. Note that the duration of time between the beginning of the *P*-wave and the end of the *T*-wave represents 0.8 seconds. It can be seen then that by dividing 8 into 60 sec (1 min) an average rate of 75 beats/min will result. The duration of time between certain segments on the EKG strip becomes very important in determining certain arrhythmias.

The height of a *P*-wave or *QRS* complex or *T*-wave is an indication of voltage.

Each stage of the cardiac cycle is characterized by very subtle changes in the electrical activity of the heart, and, therefore, is reflected by very subtle changes in the electrocardiogram recording. The basis of the electrocardiogram is simple. The electrical impulse within the heart is transmitted to the surface of the body and can be detected on the surface by the use of electrodes. By properly placing electrodes in certain regions of the body, specific leads can be created. The lead merely identifies where given electrodes have been placed. Patients in the intensive or coronary care unit will not have the same type of electrodes placed on them that

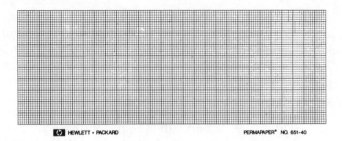

A. Standard EKG ruled paper

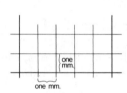

B. Each small square of the ruled paper
is 1 mm. square.

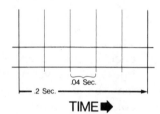

TIME ➡

C. At a paper speed of 2.5 cm./sec.,
the horizontal axis becomes a
measure of time.

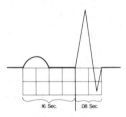

D. Duration of cardiac cycles
is found by measuring events
on the horizontal axis.

FIG. 11-3. Relationship between EKG paper and the electrical activity of the heart.

a physician would use in his office for diagnostic purposes. The cardiac monitors within the unit generally will have only a single lead that is approximately the same as a Lead II (modified Lead II). This is the most useful lead for detecting arrhythmias.

# CARDIAC ARRHYTHMIAS

## DETERMINATION OF RATE

The normal electrocardiogram consists of a repeating series of *P*-waves, *QRS* complexes, and *T*-waves that occur at a rate approximately 70–90 times each minute. The *S-A* Node discharges regularly because of the inherent automaticity. Therefore, *P*-waves will occur at regular intervals on the *QRS* complex. The conduction pathway is predictable in both the normal and the diseased heart. The impulse must travel down the *A-V* Node, and, therefore, at regular intervals a QRS, ventricular complex, will occur. There will be an interval of time between the initiation of the *P*-wave and the *QRS* complex. The time lapse from the beginning of the *P*-wave to the beginning of the *QRS* complex varies in the normal population from 0.12 to 0.20 sec. This means that an impulse, in the normal heart, will not travel at a rate faster than 0.12 sec and will not take longer than 0.20 sec. If the time lapse takes longer than 0.20 sec, this indicates a pathological change in the *A-V* Node. The process is as follows:

1. Find an *R*-wave that falls on a vertical heavy black line;
2. Count off the next six heavy black lines with the following numbers: 300, 150, 100, and then 75, 60, 50;
3. Now find where the second *R*-wave falls within these numbers. This is the rate.

When looking for and classifying arrhythmias, the rate should be determined first. In order to determine rate in the normal electrocardiogram or an electrocardiogram where an elevated heart rate is obvious, the following procedure is helpful. First, find an *R*-wave that falls exactly on one of the vertical heavy black lines of the EKG strip (see Fig. 11-4A). Remember that the *R*-wave is the high point of the *QRS* complex. It may be necessary to run a relatively long EKG strip in order to find an *R*-wave exactly on the black line (see Fig. 11-4B), however, this is necessary for concise rate determination. Second, for the three heavy black lines that follow, count off 300, 150, and 100. It is necessary to memorize these numbers. Remember, first find the *R*-wave of the *QRS* complex that falls on a vertical black heavy line; then for the three subsequent black heavy lines count off 300, 150, and 100. Next, for the three following lines count off 75, 60, and 50 (see Fig. 11-4C). This means that there are six numbers that must be remembered: 300, 150, 100, and then 75, 60, and 50. It is absolutely necessary to memorize these six numbers. The first *R*-wave fell on the line preceding our six sets of numbers. The process at

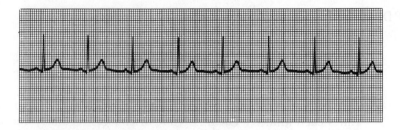

## A. Sample tracing for rate.

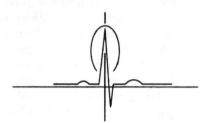

## B. Find R wave.

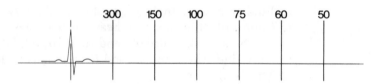

## C. Count off the subsequent heavy lines.

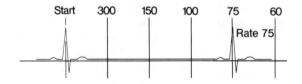

## D. Rate is 75

FIG. 11-4. Rate determination. (*Modified from Dale Dubin, M.D., Rapid Interpretation of EKGs, 3rd ed., Cover Publishing Co., 1976.*)

this point is to find where the second *R*-wave falls. Figure 11-5 shows three examples for determining rate by this method. For example if the second *R*-wave falls between 75 and 60, then the approximate rate will be between 75 and 60 beats/min. If the *R*-wave falls almost exactly between

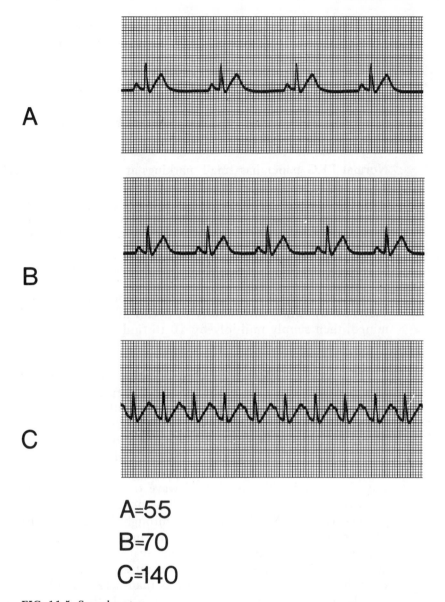

A=55
B=70
C=140

FIG. 11-5. Sample rates.

the 75 and 60 markings, then the rate is approximately 65–70 beats/min, and so forth.

When trying to determine the heart rate of very slow rates (Brady-cardia) a second method is easier. For determining low cardiac rates the process is as follows:

1. Find the 3-sec interval markings at the top of the sheet and mark off two of these 3-sec intervals, making a total 6-sec interval phase;
2. Count the number of complete heart cycles (*R*-wave to *R*-wave represents one heart cycle) that occur in this 6-sec interval time;
3. Multiply by 10 the number of heart cycles in the 6-sec strip. This is the rate.

Normal EKG paper has small markings at the top of the EKG strip (see Fig. 11-6). These markings indicate that the interval between them represents 3-sec and, therefore, they are called 3-sec interval markings. When the EKG is being operated at normal speed (2.5 cm/sec), then the distance between two of these intervals will represent 6 sec (see Fig. 11-6-b). At this point the process is simple. Simply count the number of complete cardiac cycles within the 6-sec period of time. It is easy to do this if one assumes that the distance from one wave (any corresponding wave, e.g. *T*-wave, *R*-wave, etc.) to the next wave represents one cardiac cycle (see Fig. 11-6-b). Once the number of cycles in a given 6-sec period is determined, then simply multiply by 10 to find out how many cycles or heart beats there are in one minute. Figure 11-7 provides three examples of bradycardia for determining the rate.

It is not sufficient merely to determine heart rate. The respiratory therapist also must be aware of the significance of the waves and the intervals between them. The following should be remembered about the various waves. The *P*-wave represents the electrical activity of the initial impulse originating in the *S-A* Node and should be similar in appearance. Changes in the *P*-wave indicate that the *S-A* Node may not be the originating source of that particular *P*-wave. The *P-R* interval is the period of time from the beginning of the *P*-wave to the beginning of the *QRS* complex. It represents the amount of time necessary for the original impulse coming from the *S-A* Node to pass through the atria and the *A-V* Node to the ventricles. Remember that the normal duration of time is between 0.12 sec and 0.20 sec. If the *P-R* interval is longer than 0.20 seconds, it can be assumed that a conduction defect exists in the *A-V* Node. On the other hand, if the *P-R* interval is less than 0.12 seconds, this implies that the electrical impulse is reaching the ventricle through a shorter than normal route. The *QRS* complex represents the depolarization of the ventricular wall and reflects the time necessary for the impulse to go from the Bundle of His through the right and left bundle branches, through the Purkinje system, and to complete ventricular contraction. The complex consists of a *Q*-wave (the initial downward deflection) and an *R*-wave (the large upward deflection). The normal duration of the *QRS* complex is less than 0.12 sec. When the duration is greater than 0.12 sec, this implies

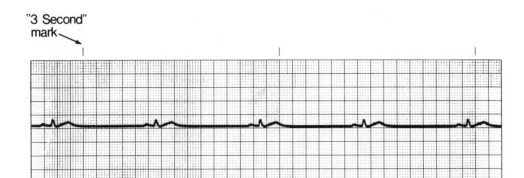

A. Sample Tracing for Rate. The straight lines at the top represent "3 second" time intervals when the paper speed is 2.5 cm./sec.

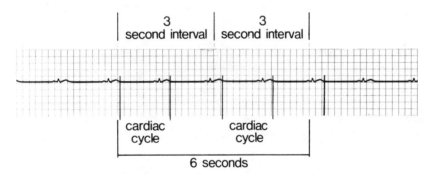

B. Count the number of complete cardiac cycles in a second period of time and multiply by 10 (remember the 6 sec. × 10 = 60 sec.)

C. Rate is 10 × 4 cardiac cycles = 40.

FIG. 11-6. Rate determination for slow rates.

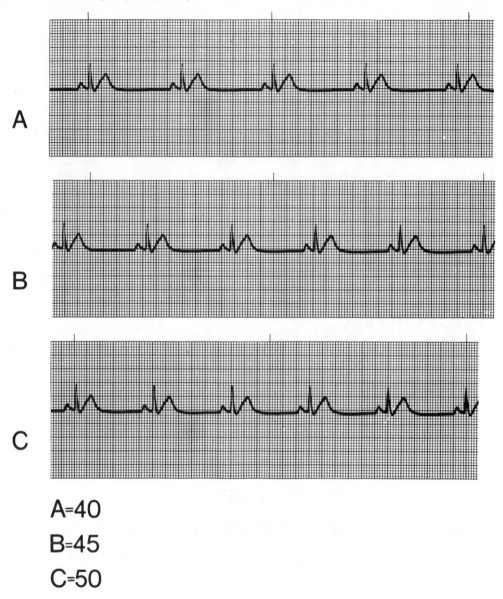

A

B

C

A=40

B=45

C=50

FIG. 11-7. Sample rates.

that there is a blockage or delay in the pathway below the Bundle of His. Generally this suggests a bundle branch block, either right or left. The *S-T* segment is the period of time between the completion of ventricular depolarization and the recovery or repolarization of the ventricle walls. This segment may be elevated or depressed if there is any injury at all to the muscle wall. Situations such as myocardial infarction and severe myo-cardial ischemia will interfere with the repolarization process and alter the normal *S-T* segment. Finally, the *T*-wave represents the recovery phase after ventricular contraction. If the repolarization process is abnormal, the wave will typically be inverted. Two considerations are necessary for ac-curate determination of abnormalities. First, one must be able to deter-mine the rate quickly and accurately, and second, one must be aware of the intervals and appearance of each of the waves found on the EKG strip.

It is possible to classify the most common cardiac arrhythmias by:

1. Site of origin and mechanism, and
2. Prognosis of the patient.

It is the purpose of this text to provide the therapist with the knowledge and skill necessary to identify the common arrhythmias; therefore, we will deal with the site of origin and the mechanism.

In the following sections, the type of arrhythmia will be given with its distinguishing characteristics and an example of how this arrhythmia ap-pears on an EKG strip. Where applicable, a statement will be made as to whether this is a minor, major, or death producing arrhythmia.

## ARRHYTHMIAS ORIGINATING FROM THE S-A NODE

### Normal Rhythm

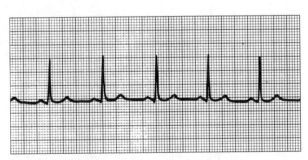

EKG pattern.

1. In the normal cardiac rhythm, the distance between successive *QRS* complexes is equal.
2. The *P*-waves are all similar in appearance thus indicating that their origin is in the *S-A* Node.
3. The *P-R* interval is between 0.12 and 0.20 sec.
4. The *S-T* segment is normal.
5. The *T*-wave is upright.

1.  Sinus Tachycardia

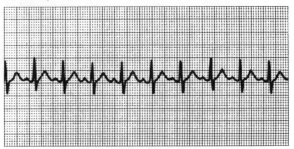

Sinus Tachycardia

a) The distance between *QRS* complexes is equal.
b) The *P*-waves are normal.
c) The rate is greater than 100 beats/min.
d) Each *P*-wave is followed by a *QRS* complex.
e) The *ST*-segment is normal.
f) The *T*-wave is upright (if the *T*-waves are inverted, this indicates myocardial ischemia).

2.  Sinus Bradycardia

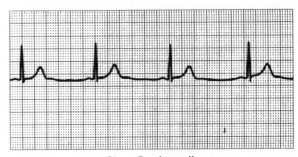

Sinus Bradycardia

a) Distance between *QRS* complexes is equal.
b) *P*-waves are similar.
c) Rate is less than 60 beats/min.
d) Each *P*-wave is followed by a *QRS* complex.
e) *S-T* segment is normal.
f) *T*-wave is upright (if the *T*-wave is inverted, this is probably a result of myocardial ischemia.

3.  Sinus Arrhythmia

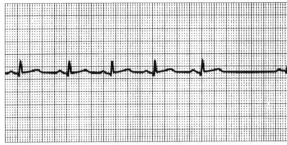

·Sinus Arrhythmia

a) The distances between successive *QRS* complexes are not equal; therefore, a varying rhythm exists.
b) *P*-waves are identical.
c) Rate is generally normal.
d) *P*-waves are followed by normal *QRS* complexes.
e) *S-T* segment is generally normal.
f) *T*-wave is upright (the *T*-wave may appear flat or inverted when myocardial ischemia is present).

**4.** *S-A* Node Block or Arrest

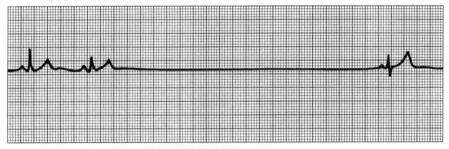

*S-A* Node Block or Arrest

a) The distance between successive *QRS* complexes is equal, except for the missing beats.
b) *P*-waves are similar.
c) The rate is generally less than 60.
d) *P*-waves are followed by normal *QRS* complexes.
e) *S-T* segment generally normal.
f) *T*-wave may be upright, flat, or inverted (however this is generally separate from the arrhythmia).

## *ATRIAL ARRHYTHMIAS*

**1.** Wandering Pacemaker

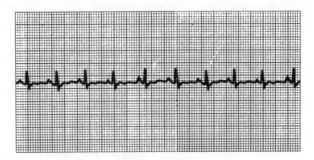

Wandering Pacemaker

a) Distance between successive $QRS$ complexes not equal.
b) The $P$-wave changes shape, thus suggesting different pacemakers in operation.
c) The rate is generally within normal limits.
d) All $P$-waves are followed by $QRS$ complexes.
e) The $S$-$T$ segment is generally normal.
f) The $T$-wave may be elevated, flat or inverted.

2. Premature Atrial Contractions (PAC)

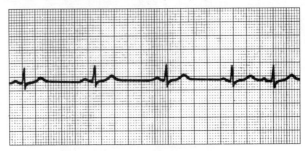

Premature Atrial Contraction

a) The distance between successive $QRS$ complexes is not equal.
b) The $P$-waves are not similar. Normally, however, a premature atrial contraction is the result of one ectopic focus creating the abnormal $P$-wave. This varies from the wandering pacemaker in that in the wandering pacemaker, very few of the $P$-waves are similar. However, in the $PAC$, one can usually identify two different $P$-waves, suggesting the $S$-$A$ Node is firing and one other pacemaker in the atrial wall is firing.
c) The rate may be normal or slightly elevated.
d) $P$-waves are followed by $QRS$ complexes.
e) The $S$-$T$ segment is generally normal.
f) The $T$-wave may be upright, flat, or inverted, depending on the disease state in the heart.

3. Atrial Flutter

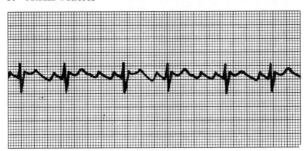

Atrial Flutter

a) The distance between successive *QRS* complexes varies. The rate may vary from 60 to approximately 150 per minute, depending on the number of atrial impulses that activate the ventricles (pass through the *S-A* Node).

b) The *P*-waves are similar in appearance, they occur in rapid succession, and they have a "saw tooth" appearance. Normally in atrial flutter, the ectopic focus in the atria is firing at a rate of 250 to 350 beats/min.

c) The rate varies from 60 to 150. Note that the atrial flutter rate and the ventricular contraction rate are not the same.

d) Each *P*-wave is not followed by a *QRS* complex. Normally, the ratio of *P*-waves to *QRS* complexes is constant. For example, every five *P*-waves may elicit one *QRS* complex or every three *P*-waves may elicit one *QRS* complex. The ratio of *P*-waves to *QRS* complexes generally is the same. The ratio may be 2:1, 3:1, or 4:1 etc.

4. Atrial Fibrillation

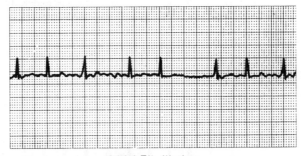

Atrial Fibrillation

a) The distance between successive *QRS* complexes varies.

b) There are no real *P*-waves, but multiple spikes appearing with no uniform appearance.

c) The rate will vary according to the ventricular response.

d) Since there are no real *P*-waves, the *QRS* complexes appear irregularly; however, they are generally normal in shape and duration.

e) The *S-T* segment may vary.

f) The *T*-wave may vary.

## ARRHYTHMIAS ORIGINATING IN THE
## A-V NODE

1. Nodal escape

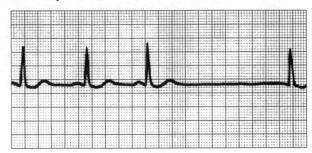

Nodal escape

a) The distance between successive QRS complexes will vary.
b) *P*-waves, when they occur, will be similar. In nodal escape, the *A-V* Node becomes the pacemaker for a given particular cardiac cycle because of the failure of the *S-A* Node or atrial wall to fire. Therefore, *P* waves may be missing.
c) The rate may vary but generally it is decreased.
d) Not all *P*-waves are followed by *QRS* complexes. In nodal escape, the beat originates at the *A-V* Node and the impulse following is generally through the normal conduction system of the Bundle of His and the right and left bundle branches. The *QRS* complex will be normal in appearance.
e) The *S-T* segment may vary.
f) The *T*-wave may vary (this is generally a result of cardiac disease and not the arrhythmia itself).

2. Nodal Tachycardia

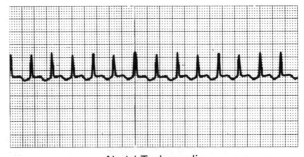

Nodal Tachycardia

a) The distance between successive *QRS* complexes is equal.
b) Because the impulse originates in the *A V*-Node, traditionally speaking there are no *P*-waves. However, an extra wave does occur either

just before or just after the QRS complex. This wave is inverted and is called a *P*-wave because it corresponds to the originating impulse.

c) The rate is generally from 100 to about 160 beats/min.

d) The *ST*-segment will vary.

e) The *T*-wave will vary.


NOTE: Paroxysmal (sudden) *A-V* Nodal tachycardia should be watched extremely carefully because of the impending danger of myocardial ischemia. This danger is related to the duration of tachycardia that occurs. High ventricular rates which occur in paroxysmal tachycardia generally result in a decreased cardiac output and predisposes the patient to left ventricular failure. Nodal tachycardia may convert into left ventricular tachycardia and ventricular fibrillation. It is an extremely dangerous arrhythmia in terms of serving as a warning of more serious, lethal, ventricular arrhythmias.

3.  First Degree Heart Block (Delayed *AV* Conduction)

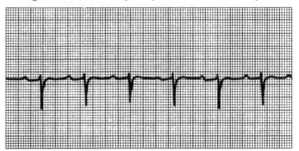

Heart Block (Delayed *AV* Conduction)

a) The distance between successive *QRS* complexes is normal.

b) The *P*-waves are normal and similar since they originate in the *S-A* Node.

c) The rate is normal.

d) *P*-waves are followed by *QRS* complexes. The distinguishing feature of first-degree heart block is that the *P-R* interval is longer than 0.20 secs. This is the only abnormality that will be noted on the EKG strip. *AV* first-degree block is not a serious arrhythmia, but it is important because it suggests injury at the *A-V* Node may be the precursor to more serious heart blocks.


4.  Second Degree *A-V* Heart Block

a) The distance between successive *QRS* complexes is equal but increased in duration.

b) There are generally two, three, or four times as many *P*-waves as *QRS* complexes. This creates a situation where there is a ratio between *P*-waves to *QRS* complexes. When there are two *P*-waves for every *QRS* complex, this is called a Two-One Block. When there are

2:1

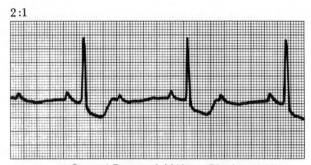

Second Degree *A-V* Heart Block

three *P*-waves for every *QRS* complex, this is called a Three-One Heart Block and so forth.

3:1

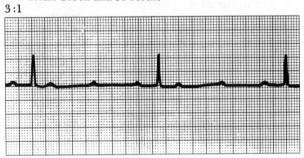

Second Degree *A-V* Heart Block

d) Not all *P*-waves are followed by *QRS* complexes.
e) The *S-T* segment may vary.
f) The *T*-wave may vary.

5. Wenckebach Phenomenon
The Wenckebach Phenomenon is a type of second degree heart-block. The Wenckebach Phenomenon occurs when the *P-R* interval becomes increasingly longer until the *A-V* Node is not stimulated at all and therefore no *QRS* complex is seen at that particular point.

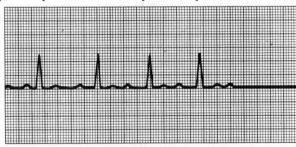

Wenckebach Phenomenon

a) The distance between *QRS* complexes becomes increasingly longer from cardiac cycle to cardiac cycle until a *QRS* complex is missed.
b) The *P*-waves are all normal in appearance.
c) The rate is generally less than normal.

d) Not all *P*-waves are followed by a *QRS* complex (the missing *QRS* complex). The *P-R* interval becomes increasingly longer.
e) The *S-T* segment may vary.
f) The *T*-wave may vary.

6. Third Degree Heart Block (Complete)

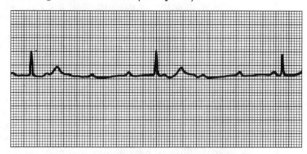

Third Degree Heart Block (Complete)

a) The distance between successive *QRS* complexes is equal.
b) The *P*-waves are normal according to size and shape; however, there are more *P*-waves than *QRS* complexes.
c) The rate is generally less than 50 beats/min, while the atrial rate is generally normal.
d) Not all *P*-waves are followed by *QRS* complexes. This means that no atrial impulses are getting through the *A-V* Node. Therefore, the *A-V* Node becomes the pacemaker for the ventricles while at the same time the *S-A* Node is the pacemaker for the atria. It is important to note here that the atria and ventricles are beating independent of one another. When the *QRS* complexes occur they are generally normal in appearance if the impulse is originating at the *A-V* Node; however, the complex may vary if the ventricular pacemaker is not at the site of the *A-V* Node.
e) The *S-T* segment rate may vary.
f) The *T*-wave may vary.

## VENTRICULAR ARRHYTHMIAS

1. Premature Ventricular Contractions (PVC)

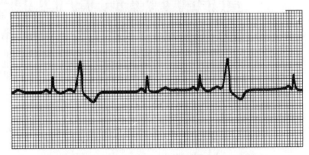

Premature Ventricular Contractions (PVC)

a) The distance between successive $QRS$ complexes will be equal except when the $PVC$ occurs. There is a long pause after a $PVC$ before the following $P$-wave exists.
b) The $P$-wave will be normal in appearance and similar except when $PVC$ occurs. Because the beat is originating within the ventricular wall, no $P$-wave will be observed. Also, since the originating impulse is within the ventricular wall the $PVC$ will be a very wide complex and look very different from a normal $QRS$ complex.
c) The rate is generally normal; however, $PVC$'s can occur at any cardiac rate—both in bradycardia and tachycardia.
d) Where $P$-waves occur, they are generally followed by a $QRS$ complex.
e) $PVC$ may be coupled with one or more normal beats. When PVC's occur with one normal $QRS$ complex, this is called bigeminy. When $PVC$ occurs in conjunction with every two normal beats, this is called trigeminy, and so forth. $PVC$'s are extremely important because they suggest severe myocardial ischemia and an increased irritability or excitability that may produce ventricular contractions and are especially dangerous when they occur in the following situations:

   (1) When $PVC$'s occur in runs or series of successive impulses greater than six per minute.
   (2) When bigeminy or trigeminy become a regular part of the EKG pattern.
   (3) When the $PVC$ falls on or near $T$-wave of the preceding cardiac complex.
   (4) When $PVC$'s originate from more than one point in the ventricular wall. Isolated $PVC$'s seldom pose a threat to the patient; however they should be considered a warning of an underlying disease process.

2. Ventricular Tachycardia

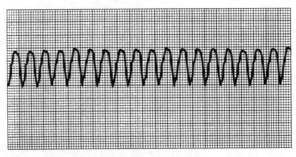

Ventricular Tachycardia

a) The distance between successive $QRS$ complexes is generally equal.
b) $P$-waves are generally hidden within the $QRS$ complex and cannot be observed.
c) The rate is generally greater than 140 beats/min.

Because the impulses are originating within the ventricular wall, the complexes are very wide and large. Runs of ventricular tachycardia generally signify extensive coronary artery disease. Runs of ventricular tachycardia often set up the heart for the possibility of ventricular fibrillation.

3. Ventricular Fibrillation

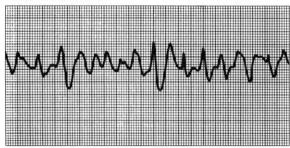

Ventricular Fibrillation

Ventricular fibrillation is characterized by chaotic waves occurring in rapid succession and originating from the ventricles. There is no uniform or predictable sequence of the waves. It is not possible to distinguish *P*-waves, *QRS* complexes, or *T*-waves from the electrocardiogram. Ventricular fibrillation is the result of stimuli from numerous ventricular ectopic foci causing the chaotic contraction of the ventricles. At this point, the ventricles are doing no work and essentially pumping no blood. Ventricular fibrillation is a lethal cardiac arrhythmia and represents a major medical emergency. Death will occur within minutes after the onset of ventricular fibrillation unless the arrhythmia is corrected. In ventricular fibrillation, cardiopulmonary resuscitation is absolutely necessary in order to prevent death of the patient. Ventricular fibrillation will never convert into a less serious arrhythmia without direct medical intervention.

# MYOCARDIAL INFARCTION

Myocardial infarction is the formation of a localized area of ischemic necrosis in the heart muscle resulting from an interruption of the blood supply to that area. Nearly 90 percent of myocardial infarctions are secondary to coronary occlusion that results from progressive coronary atherosclerosis. In most patients with myocardial infarction, the initial signs are chest pains. The pain occurs suddenly, is severe, and is of a crushing quality. Quite often the patient describes the chest pain as being like a "vice" and crushing the chest like an "elephant stepping" on the chest. The pain is generally directly beneath the sternum and radiates across the chest to the arm and neck. In a myocardial infarction, the pain does not necessarily have to be related to exercise. In fact, in many patients the pain begins during the night while the patient is sleeping. In a true myocardial infarction, the chest pain in continuous and will not be relieved by lying down, changing body position, or taking medication. Nausea, vomiting, and sweating occur shortly after the onset of the pain. Fear, apprehension, weakness, and dyspnea are observed. In a small number of patients, a myocardial infarction may occur without any symptoms of chest pain. These are often called silent infarctions. Generally they are noted during the patient's history when the EKG is observed.

Myocardial infarction can be broken down into two categories: (1) A transmural myocardial infarction that is generally the result of the atherosclerotic process of the coronary artery; and (2) A subendocardial infarction that involves the subendocardial wall of the left ventricle, septum, and papillary muscles. The etiology of subendocardial infarction is not well understood. The clinical appearance and prognosis of a patient suffering acute myocardial infarction will vary considerably depending on the size of infarction and the general condition of the patient. If the infarction is relatively small in size and does not totally cut off the blood supply as a result of collateral circulation, the myocardium may continue to function adequately. This type of situation generally occurs in those patients who have silent infarction. In addition, if the infarction is very small, the initial symptoms of pain may gradually subside. If the infarction is large enough to involve a significant portion of the myocardium, the function of the heart may be impaired. The heart may decrease its pumping action and cardiac failure may occur or disturbances in the conduction system may occur and arrhythmias may be observed. If the pumping ability of the heart is sufficiently modified by the myocardial infarction, the left ventricle may go into failure, resulting in a drop of arterial blood pressure, a reflexive increase in heart rate, a reduction in urinary output, and generalized peripheral vasoconstriction leading to a cold, clammy feeling of the skin. This situation is called cardiogenic shock and suggests massive infarction. Finally, in some patients death may occur almost instantaneously after occlusion has occurred. The sudden death is a result of the lethal arrhythmias that have resulted from the infarction. In such cases, the heart either goes into ventricular standstill or ventricular fibrillation. It is estimated that nearly 60 percent of all patients who die from myocardial infarction do so within the first two hours after the infarction has occurred.

The diagnosis of acute myocardial infarction can be made by the electrocardiogram. Significant electrocardiographic changes of myocardial infarction can be observed because of the injury and death of the myocardial tissue that occurs. However, the electrocardiogram will not demonstrate the extent of the damage. It is merely an indication of the extent. A complete diagnosis must be made on the basis of the patient's history, the electrocardiogram, and enzyme studies. In patients suffering from acute myocardial infarction, there will be significant changes in the $Q$-wave, the

*S-T* segment, and the *T*-wave. It is important to remember that it is the thick left ventricle of the heart that suffers serious myocardial infarction. In an area of infarction, there is no electrical activity, and it is this disruption of the electrical activity that is observed on the electrocardiogram. In areas of the myocardium where ischemia is occurring, this will be characterized by an inverted *T*-wave. When the *ST* segment is elevated, there is injury to the myocardium. This should serve as a warning that an infarction is acute or recent. In some clinical situations, the *ST* segment may be depressed. This occurs when the patient is on digitalis, if there is a subendocardial infarction, or when a patient with coronary ischemia is being exercised. The diagnosis of the myocardial infarction is made on the basis of the *Q*-wave. Remember that the *Q*-wave is the first downward part of the *QRS* complex. In the normal individual, the *Q*-wave is hidden within the *QRS* complex and is not observed; however, when the *Q*-wave is significant and readily observable, this serves as the criteria for the diagnosis of myocardial infarction. *Q*-waves can be considered significant if they are of sufficient amplitude so that the height of the *Q*-wave is greater than one-third of the height of the *QRS* complex, or if the *Q*-wave is increased in amplitude but wider than one millimeter. Remember that each small square on the EKG strip is one millimeter wide.

The following are lethal complications of acute myocardial infarction:

1. The occurrence of lethal arrhythmias. Remember that arrhythmias may occur at any time during the patient's hospitalization;
2. Acute heart failure can occur following an infarction because of the failure of the heart to pump blood. The failure can occur suddenly associated with pulmonary edema or may occur gradually. More than 60 percent of the patients suffering myocardial infarction show clinical signs of heart failure;
3. Cardiogenic shock can occur if the heart is unable to circulate adequate oxygen. This is the most serious complication of infarction today. Cardiogenic shock generally occurs within the first four to six hours after the infarction;
4. Thromboembolism (blood clot) may occur on the inner wall of the left ventricle after a myocardial infarction. These clots may then break loose, leave the heart, and block the arterial supply to other vital organs of the body such as the brain. This type of thromboembolism, because of the use of anticoagulants and drug therapy, are not as serious a problem as once. However, emboli may form in the deep veins of the legs, generally from the statis of blood, and these may find their way to the lungs, thus producing pulmonary infarction. Sudden death as a result of thromboembolism is relatively uncommon in the unit today;

however, it does account for a small percentage of deaths and should be considered a possibility;

5. Rupture of the ventricular wall can occur when the infarction produces necrosis in the tissue area of sufficient size to weaken the ventricle. When this occurs, the blood from the ventricle fills the pericardial sac instantly causing cardiac tamponade and death within minutes. Ventricular rupture can occur from five to ten days after the infarction. Like thromboembolism, ventricular rupture is relatively uncommon.

Because of the improved methods of treating myocardial infarction and the ability to do corrective surgery of the coronary vessels, life expectancy after a myocardial infarction has improved and continues to do so. Studies vary considerably in their data; however, more than 50% of the patients suffering from myocardial infarction will survive for at least a five year period of time post infarction. At the present time, there is a great controversy among physicians and researchers as to how to protect the general population from developing myocardial infarction secondary to the atherosclerotic process and how to prevent its reoccurrence in infarction patients. There is no definitive answer; however, several factors are well documented: obesity, hypertension, exercise, smoking, cholesterol and triglycerides, and stress are all vital factors in the development of myocardial infarction.

## BIBLIOGRAPHY

Berne, Robert, M. and Matthew N. Levy., *Cardiovascular Physiology*, C.V. Mosby, Saint Louis, 1972.

Chung, Edward, K., *Cardiac Emergency Care*. Lea & Febiger, Philadelphia, 1975.

Dubin, Dale., *Rapid Interpretations of EKG's,* 3rd edition, Cover, Tampa, 1976.

Goldberger, Emanuel., *Treatment of Cardiac Emergencies*, C.V. Mosby, Saint Louis, 1974.

Guyton, Arthur, C. and Allen W. Coraley, *Cardiovascular Physiology II*, University Park Press, Baltimore, 1976.

Lindsay, Alan, E. and B. Alberto, *The Cardiac Arrhythmias*, 2nd edition. Year Book Medical Publishers, Chicago, 1975.

Meltzer, Lawrence, E., Pinneo, Rose, and J. Roderick Kitchell, *Intensive Coronary Care*, The Charles Press, Philadelphia, 1970.

Phibbs, Brenden, *The Cardiac Arrhythmias*, 2nd edition, C.V. Mosby, Saint Louis, 1973.

Schamroth, Leo, *An Introduction to Electrocardiography*, 4th edition, Blackwell Scientific Publications, London, 1971.

# CHAPTER

# 12

# Considerations for Equipment Sterilization and Cleaning

The equipment used by respiratory therapy personnel in clinical areas is a potential source of nosocomial (hospital-acquired) infections and diseases. The proper sterilization and disinfection of respiratory therapy equipment represents one of the most vital functions of the respiratory therapy department. The hospital environment is continually contaminated with microorganisms and can be the source of an initial infection of a healthy patient, the reinfection of a recently recovered patient, or a reinforcing infection to a patient not fully recovered. Infection can be the result of cross-contamination between patients, cross-contamination between the therapist and the patient, or the transmission of an infection by contact with inanimate objects.

The importance of using proper aseptic techniques while handling equipment along with the awareness of the processes of cross-contamination must be applied to achieve a safe working environment for the cleaning and processing of respiratory therapy equipment. It is important for respiratory care personnel to have a working knowledge of nosocomial infections associated with respiratory care.

In order to understand the various processes utilized in the cleaning and sterilization of respiratory therapy equipment, it is necessary to have a basic understanding between terminology and processes associated with the cleaning of equipment. The following are common definitions used in equipment sterilization and cleaning:

| | |
|---|---|
| *Sterile:* | If an item is said to be sterile, this means that it is free of any living organisms. The process of making an item sterile is called *sterilization*. Sterilization involves killing all microorganisms, both pathogenic and non-pathogenic, and implies an absolute freedom from living organisms. Sterilization will kill both the spore (resistant-resting form of microorganism) and the vegetative (active growth form of microorganism) form of microorganism. |
| *Disinfect:* | To disinfect a piece of equipment or object implies the elimination of those organisms that might cause disease. Disinfection is the process that destroys the pathogenic or vegetative form of the microorganisms and it generally uses a substance or chemical called a *disinfectant*. |
| *Antiseptic:* | Antisepsis uses a chemical or substance called an *antiseptic* for the removal of pathogenic and other organisms from the surface of the body (i.e. skin). Antisepsis and disinfection differ from sterilization in that in the former, the number and kinds of microorganisms are reduced to a safe or minimal level, while in sterilization, all organisms are destroyed. |
| *Bacteriocidal:* | The term bacteriocidal means that the substance has the ability to kill bacteria. |
| *Bacteriostatic:* | The term bacteriostatic means that the substance has the ability to prevent or inhibit the growth of bacteria. |

Much attention should be given to the mechanisms responsible for the transmission of organisms from the interior of equipment set-ups such as IPPB equipment, humidity and aerosol reservoirs, and tubing. The transmission of microorganisms increases with:

1. Direct personal contact,
2. Elevated levels of pathogens in confined areas,
3. Elevated levels of pathogens on materials or objects,
4. Airborne microorganisms.

To control these modes of transmission, general medical aseptic techniques should be used on an everyday basis. These include:

1. Hand washing between patients,
2. Use of disposable equipment,
3. Improved house cleaning procedures,
4. Improved laundry systems,
5. Control of airborne pathogens utilizing improved ventilation and filtration systems,
6. The use of filters in equipment systems such as mechanical ventilators,
7. Isolation of patients.

The equipment used in medical practice can be ranked on the basis of its potential source of nosocomial infections. Those items that are inserted beneath the body surface or broken skin are called *critical items* and must always be sterilized. Such items include hypodermic needles, surgical instruments, indwelling cannulae, etc. The next category of equipment includes those items that are inserted into body orifices or come in contact with broken skin adjacent to such areas. These items are called *semicritical* items and preferably are sterilized, but at least must be disinfected. Such items include oral airways, nasogastric tubes, rectal tubes, instruments used in the nose or ear, dental instruments, etc. The third type of equipment includes those items which come into contact with the unbroken skin. It is preferable that such items have been disinfected; however, they at least should be clean. The term *clean* here means that the item has been washed and packaged appropriately until use. It is quite often very difficult to estimate the significance of these noncritical items of equipment that would include such things as stethoscopes, EKG electrodes, sphygmomanometers, etc. It is in the area of noncritical items that the likelihood of cross-contamination is greatest.

## METHODS OF STERILIZATION

### *AUTOCLAVING (STEAM UNDER PRESSURE)*

Heat, either in a moist or dry form, is a very effective means of sterilization used in hospitals today. An autoclave is a chamber which is double insulated and utilizes steam under pressure to reach high thermal levels. The temperature necessary to destroy all spores and thus insure sterility cannot be reached under normal ambient conditions. For this reason, sterilization by the use of the autoclave is the most prevalent. The high pressure of the steam autoclave is the most prevalent. The high pressure of the steam autoclave does not have a detrimental effect on bacteria in and of itself; however, it does allow for rapid heating and high temperature, which facilitates the steam penetrating any spores that may be present. Heat (high pressure steam) kills organisms by coagulation of the cell protein. The general procedure of steam autoclave is to create a pressure of 15 pounds per square inch at 120°C and maintain it for 15 min. The exposure time required can vary for different materials depending upon the size and substance of which it is made. For the effective operation of the steam autoclave, it is necessary that the chamber be saturated with steam. If residual air is left in the chamber, it will reduce the absolute temperature. It is important to remember that it is the heat that kills the microorganisms and not the pressure.

Equipment that is to be steam autoclaved must be cleaned and dried and wrapped properly before the sterilization process. It is also important not to overpack the sterilizer with materials, because this will reduce the penetrating ability of the steam and require longer sterilization time. A drying time within the sterilizer is also necessary to prevent recontamination of the material with bacteria which is facilitated when the bundles are moist. The overall time for sterilization process is approximately 30–45 min during which material is held at 120°C for 15 min and the remainder of the time for drying. Because of the variation in time at which the sterilizer must be maintained at high temperatures, the only reliable way to assure sterilization is through the use of various indicators.

The use of steam autoclave has limited application in respiratory therapy because many of the materials that are utilized are distorted or melt at high temperatures. In addition, it is not possible to sterilize electrical devices, machines, or other pieces of equipment which are sensitive to high temperature and/or high pressures. Steam autoclave is an effective method of sterilization for both gram-positive and gram-negative bacteria, tubercle bacilli, spores, and viruses.

## GAS STERILIZATION (ETHYLENE OXIDE)

Ethylene oxide $(C_2H_4O)$ is the simplest of the cyclic ethers. It is a sterilizing agent that will readily kill both the spore form and vegetative form of microorganisms and viruses. It is flammable both in the liquid and gas phases. The mode of action is alkylation in which the nucleic acids, enzyme systems, and vitamin complexes are inactivated. This causes inhibition of critical molecular sites within the microorganisms' cellular processes and thus alters the microorganism in such a way that normal metabolic and reproductive processes will cease.

Ethylene oxide (ETO) is used as a sterilizing agent in its gaseous form in a mixture with other gases such as carbon dioxide or the fluorinated hydrocarbons (for example, freon). ETO must be used with noncombustible gases; therefore, it is never used with oxygen. There are three variables that affect the rate at which the microorganisms are killed in ETO sterilization:

1. The concentration of ETO,
2. Temperature,
3. Relative humidity.

The optimal conditions for sterilization are:

1. A gas concentration of ETO from 450 mg/l to 1500 mg/l (the most common range being 800 to 1000 mg/l).
2. A relative humidity of 20–50 percent,
3. Exposure time of 1–4 hr.

In order for sterilization of the microorganisms to be complete, it is necessary that the microorganism itself contain moisture but that the equipment itself must be dry. If water remains on the equipment, the ethylene oxide will combine with the water to form ethylene glycol, which is toxic to the respiratory tract.

Ethylene oxide has proven to be an excellent sterilization method for most types of equipment used in respiratory therapy. Proper precautions must be taken to see that the equipment is prepared properly for sterilization and that an adequate aeration time is provided following the sterilization process. ETO sterilization is a safe, reliable and practical method for the greatest amount of respiratory therapy equipment.

Sterilization systems for ethylene oxide are initially expensive, and the time needed for proper aeration before the equipment can be reused may be a significant cost factor to the department. This can be reduced by the use of an aeration chamber.

Items which have been previously gamma-radiated at the factory should never be ethylene oxide sterilized because a significant amount of ethylene chlorohydrin, which is very toxic, will be formed. This is particularly true of items made of polyvinylchloride since these items have been gamma-radiated at the factory. Such items include tracheostomy tubes, certain cannulae, and disposable mouth pieces. These items should be considered disposable and thrown away after use.

It is possible to gas sterilize an entire ventilation unit such as the Bennet PR2 or Bird Mark 7. When doing so, care needs to be taken to insure that the correct ventilator settings exist when putting the unit into the gas sterilizer. For gas sterilizing a Bennett PR2, the pressure control setting should be increased all the way, the rate should be on the maximum setting, the expiration time, terminal flow, and sensitivity control all should be placed at their maximum open position, and the air mix control should be open for maximum dilution. Next, the high pressure hose of the ventilator should be connected to the gas outlet inside the sterilization unit. If the unit is large enough and several ventilators are being sterilized, this may be accomplished by using a *Y*-connector or a series of connectors hooked into the gas outlet. Following sterilization of the PR2 unit, the recommended aeration time in a chamber should not be less than 3 hours and not less than 48 hours when aeration is accomplished in ambient conditions. For sterilization of a Bird Mark 7, the settings should be as follows for a calibrated unit: the flow rate control should be open counter-clockwise to 40, the sensitivity should be set at 5, the apneustic control should be open counter-clockwise for approximately 2 complete turns, the inspiratory pressure controls should be set for approximately 40 centimeters of water, the negative pressure generator should be open counter-clockwise for approximately 2 complete turns, and for a Bird Mark 10, 14, or 17, the flow accelerator control should be open approximately 1/2 of a turn. The high pressure hose should be then set to the gas outlet within the sterilization chamber as the PR2. Once sterilization is complete, the aeration chamber time should be not less than 3 hours and not more than 48 hours under ambient conditions.

Other mechanical ventilators can be sterilized in a similar manner. The important aspect is that the ventilator settings should be set so the ethylene oxide is able to penetrate all gas passages that connect with the patient.

### PASTEURIZATION

Pasteurization is a method of disinfection developed by Louis Pasteur, and it is not a sterilization procedure. The process of pasteurization uses high temperatures in a water bath for specific intervals of time. Pasteurization is effective for instruments and solutions that would be destroyed by various high temperatures, such as wine, sugar solutions, and milk. Pasteurization will kill many pathogenic organisms but is ineffective against spores. The procedure is to use a waterbath heated to approximately 63 degrees centigrade for 30 minutes. This is effective for many common pathogens found in the hospital. The mode of action is the coagulation of the cell protein in the microorganism. The advantages of pasteurization are: the minimal cost of disinfecting procedure, no aeration time is necessary, the equipment is simple to operate, and because of the relatively short time necessary, a reduced inventory of equipment is possible. The primary disadvantage of pasteurization is that it does not provide a sterilization process but only a disinfecting one. For this reason, departments using pasteurization as a mode of cleaning equipment will also have to invest in a sterilization procedure as well.

## Ultrasonic Sterilization

Ultrasonic sterilization uses the principle of high energy sound waves (ultrasonic waves) that cause cavitation of the cell walls of microorganisms forcing them to tear apart or explode. As a sterilizing procedure, the use of ultrasonic waves has had limited value. It is effective against many of the gram-negative and gram-positive organisms; however, spores seem to be resistant to cavitation by ultrasound. It has also been very difficult to determine proper sterilization times, frequencies, and amounts of equipment which can be sterilized at a given time; therefore, ultrasound has not been a popular mode of sterilization for respiratory therapy equipment.

The vibration developed in ultrasonic waves enables pieces of equipment to be easily cleaned in inaccessible areas where scrubbing or washing by hand would be very difficult. The advantages of using ultrasonic cleaners in the respiratory therapy department are: more effective than scrubbing, increase the efficiency of the cleaning process, and has potential sterilization value for limited situations. The disadvantages are: only a small amount of equipment can be cleaned at a time, may not kill all organisms during the "sterilization process," and spores and certain other microorganisms are resistant to the process.

## Gamma Radiation

Gamma radiation uses the process of high-energy short-wave lengths of light (called gamma rays) that are absorbed by cellular proteins and nucleic acids within the microorganisms. This causes ionization within the cells or the microorganisms which results in the formation of hydrogen peroxide which is a strong bacteriocidal and virucidal agent.

Gamma radiation is an effective and a rapid means of sterilization and is used most often by industry for the sterilization of prepackaged materials. Gamma radiation has little value in respiratory therapy because of the extremely expensive equipment necessary for radiation sterilization. Items that have been gamma radiated cannot be resterilized using ethylene oxide because of the development of ethylene chlorohydrin which is a toxic substance.

## Cold Sterilization and Disinfection

Many cold solutions are used for either sterilization or disinfection processes. Of these, the two most commonly utilized sterilizing solutions are aqueous buffered glutaraldehyde (Cidex) and acid glutaraldehyde (Sonacide). Aqueous buffered glutaraldehyde is a two percent aqueous solution in the pH range of 7.5-8.5. Glutaraldehyde loses its activity in the alkaline pH range and is considered an active sterilizing solution for approximately two weeks. The solution is bacteriocidal in 10 minutes and

**TABLE 12-1**

**Methods of Sterilization and Disinfection**

| Method | Effectiveness Against Selected Microorganisms | | | | | Mode of Action | Application to Respiratory Therapy |
|---|---|---|---|---|---|---|---|
| | Gram+ | Gram− | Spores | T.B. | Viruses | | |
| Steam Autoclave | yes | yes | yes | yes | yes | Denaturation of protein and cause cell coagulation | Allows rapid and complete sterilization of limited equipment. Can deform plastics, some rubber items, and will damage electrical items. Generally, not practical for most *RT* equipment |
| Ethylene Oxide | yes | yes | yes | yes | yes | Inhibition of metabolic processes and enzyme action in microorganisms | Use in respiratory therapy excellent. Equipment must be dry and an aeration time is necessary. Ethylene glycol and ethylene chlorohydrin are toxic substances which can be formed in sterilizing process if not performed correctly. |
| Pasteurization | yes | yes | no | yes | yes | Coagulation of cell protein | The use in respiratory therapy is somewhat limited. The equipment is simple to operate, not expensive after initial investment, no aeration time needed, and no toxic residual possible. Not truly a sterilization process but only disinfecting. |

| Agent | gram+ | gram- | resistent | | | Mode of Action | Comments |
|---|---|---|---|---|---|---|---|
| Ultrasonic (Greater than 9000 cycles/sec) | less effective | more effective | | yes | yes | Cavitation | Little use in respiratory therapy as a sterilization process-more value as a cleaning process. Difficult to determine effectiveness. Many variables. |
| Gamma Radiation | yes | yes | yes | yes | yes | Breakdown of cell structures: proteins and nucleic acids | Little use in respiratory therapy. Can not resterilize with ETO. |
| Aqueous buffered glutaraldehyde (Cidex) and acid glutaraldehyde (Sonacide) | yes | yes | yes | yes | yes | Denaturization of cell proteins | Use in respiratory therapy excellent. Obviously can not sterilize ventilators, etc. Can cause skin reactions. |

sporicidal in 10–20 hr. The acid glutaraldehyde (Sonacide) has a pH range of 2.7–3.7. Sonacide is most effective as a sterilizing agent at elevated temperatures of approximately 60 degrees centigrade (140°F) and will kill all microorganisms including spores within one hour at this temperature and pH. The solution is a disinfectant in 5 min. at this temperature. Both the buffered and acid forms of Glutaraldehyde have similar disadvantages and advantages. The advantages include: both are effective sterilizing agents within a relatively short period of time, they are simple and easy to use, they are suitable for many types of respiratory therapy equipment, and they are a relatively new form of sterilization. The disadvantages include: the equipment requires thorough rinsing to eliminate residual toxins, a chemical can cause skin reactions on contact, recontamination is easy, and may etch or dull certain pieces of equipment.

Many chemical solutions exist that serve as disinfectants for equipment or for aseptic procedures on the skin. These solutions are used to disinfect the external surfaces of equipment. They include alcohols, hexachlorophene, formaldehyde, betadine, iodine solutions, mercury compound, and detergents.

In summary, chemical solutions can be divided into the sterilizing agents: aqueous buffered glutaraldehyde and acid glutaraldehyde and disinfecting agents listed above. Table 12-1 provides an overview of the methods of sterilization and disinfection.

# Index

## E

## F